P9-DHP-040

## Seventh Edition

# RADIATION PROTECTION

## IN MEDICAL RADIOGRAPHY

Mary Alice Statkiewicz Sherer, AS, RT(R), FASRT

Paula J. Visconti, PhD, DABR

E. Russell Ritenour, PhD, DABR, FAAPM, FACR

Kelli Welch Haynes, MSRS, RT(R)

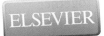

# ELSEVIER
MOSBY

3251 Riverport Lane
Maryland Heights, MO 63043

RADIATION PROTECTION IN MEDICAL RADIOGRAPHY,      ISBN: 978-0-323-17220-2
SEVENTH EDITION
Copyright © 2014 by Mosby, an imprint of Elsevier Inc.

**All rights reserved.** No part of this publication may be reproduced or transmitted in any form or by any means, electronic or mechanical, including photocopying, recording, or any information storage and retrieval system, without permission in writing from the publisher.

---

### Notice

Knowledge and best practice in this field are constantly changing. As new research and experience broaden our knowledge, changes in practice, treatment and drug therapy may become necessary or appropriate. Readers are advised to check the most current information provided (i) on procedures featured or (ii) by the manufacturer of each product to be administered, to verify the recommended dose or formula, the method and duration of administration, and contraindications. It is the responsibility of the practitioner, relying on their own experience and knowledge of the patient, to make diagnoses, to determine dosages and the best treatment for each individual patient, and to take all appropriate safety precautions. To the fullest extent of the law, neither the Publisher nor the Author assumes any liability for any injury and/or damage to persons or property arising out of or related to any use of the material contained in this book.

The Publisher

---

Previous editions copyrighted 2011, 2006, 2002, 1998, 1993, 1983

**Library of Congress Cataloging-in-Publication Data**

Statkiewicz-Sherer, Mary Alice, 1945- author.
  Radiation protection in medical radiography / Mary Alice Statkiewicz Sherer, Paula J. Visconti, E. Russell Ritenour, Kelli Welch Haynes.—Seventh edition.
    p. ; cm.
  Includes bibliographical references and index.
  ISBN 978-0-323-17220-2 (pbk. : alk. paper)
  I. Visconti, Paula J., author.   II. Ritenour, E. Russell, 1953- author.   III. Haynes, Kelli (Kelli Welch), author.   IV. Title.
  [DNLM: 1. Radiation Protection—methods.   2. Radiation Effects.   3. Radiation Monitoring—methods.   4. Radiography—adverse effects.   WN 650]
  RC78.3
  616.07′570289—dc23

                                                      2013025952

*Executive Content Strategist:* Sonya Seigafuse
*Content Development Specialist:* Amy Whittier
*Publishing Services Manager:* Julie Eddy/Hemamalini Rajendrababu
*Senior Project Manager/Project Manager:* Rich Barber/Kamatchi Madhavan
*Design Direction:* Paula Catalano

Printed in the United States of America

Last digit is the print number:   9   8   7   6   5   4   3

Working together
to grow libraries in
developing countries

www.elsevier.com • www.bookaid.org

*In memory of my parents,*
*Felix J. and Elizabeth M. Krohn,*
*To my sons,*
*Joseph F. Statkiewicz, Christopher R. Statkiewicz,*
*and Terry R. Sherer, Jr., with love,*
*And*
*To all with whom I may share my knowledge.*

# REVIEWERS

**Susan Anderson, MAED, RT(R)**
Associate Professor
Central Virginia Community College
Lynchburg, Virginia

**Deanna Butcher, MA, RT(R)**
Program Director
St. Cloud School of Diagnostic Imaging
St. Cloud, Minnesota

**Gail Faig, BS, RT(R) (CV) (CT)**
Clinical Coordinator
Shore Medical Center
Somers Point, New Jersey

**Joe A. Garza, MS, RT(R)**
Professor
Lone Star College, Montgomery
Conroe, Texas

**Cory J. Neill, BS, RT(R)(T), CMD**
Certified Medical Dosimetrist
Truckee Meadows Community College
Reno, Nevada

# FOREWORD

Since 1983, the authors of *Radiation Protection in Medical Radiography* have delivered one of the most comprehensive texts on the subject. Users can always count on the most timely coverage of each topic. This seventh edition appropriately comes at a time of increasing public awareness of the risks of man-made radiation exposure. It is designed to provide students with the current information they need to prepare for the ever-changing requirements of the profession they are about to enter. The radiographers they will become face increasing responsibilities to help patients understand the risks and for reporting patient radiation exposure to governmental and accrediting agencies.

These challenges are faced by currently practicing radiographers, as well as the students they supervise in the clinical setting. Both of these groups count on current, timely information on all aspects of radiation protection. This latest edition has been extensively revised to address these needs. The section on BERT has been expanded to assist radiographers when explaining radiation risks to patients. The Tools for Radiation Awareness and Community Education (TRACE) program and the Standardized Dose Reporting initiative, jointly sponsored by the Food and Drug Administration and the Medical Imaging and Technology Alliance, are introduced.

Knowledge of these tools and soon-to-be mandated practices are essential for both students and radiographers as they work to improve future practices in their departments. All relevant material has been updated to reflect information and recommendations found in current reports of the National Council on Radiation Protection and Measurements.

Educators, students, and practicing radiologic professionals can count on complete coverage of current and relevant information, in an easy-to-read and understand format. In addition, this book will be very useful to newly appointed radiation safety officers and radiation safety committee chairs, including radiation physicists, radiologists, and radiology residents. The text is richly illustrated with tables, art, and photography that improve understanding of complex concepts. The considerable efforts of the author team are readily apparent in this new edition. I will use this text in my courses with confidence, knowing that my students will have the most current information available.

**Bruce W. Long, MS, RT(R) (CV), FASRT**
Director and Associate Professor
Indiana University Radiologic and Imaging
    Sciences Programs
Indianapolis, Indiana

# PREFACE

## CONTENT

Extensively revised, and expanded, the seventh edition of *Radiation Protection in Medical* *Radiography* continues to offer student and practicing radiographers essential information on the biologic effects of ionizing radiation and radiation protection to ensure the safe use of x-rays in diagnostic imaging. The book also presents radiation physics relevant to radiation protection; information on radiation types, sources, and doses received; cell structure; effects of radiation on humans at the molecular, cellular, and systemic levels; radiation quantities and units with emphasis on metric measurements; regulatory and advisory limits for human exposure to radiation; equipment design for radiation protection; the implementation of patient and personnel radiation protection practices for diagnostic x-ray procedures; radiation monitoring; and radioisotopes and radiation protection.

The seventh edition contains practical material that describes the way radiographers handle day-to-day implementation of radiation safety, regulations, and theory. The latest information concerning regulations and guidelines from the major standards-setting and advisory agencies, including the National Council on Radiation Protection and Measurements (NCRP) and the International Commission on Radiological Protection (ICRP), are discussed. The authors have endeavored to present this material in a succinct but reasonably complete fashion to meet the needs of the various members of the health care sector. With each new edition, the authors have also expanded the scope of the material covered in the text to provide the reader with a broader base of knowledge.

## New to This Edition

Although the format of each chapter remains the same as in previous editions, bullets are now being used to enhance readability by calling attention to specific information in each chapter.

The number of chapters in the textbook has increased from 13 to 14 and the order of certain materials in some chapters has also been rearranged to facilitate more effective and efficient delivery of information. Subject matter includes discussion of effective radiation protection, justification and responsibility for imaging procedures, the ALARA principle, and several topics relating to patient protection and patient education. Within the latter, the discussion of

Background Equivalent Radiation Time (BERT) has been expanded to aid radiographers in explaining radiation risks to patients. New to this section of material is the inclusion of information on the Tools for Radiation Awareness and Community Education (TRACE) program and also a discussion concerning the process of Standardized Dose Reporting. Cardinal Rules of Radiation Protection are also briefly presented in this chapter.

Chapter 2 is now dedicated to an explanation of radiation, including its various types and sources and doses received from its presence. Both ionizing and nonionizing radiations are covered. The concepts of equivalent dose (EqD) and effective dose (EfD) are briefly introduced. Biologic damage potential, resulting from ionizing radiation penetrating human body tissue, is also addressed. To expand the reader's knowledge of general information about radiation, both natural and man-made sources of radiation are examined. The latter includes follow-up information on the 1986 Chernobyl Nuclear Power Plant accident and the 2012 Fukushima Daiichi Nuclear Plant crisis. The effect of increasing medical radiation exposure for the US population is also addressed. Interaction of x-radiation with matter is covered in Chapter 3. The revision of this chapter resulted in some change in the sequence in which the material in this chapter is presented.

Radiation quantities and units are covered in Chapter 4, which provides a historical overview of radiation quantities and units. Conversion to metric units of measure and the gradual phasing out of traditional units are emphasized. New information includes discussion of the radiation quantity, air kerma, and its respective metric unit of measure. Discussions of dose area product (DAP), surface integral dose (SID), total effective dose equivalent (TEDE), and committed effective dose equivalent (CEDE) have also been added.

Radiation monitoring for personnel and the use of radiation survey instruments for area monitoring are now covered in Chapter 5. Chapter 6 gives an overview of cell biology. Some new information on structural differences between DNA and RNA has been added. Molecular and cellular radiation biology is covered in Chapter 7. In this chapter, discussion on the target theory has been enhanced.

Chapter 8 is now dedicated to covering subject matter on early deterministic radiation effects on organ systems. Some changes have been made in the sequence of information in this chapter to facilitate greater understanding of the material. Late deterministic and stochastic radiation effects on organ systems are now included in Chapter 9. Several topics in this chapter have been enhanced with additional or updated information.

Chapter 10 addresses the subject of dose limits for exposure to ionizing radiation. The FDA White Paper contributes new information in this chapter, and other topics have been expanded or updated.

Equipment design for radiation protection is covered in Chapter 11. The treatment of digital radiography has been enhanced. Again, the use of metric units is stressed.

Chapter 12 describes management of patient radiation dose during diagnostic x-ray procedures. Many subjects in this chapter have been expanded and updated. Emphasis continues to be placed on the use of metric units in the clinical setting. The subject of fluoroscopic guided positioning (FGP) represents new information in this chapter. Also new is discussion of the Image Wisely Campaign.

Management of imaging personnel radiation dose during diagnostic x-ray procedures is discussed in Chapter 13. Again, several topics have been expanded and updated, including discussion of lead equivalency for protective apparel. The section on diagnostic x-ray suite protection design has been revised to comply with NCRP Report No. 147. Finally, radioisotopes and radiation protection are covered in Chapter 14, with revision of some material.

To correspond with some of the changes in position of chapter materials, the order of appendices in the book has also slightly changed. The glossary from the book, which itself has been revised and extended, and the answers to the review questions at the end of each chapter may now be found on Evolve.

Several new illustrations (diagrams, photos, information boxes and tables) have been added to complement new, updated, or expanded material. Extra tables have been inserted in some chapters, and some existing tables have been updated to reflect the most current data. Additional information boxes have been created to call attention to important information, and some existing boxes have also been updated. Throughout the book, subheadings were either added or revised to aid the reader in locating specific material.

## LEARNING ENHANCEMENTS

Each chapter begins with a list of objectives, followed by a chapter outline and learning objectives. An introductory paragraph provides an overview of the material to be covered in each chapter. Bullets have been added throughout the contents of each chapter to facilitate readability and call attention to specific information.

Chapter content is followed by a bulleted summary, references, general discussion questions, and multiple-choice review questions, all of which can be used by the reader to assess acquired knowledge or by the instructor to stimulate discussion. Bold print has been used to focus the reader's attention on the key terms in each chapter. These key terms are defined in the individual chapter itself or they may be found in the glossary that is now located on the Evolve website, along with other relevant ancillary materials. Throughout the text, information boxes are present to direct the reader to important information. The back matter of the book contains a series of updated and previously existing appendices that provide support material for the text and additional relevant information. Answers to the multiple-choice review questions at the end of each chapter are now found on Evolve.

Information has been presented as clearly and concisely as possible in a style that builds from basic to more complex concepts. Radiographic images, photographs, tables, information boxes, and graphs reinforce and enhance learning and retention of material. Many examples are included after discussions of difficult concepts to aid comprehension.

## Ancillaries

**Workbook.** A workbook to accompany the text is also available. The workbook contains a variety of exercises for each of the 14 chapters in the book. Examples include: crossword puzzles, matching terms with their definitions, labeling of diagrams, true-or-false statements, fill-in-the-blanks, short-answer questions, multiple-choice review questions, general discussion or opinion questions, and a chapter post-test. Use of the workbook will provide a challenging experience for the learner. It will reinforce learning and help students to remember important concepts and material covered in each chapter of the book. The answers for the exercises are located in the back of the workbook. Use of the workbook in conjunction with the textbook will be of significant value in helping the student learner prepare for credentialing examinations, such as the American Registry of Radiologic Technologists (ARRT) certification examination for full-scope radiographers.

**Instructor's Ancillaries.** Instructor's ancillaries are also available with this edition to assist the educator in preparing lesson plans and presenting material. Ancillaries include a test bank containing multiple-choice questions, an image collection from the textbook, and a PowerPoint lecture presentation available at http://evolve.elsevier.com.

**Evolve.** Evolve is an interactive learning environment designed to work in conjunction with *Radiation Protection in Medical Radiography,* seventh edition. Instructor's ancillary materials, an updated glossary, the About the Authors section, and the acknowledgments section and bibliography are all available on Evolve. Instructors using the textbook may use Evolve to provide an Internet-based course component that reinforces and expands the concepts presented in class. Evolve may be used to publish the class syllabus, outlines, and lecture notes; to set up "virtual office hours" and e-mail communication;

to share important dates and information through the online class calendar; and to encourage student participation through chat rooms and discussion boards. Evolve allows instructors to post examinations and manage their grade books online. For more information, visit http://evolve.elsevier.com/Sherer/radiationprotection or contact an Elsevier sales representative.

**Using the Book.** In general, the presentation of the seventh edition presumes that the reader has some background in physics, human anatomy, and medical and imaging terminology. Basic knowledge of simplified mathematics, units of measurement (metric and English), basic atomic structure, the physical concepts of energy, electric charge, subdivision of matter, electromagnetic radiation, x-ray production (both quality and quantity), and the process of ionization is useful but not mandatory. The reader may build on this knowledge by assimilating information presented in this text.

To facilitate a working knowledge of the principles of radiation protection, study materials presented in the seventh edition remain sophisticated enough to be true to the complexity of the subject, yet simple and concise enough to permit comprehension by all readers. For student radiographers and radiology residents, this text is best used in conjunction with formal instruction from a qualified instructor. Practicing radiographers, new medical physicists, newly appointed radiation safety committee chairs, and radiologists may use this book as a self-teaching instrument to broaden and reinforce existing knowledge of the subject matter and also as a means to acquaint themselves with changing concepts and new material. The book can serve as a resource for continuing education because it provides an extensive range of information.

By mastering the material covered in this radiation protection text and its ancillaries and by applying this knowledge in the performance of radiologic procedures, the reader will help to ensure the safety of patients and all diagnostic imaging personnel.

**Mary Alice Statkiewicz Sherer**

# CONTENTS

# Introduction to Radiation Protection

## OBJECTIVES

*After completing this chapter, the reader will be able to perform the following:*

- Identify the consequences of ionization in human cells.
- Give examples of how radiologic technologists and radiologists can exercise control of radiant energy while performing imaging procedures.
- Discuss the concept of effective radiation protection.
- Discuss the need to safeguard against significant and continuing radiation exposure.
- Explain the justification and responsibility for imaging procedures.
- Explain how diagnostic efficacy of an imaging procedure can be maximized.
- Explain how imaging professionals can help ensure that both occupational and nonoccupational dose limits remain well below maximum allowable levels.
- State the ALARA principle and discuss its significance in diagnostic imaging.
- List employer requirements for implementing and maintaining an effective radiation safety program in a facility that provides imaging services.
- List the responsibilities that radiation workers must fulfill to maintain an effective radiation safety program.
- Describe the importance of patient education as it relates to medical imaging.
- Explain how radiographers should answer patients' questions about the risk of radiation exposure from an imaging procedure, and give some examples.
- Define the terms *sievert* (Sv) and *millisievert* (mSv).

## CHAPTER OUTLINE

## KEY TERMS

as low as reasonably
  achievable (ALARA)
background equivalent
  radiation time (BERT)
biologic effects
diagnostic efficacy
entrance skin exposure (ESE)

ionizing radiation
millisievert (mSv)
occupational and
  nonoccupational doses
optimization for radiation
  protection (ORP)
radiation protection

risk
sievert (Sv)
standardized dose reporting
Tools for Radiation Awareness
  and Community Education
  (TRACE Program)

Although radiation in all its manifestations has been present on our planet since its beginnings, the use of radiation in the healing arts did not begin until the discovery of x-rays in 1895. Scientists experimenting with the newly discovered mysterious rays gradually became aware of their value to the medical community both as a diagnostic and as a therapeutic tool. The ability of x-rays to cause injury in normal biologic tissue soon became apparent as well. Hence, since the early 1900s both the beneficial and destructive potentials of x-rays have been known. X-rays are a form of **ionizing radiation.** When passing through matter, ionizing radiation produces positively and negatively charged particles (ions). The production of these ions is the event that may cause injury in normal biologic tissue. Consequences of ionization in human cells are listed in Box 1-1 and are discussed in Chapter 7 of this text.

By using the knowledge of radiation-induced hazards that has been gained over many years and by employing effective methods to limit or eliminate those hazards, humans can safely control the use of "radiant energy." An example of controllable radiant energy is the radiation produced from an x-ray tube (Fig. 1-1).

Radiologic technologists and radiologists:

- Are educated in the safe operation of radiation-producing imaging equipment.
- Use protective devices whenever possible.
- Follow established procedures.
- Select technical exposure factors that significantly reduce radiation exposure to patients and to themselves.

Through these good practices, technologists and radiologists minimize the possibility of causing damage to healthy biologic tissue.

## EFFECTIVE RADIATION PROTECTION

Diagnostic imaging professionals have an ongoing responsibility to ensure radiation safety during all medical radiation procedures. They fulfill this obligation by adhering to an established radiation protection program. **Radiation protection** may be defined simply as effective measures employed by radiation workers to safeguard patients, personnel, and the general public from *unnecessary* exposure to ionizing radiation. This is any radiation exposure that does not benefit a person in terms of diagnostic information obtained for the clinical management of medical

| BOX 1-1 | Consequences of Ionization in Human Cells* |
|---|---|

- Creation of unstable atoms
- Production of free electrons
- Production of low-energy x-ray photons
- Creation of reactive free radicals capable of producing substances poisonous to the cell
- Creation of new biologic molecules detrimental to the living cell
- Injury to the cell that may manifest itself as abnormal function or loss of function

*Each of these consequences is fully discussed in subsequent chapters.

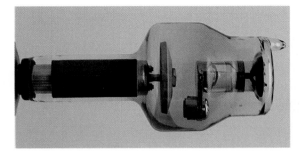

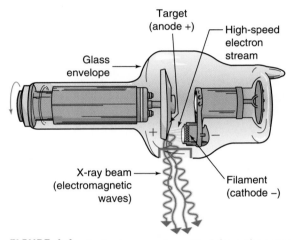

**FIGURE 1-1** Radiant energy is emitted from the x-ray tube in the form of waves (or particles). This manmade energy can be controlled by the selection of equipment components and devices made for this purpose and by the selection of appropriate technical exposure factors.

needs or any radiation exposure that does not enhance the quality of the study. Effective protective measures take into consideration both human and environmental physical determinants, technical elements, and procedural factors. They consist of tools and techniques primarily designed to minimize radiation exposure while producing optimal-quality diagnostic images. To comprehend that process more fully, this textbook has been designed to introduce to its readers at appropriate times in the following chapters the relevant scientific principles that underlie those tools and techniques. In science, fundamental pieces of information are necessary to describe physical processes correctly. Some basic examples are the concepts of length, force, energy, and

time. To know these concepts in a quantitative way, which is what scientific reality demands, units have been constructed to quantify every such concept uniquely. Unfortunately, there is not just one unique set or system of these units. Rather, three such unit systems are currently in existence, and each one has a significant area of usage. Appendix A contains detailed lists of all the major units comprising each of the three systems and furthermore gives the numeric relationships among the corresponding units of each system.

## Need to Safeguard against Significant and Continuing Radiation Exposure

**Biologic Effects.** The need for safeguarding against significant and continuing radiation exposure is based on evidence of harmful **biologic effects** (i.e., damage to living tissue of animals and humans exposed to radiation). Various methods of radiation protection may be applied to ensure safety for persons employed in radiation industries, including medicine, and for the population at large. In medicine, when radiation safety principles are correctly applied during imaging procedures, the energy deposited in living tissue by the radiation can be limited, thereby reducing the potential for adverse biologic effects. This book focuses on radiation protection for patients, diagnostic imaging personnel, and the general public. Biologic effects are also discussed extensively in Chapters 7, 8, 9, and 10.

## JUSTIFICATION AND RESPONSIBILITY FOR IMAGING PROCEDURES

### Benefit versus Risk

Radiation exposure should *always* be kept at the lowest possible level for the general public. However, when illness or injury occurs or when a specific imaging procedure for health screening purposes is prudent, a patient may elect to assume the relatively small risk of exposure to ionizing

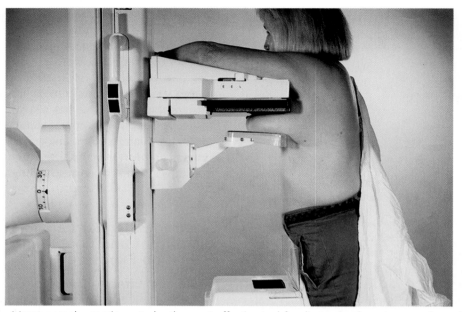

**FIGURE 1-2** Mammography continues to be the most effective tool for diagnosing breast cancer. It can be used as a screening tool or a diagnostic procedure. In either instance, the directly realized benefit, in terms of medical information obtained, far outweighs any slight risk of possible biologic damage.

radiation to obtain essential diagnostic medical information. A prime example of such a voluntary assumption of risk occurs when women elect to undergo screening mammography to detect breast cancer in its early stages (Fig. 1-2). Because mammography continues to be the most effective tool for diagnosing breast cancer early, when the disease can best be treated,[1] its use contributes significantly to improving the quality of life for women. When ionizing radiation is used in this fashion for the welfare of the patient, the directly realized benefits of the exposure to this radiant energy far outweigh any slight risk of inducing a radiogenic malignancy or any genetic defects (Fig. 1-3).

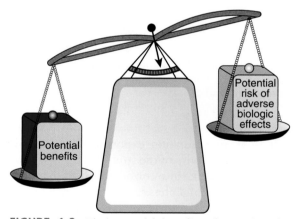

**FIGURE 1-3** The potential benefits of exposing the patient to ionizing radiation must far outweigh the potential risk of adverse biologic effects.

## Diagnostic Efficacy

**Diagnostic efficacy** is the degree to which the diagnostic study accurately reveals the presence or absence of disease in the patient. It is maximized when essential images are produced under recommended radiation protection guidelines.

Efficacy is a vital part of radiation protection in the healing arts. It provides the basis for determining whether an imaging procedure or practice is justified (Box 1-2). The referring physician carries the responsibility for determining this medical necessity for the patient. After ordering

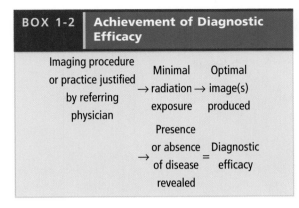

**BOX 1-2** | **Achievement of Diagnostic Efficacy**

Imaging procedure or practice justified by referring physician

→ Minimal radiation exposure → Optimal image(s) produced

→ Presence or absence of disease revealed = Diagnostic efficacy

an x-ray examination or procedure, the referring physician must accept basic responsibility for protecting the patient from nonuseful radiation exposure. The physician exercises this responsibility by relying on qualified imaging personnel. As health care professionals, radiographers accept a portion of the responsibility for the patient's welfare by providing high-quality imaging services. The radiographer and participating radiologist share in keeping the patient's medical radiation exposure at the lowest level possible. In this way imaging professionals help ensure that both **occupational and nonoccupational doses** remain well below maximum allowable levels, that is, the upper boundary doses of ionizing radiation for which there is a negligible risk of bodily injury or genetic damage. This can best be accomplished by using the *smallest* radiation exposure that will produce useful images and by producing optimal images with the *first* exposure. Repeated examinations made necessary by technical error or carelessness (Fig. 1-4) must be avoided because they significantly increase radiation exposure for both the patient and the radiation worker.

## AS LOW AS REASONABLY ACHIEVABLE (ALARA) PRINCIPLE

### Concepts of Radiologic Practice

**ALARA** is an acronym for **as low as reasonably achievable.** This term is synonymous with the term **optimization for radiation protection (ORP).** The intention behind these concepts of radiologic practice is to keep radiation exposure and consequent dose to the lowest possible level (Fig. 1-5). The rationale for this intention comes from evidence compiled by scientists over the past century.[2] At the time of this publication, radiation protection guidelines are rooted in the philosophy of ALARA. Therefore, this philosophy, *as low as reasonably achievable,* should be a main part of every health care facility's personnel radiation control program. In addition, because no dose limits have been established for the amount of radiation that patients may receive for individual imaging procedures, the ALARA philosophy should be established and maintained and must show that we have considered reasonable actions that will reduce doses to patients and personnel below required limits. Radiation-induced cancer does not have a fixed threshold, that is, a dose level below which individuals would have no chance of developing this disease. Therefore, because it appears that no safe dose levels exist for radiation-induced malignant disease, radiation exposure should always be kept ALARA for all medical imaging procedures, and ALARA should serve as a guide to radiographers and radiologists for the selection of technical exposure factors.

For many radiation regulatory agencies (see Chapter 10), the ALARA principle provides a method for comparing the amount of radiation used in various health care facilities in a particular area for specific imaging procedures. An example using this method is provided in Box 1-3.

## Cardinal Rules of Radiation Protection

The three basic principles of radiation protection are as follows:

- Time
- Distance
- Shielding

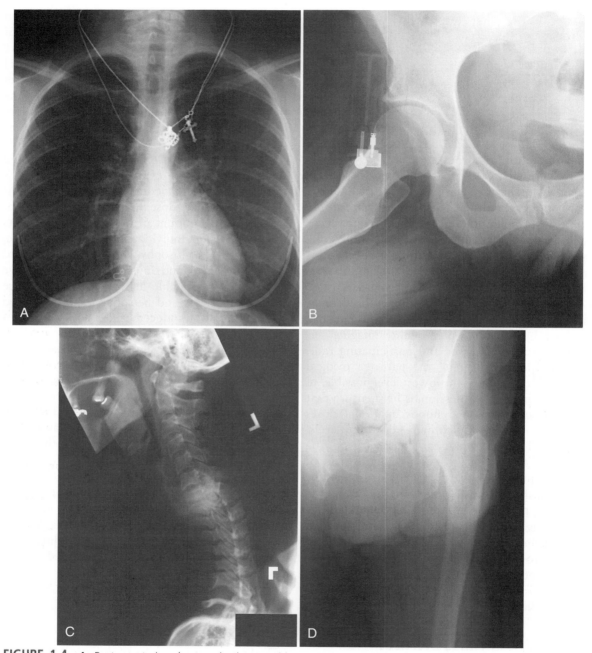

**FIGURE 1-4**   **A,** Posteroanterior chest projection requiring repeat examination because of multiple external foreign bodies (several necklaces and an underwire bra) that should have been removed before the x-ray examination. **B,** Antero-posterior projection of a right hip requiring a repeat examination because of poor collimation and the presence of an external foreign body (a cigarette lighter) overlying the anatomy of concern. The patient's slacks with the pocket containing the lighter should have been removed before the x-ray examination. **C,** Double exposure (two lateral projections of the cervical spine) requiring a repeat examination. **D,** Conventional radiograph of left hip demonstrating an "off-level" grid error. This occurs when the patient's weight is not evenly distributed on the grid, thus causing the grid to tilt so that it is not properly aligned with the x-ray tube.

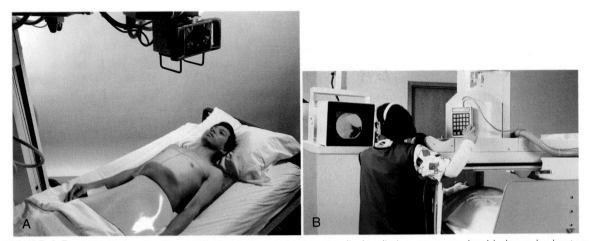

**FIGURE 1-5** **A,** Patient protection. **B,** Radiographer protection. Medical radiation exposure should always be kept as low as reasonably achievable (ALARA) for the patient and for imaging personnel.

| BOX 1-3 | **Example of ALARA Method to Compare the Amount of Radiation That Various Health Care Facilities in a Particular Area Use for Specific Imaging Procedures** |
|---|---|

If patients in a particular location were receiving on average approximately the same **entrance skin exposure (ESE)** for a specific imaging procedure in every health care facility in that same area, then that ESE would represent the radiation exposure and consequent dose that is reasonably achieved within that specific location. However, if one of the health care facilities in this same area began giving its patients higher-radiation ESEs and subsequent doses, that institution would no longer be in compliance with ALARA (as low as reasonably achievable) standards. The noncompliant facility would have to take the necessary action to bring the ESE values and subsequent doses back to a level that would comply with regulatory standards.

These principles can be applied to the patient and the radiographer. To reduce the exposure to the patient:

- Reduce the amount of the x-ray "beam-on" time.
- Use as much distance as warranted between the x-ray tube and the patient for the examination.
- Always shield the patient with appropriate gonadal and/or specific area shielding devices.

Occupational radiation exposures of imaging personnel can be minimized by the use of these cardinal principles:

- Shortening the length of time spent in a room where x-radiation is produced
- Standing at the greatest distance possible from an energized x-ray beam
- Interposing a radiation-absorbent shielding material between the radiographer and the source of radiation

These principles are discussed in greater detail in Chapter 13.

## Responsibility for Maintaining ALARA in the Medical Industry

Both employers of radiation workers and the workers themselves have a responsibility for radiation safety in the medical industry. For the welfare of patients and the workers, facilities providing imaging services must have an effective radiation safety program. This requires a firm commitment to radiation safety by all participants. It is the responsibility of the employer to provide the necessary resources and appropriate environment in which to execute an ALARA program. A written policy statement describing this program and identifying the commitment of management to keeping all radiation exposure ALARA must be available to all employees in the workplace. In a hospital setting, an individual called the Radiation Safety Officer (RSO) is expressly charged by the hospital administration to be directly responsible for the

- Execution
- Enforcement
- Maintenance

of the ALARA program. In Chapter 10, pp. 211-212, the duties of the RSO are described in much more detail.

To determine how radiation exposure in the workplace may be lowered, management should perform periodic exposure audits.[3] Radiation workers with appropriate education and work experience must function with awareness of rules governing the work situation. They are required to perform their occupational practices in a manner consistent with the ALARA principle (Box 1-4). When radiation is safely and prudently used in the imaging of patients, the benefit of the exposure can be maximized while the potential risk of biologic damage is minimized. Additional information on the ALARA concept can be found in Chapter 10.

## PATIENT PROTECTION AND PATIENT EDUCATION

### Educating Patients about Imaging Procedures

Facilities that provide imaging services have a responsibility to ensure the highest quality of service. An important aspect is education of patients about imaging procedures. Patients not only should be made aware of what a specific procedure involves and what type of cooperation

---

| BOX 1-4 | **Responsibilities for an Effective Radiation Safety Program** |
|---|---|

**Employers' Responsibilities**
- Implement and maintain an effective radiation safety program in which to execute ALARA* by providing the following:
  - Necessary resources
  - Appropriate environment for ALARA program
- Make a written policy statement describing the ALARA program and identifying the commitment of management to keep all radiation exposure ALARA available to all employees in the workplace.
- Perform periodic exposure audits to determine how to lower radiation exposure in the workplace.

**Radiation Workers' Responsibilities**
- Be aware of rules governing the workplace.
- Perform duties consistent with ALARA.

*ALARA, As low as reasonably achievable.

---

is required, but also they must be informed of what needs to be done, if anything, as a follow-up to their examination. Through appropriate and effective communication, patients can be made to feel that they are active participants in their own health care (Fig. 1-6).

### Risk of Imaging Procedure versus Potential Benefit

In general terms, risk can be defined as the probability of injury, ailment, or death resulting from an activity. In the medical industry with reference to the radiation sciences, **risk** is the possibility of inducing radiogenic cancer or a genetic defect after irradiation. Typically, people are more willing to accept a risk if they perceive that the potential benefit to be obtained is greater than the risk involved. Regarding exposure to ionizing radiation, patients who understand the medical benefit of an imaging procedure because they received factual information about the study before the examination are more likely to overcome any radiation phobia and be willing to assume a small risk of possible biologic damage. Greater understanding of biologic effects

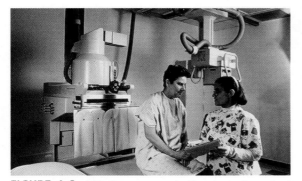

**FIGURE 1-6** Effective communication is an important part of the patient-radiographer relationship. Patients need to be educated about imaging procedures so that they can understand what the procedure involves and what type of cooperation is required. The radiographer must answer patient questions about the potential risk of radiation exposure honestly. To create understanding and reduce fear and anxiety for the patient, the radiographer can provide an example that compares the amount of radiation received for a specific procedure with natural background radiation received over a given period of time.

associated with diagnostic radiology was gained throughout the twentieth century. The medical imaging industry currently continues to build on this knowledge. This information, coupled with better design of medical imaging equipment and improved radiation safety standards, has greatly reduced risk from imaging procedures for both patients and radiographers. When radiographers use their intelligence and knowledge to answer patients' questions about the risk of radiation exposure honestly, they can do much to alleviate patients' apprehension and fears during a routine radiologic examination.

## Background Equivalent Radiation Time

Another way that radiographers can improve understanding and reduce fear and anxiety for the patient is to use the **background equivalent radiation time** (BERT) method. On occasion, a patient will ask the radiographer, "Are x-rays safe?" Radiologic technologists have a responsibility to give a reasonable, honest, and understandable answer to the patient. Radiographers correctly tell patients that for normal diagnostic examinations there are no existing data of any unsafe effects from the x-rays used in the examination. The question about the amount of radiation to the patient is difficult to answer in an understandable way because (1) the received dose is measured in a number of different units and (2) scientific units for radiation dose are not comprehensible by the patient. The purpose is not to provide high scientific accuracy but to relieve anxiety about radiation by giving an understandable and reasonable correct answer. The BERT method compares the amount of radiation received, for example, from a patient's chest x-ray examination or from radiography of any other part of the anatomy, with natural background radiation received over a specified period of time such as days, weeks, months, or years (Table 1-1). This method is also recommended by the U.S. National Council on Radiation Protection and Measurements (NCRP).[4] For example, a patient is having a chest x-ray study and asks the radiographer, "How much radiation will I receive from this x-ray?" The radiographer can respond by using an estimation based on the comparison of radiation received from the x-ray to natural background radiation received, for example, over a certain number of days. Thus the radiographer can reply, "The radiation received from having a chest x-ray is equivalent to what would be received while spending approximately 10 days in your natural surroundings" (see Table 1-1).

BERT is based on an annual U.S. population exposure of approximately 3 millisieverts per year.* Using the BERT method in this context has the following advantages:

- BERT does not imply radiation risk; it is simply a means for comparison.
- BERT emphasizes that radiation is an innate part of our environment.
- The answer given in terms of BERT is easy for the patient to comprehend.

---

*The **millisievert** (**mSv**), a subunit of the sievert (Sv), is equal to $\frac{1}{1000}$ of a sievert. The **sievert** (**Sv**) is the International System of Units (SI) unit of measure for the radiation quantity "equivalent dose."

| TABLE 1-1 | Typical Adult Patient Effective Dose (EfD) and Background Equivalent Radiation Time (BERT) Values | |
|---|---|---|
| Radiologic Procedure | EfD (mSv) | BERT (Amount of Time to Receive the Same EfD from Nature) |
| Dental, intraoral | 0.06 | 1 wk |
| Chest radiograph | 0.08 | 10 days |
| Cervical spine | 0.1 | 2 wk |
| Thoracic spine | 1.5 | 6 mo |
| Lumbar spine | 3.0 | 1 yr |
| Upper GI series | 4.5 | 1.5 yr |
| Lower GI series | 6.0 | 2 yr |
| Skull | 0.07 | 11 day |
| Hip | 0.3 | 7 wk |
| Pelvis | 0.7 | 4 mo |
| Abdomen | 0.7 | 4 mo |
| Limbs and joints (except hip) | <0.01 | <1.5 days |
| CT brain | 2.0 | 1 yr |
| CT chest | 8.0 | 3.6 yr |
| CT abdomen/pelvis | 10.0 | 4.5 yr |

Adapted from BF Wall: *Patient dosimetry techniques in diagnostic radiology,* York, UK, 1988, Institute of Physics and Engineering in Medicine, pp 53, 117; Cameron JR: *Med Phys World,* 15:20, 1999; Stabin MG: *Radiation protection and dosimetry: an introduction to health physics,* New York, 2008, Springer.
*CT,* Computed tomography; *GI,* gastrointestinal; *mSv,* millisievert.

Patients may mistakenly think that manmade radiation is more dangerous than an equal amount of natural radiation. Most patients are unaware that most of their background radiation comes from natural radioactivity in their own body. Radiation phobia can be greatly reduced by explaining the diagnostic radiation dose to the patient by using the BERT method. Radiologic technologists have a responsibility to educate patients and others who ask them about radiation. The BERT concept is understandable. BERT is not a radiation quantity. It is a method of explaining radiation to the public. The word *BERT* is never used in the explanation.[5]

## Tools for Radiation Awareness and Community Education (TRACE) Program

In 2010 Toshiba American Medical Systems awarded six "Putting Patients First Grants" to individual hospitals throughout the United States to create a radiation dose awareness and dose reduction program for patients through the process of education for these individuals, for the community, for health care workers employed in the medical imaging profession, and for physicians.[6,7] The main components of the program include technologic enhancements such as embedded software capable of recording and reporting dose, timely notification of the patient and the referring physician when the radiation dose is greater than 3 Gy, and substantial lowering of computed tomography (CT) doses through improved technology and alterations to existing protocols.[7] This process is known as the **Tools for Radiation Awareness and Community Education (TRACE) Program.** It consists of two phases:

1. Formulating new policies and procedures to promote radiation safety and the implementation of patient and community education
2. Technologic enhancements

During phase one of the TRACE Program, after new and more definitive radiation safety policies and procedures have been written, some ways of providing patient and community education are through the use of:

1. Informational posters placed strategically throughout the health care facility.
2. Brochures that describe imaging procedures in simple terms.
3. Basic information on a specific website designed for patient education.
4. Use of a wallet-size card on which a person's radiation exposure can be recorded and tracked.

Some ways of providing education for imaging department staff are:

1. Providing in-service education on various radiation safety topics to accommodate individual needs of staff members.
2. Handing out a facts-to-remember sheet at the end of an in-service program.
3. E-mails highlighting the most important topics covered in a staff in-service program to imaging staff members to help reinforce and retain vital information.

Some ways of providing education for nonradiologist physicians who perform fluoroscopic procedures can include:

1. Creating increased awareness of radiation dose for specific procedures through discussion.
2. Establishing goals for lowering radiation dose for patients, assisting personnel, and themselves.
3. Radiographers helping physicians performing fluoroscopic procedures by informing them "that they have reached a specific dose,"[7] thereby giving fluoroscopists the opportunity to decide to continue or stop a procedure.

During phase two of the TRACE Program, to accommodate technologic enhancements, the following items are required:

1. "An operational or capital budget, such as acquiring CT dose reduction technology"[7]

2. "Utilization of tools for recording and reporting dose"[7]
3. "Providing notification for excessive radiation dose"[7]

Introducing and implementing the TRACE Program in a medical imaging department can lead to greater radiation safety through patient and community education. Patients become empowered and benefit through their inclusion in decisions concerning their own radiologic care. Physicians become better able to make decisions involving the use of ionizing radiation because the TRACE Program creates "greater awareness of radiation doses."[6] The end result of this program is a reduction in dose to the patient.

## Standardized Dose Reporting

Standardization of dose reporting can also lead to a reduction in radiation dose for patients. A large variability in radiation dose still exists for many procedures. The radiation dose to the patient for individual procedures, such as those involving general fluoroscopy, CT, and interventional procedures, needs to be dictated into every radiologic report. Many newer CT systems and interventional fluoroscopic units possess the technical capability for standardized dose structured reporting.[8] However, other ionizing radiation equipment may not as yet have such a capability.

The benefit to the referring physician in having direct access to a patient's radiation dose history is the option of knowing whether ordering an additional radiologic procedure is advisable. The need to develop a way for each radiation-producing modality to record a patient's radiation dose persists.

## SUMMARY

- Ionizing radiation has both a beneficial and a destructive potential.
- Healthy normal biologic tissue can be injured by ionizing radiation; therefore, it is

necessary to protect humans against significant and continuous exposure.

- X-rays are a form of ionizing radiation; therefore, their use in medicine for the detection of disease and injury requires protective measures.
- To safeguard patients, personnel, and the general public, effective radiation protection measures should always be employed when diagnostic imaging procedures are performed.
- Radiation exposure should always be kept as low as reasonably achievable (ALARA) to minimize the probability of any potential damage to people.
- Referring physicians should justify the need for every radiation procedure and accept basic responsibility to protect the patient from excessive ionizing radiation.
- The benefits of exposing patients to ionizing radiation should far outweigh any slight risk of inducing radiogenic cancer or genetic effects after irradiation.
- Radiographers should select the smallest radiation exposure that produces the best radiographic results and should avoid errors that result in repeated radiographic exposures.
- Imaging facilities must have an effective radiation safety program that provides patient protection and patient education.
- Background equivalent radiation time (BERT) is used to compare the amount of radiation a patient receives from a radiologic procedure with natural background radiation received over a specific period of time.
- The millisievert (mSv) is equal to $\frac{1}{1000}$ of a sievert (Sv).
- The Tools for Radiation Awareness and Community Education (TRACE) Program helps patients and the community to enhance understanding for using radiation safely and for enabling these people to participate in their own medical decisions more actively.
- Methods for standardized patient radiation dose reporting must be developed and implemented.

# REFERENCES

1. Women's breast health: annual reminder needed for mammography. *RT Image* 17:35, 2004.
2. National Research Council, Commission of Life Sciences, Committee on Biological Effects on Ionizing Radiation (BEIR V), Board on Radiation Effects Research: *Health effects of exposure to low levels of ionizing radiations*, Washington, DC, 1989, National Academy Press.
3. Gollnick DA: *Basic radiation protection technology*, ed 4, Altadena, Calif, 2000, Pacific Radiation Corporation.
4. National Council on Radiation Protection and Measurements (NCRP): *Research needs for radiation protection*, Report No. 117. Bethesda, MD, 1993, NCRP, p 51.
5. Ng K-H, Cameron JR: Using the BERT concept to promote understanding of radiation, International conference on the radiological protection of patients organized by the International Atomic Energy Agency, Malaga, Spain, 26-30 March 2011. C&S Paper Series 7/P, Austria, Vienna. 784-787.
6. *Radiation Safety Awareness*. Available at: http://healthoutlook.com/summer-2011/106-radiation-safety-awareness. Accessed September 8, 2012.
7. Rinehart B: TRACE Program: improving patient safety. *Radiol Manage* 33:35, 2011.
8. Center for Devices and Radiological Health, U.S. Food and Drug Administration: White Paper: initiative to reduce unnecessary radiation exposure from medical imaging, Washington, DC, U.S. Government Printing Office, February 2010.

# GENERAL DISCUSSION QUESTIONS

1. What are the consequences of ionization in the human cell?
2. When is medical radiation exposure considered unnecessary?
3. How can the background equivalent radiation time (BERT) method be used to eliminate a patient's fears about medical radiation exposure?
4. Describe how radiographers can use the ALARA concept in the performance of their daily responsibilities.
5. How does implementation of the TRACE Program improve patient safety?
6. How will a patient benefit from standardized radiation dose reporting?

7. Why should the ALARA philosophy be established and maintained as a main part of every health care facility's radiation safety program?
8. When are patients more likely to overcome any radiation phobia and be willing to assume a small risk of possible biologic damage?
9. On what premise is BERT based?
10. In the medical industry with reference to the radiation sciences, how is risk defined?

## REVIEW QUESTIONS

1. A patient may elect to assume the relatively small risk of exposure to ionizing radiation to obtain essential diagnostic medical information when:
   1. Illness occurs
   2. Injury occurs
   3. A specific imaging procedure for health screening purposes is prudent
   A. 1 and 2 only
   B. 1 and 3 only
   C. 2 and 3 only
   D. 1, 2, and 3
2. Effective measures employed by radiation workers to safeguard patients, personnel, and the general public from unnecessary exposure to ionizing radiation define:
   A. Diagnostic efficacy.
   B. Optimization.
   C. Radiation protection.
   D. The concept of equivalent dose (EqD).
3. Which of the following is a method that can be used to answer patients' questions about the amount of radiation received from a radiographic procedure?
   A. ALARA concept
   B. BERT
   C. BRET
   D. EPA

4. The term *optimization for radiation protection* (ORP) is synonymous with the term:
   A. As low as reasonably achievable (ALARA).
   B. Background equivalent radiation time (BERT).
   C. Equivalent dose (EqD).
   D. Diagnostic efficacy (DE).
5. Standardized dose reporting for radiologic procedures can lead to:
   A. An invasion of patient privacy.
   B. An increase in patient radiation dose.
   C. A reduction in patient radiation dose.
   D. Elimination of the need for imaging equipment radiation safety features.
6. Which of the following is a two-phase program to create radiation awareness and community education?
   A. ALARA
   B. BERT
   C. DE
   D. TRACE
7. The degree to which the diagnostic study accurately reveals the presence or absence of disease in the patient defines which of the following terms?
   A. Radiation protection
   B. Radiographic pathology
   C. Effective diagnosis
   D. Diagnostic efficacy
8. The millisievert (mSv) is equal to:
   A. $\frac{1}{10}$ of a sievert.
   B. $\frac{1}{100}$ of a sievert.
   C. $\frac{1}{1000}$ of a sievert.
   D. $\frac{1}{10,000}$ of a sievert.
9. An effective radiation safety program requires a firm commitment to radiation safety by:
   1. Facilities providing imaging services
   2. Radiation workers
   3. Patients
   A. 1 and 2 only
   B. 1 and 3 only
   C. 2 and 3 only
   D. 1, 2, and 3

**10.** If patients in facilities in the same location are receiving on average approximately the same entrance skin exposure (ESE) in every health care facility for a specific imaging procedure with the exception of one facility, in which higher-radiation ESEs and subsequent doses are being received for the same procedure, that institution would:
   A. Be excluded from the group of compliant facilities for comparison purposes.
   B. No longer be in compliance with ALARA standards and would have to take the necessary action to bring the ESE values and subsequent doses back to a level that would comply with regulatory standards.
   C. Simply establish their own ESE values for the specific procedure in question and ignore ALARA standards.
   D. Be required to close down the facility immediately.

## CHAPTER 2

# Radiation: Types, Sources, and Doses Received

## OBJECTIVES

*After completing this chapter, the reader will be able to perform the following:*

- Define the term radiation and give some examples of different types of radiation.
- Draw a diagram to illustrate the electromagnetic spectrum and explain how the spectrum can be divided for the purpose of studying radiation protection.
- List the different forms of electromagnetic and particulate radiations, and identify those forms that are classified as ionizing radiation.
- Explain the concepts of equivalent dose and effective dose.
- Discuss the significance of the sievert as a unit of measure for equivalent dose.
- Describe the potential for ionizing radiation to cause biologic damage.
- List and describe three sources of natural background ionizing radiation and seven sources of manmade, or artificial, ionizing radiation.
- Discuss the local and global consequences of radiation exposure resulting from accidents in nuclear power plants.
- Discuss the responsibility and need for radiation protection in medical imaging.
- Discuss the modalities used in medical imaging that have caused an increase in radiation dose for patients from 1980 until the present time.

## CHAPTER OUTLINE

**Radiation**
   Types of Radiation
   The Electromagnetic
     Spectrum
   Ionizing and Nonionizing
     Radiation

Particulate Radiation
Radiation Dose Specification:
   Equivalent Dose

Biologic Damage Potential
Sources of Radiation
**Summary**

## KEY TERMS

biologic damage
cellular damage
effective dose (EfD)
electromagnetic radiation
electromagnetic spectrum
electromagnetic wave

equivalent dose (EqD)
genetic damage
ionization
manmade, or artificial, radiation
natural background radiation
organic damage

particulate radiation
radiation
radiation dose
radionuclide
radon
sievert (Sv)

Copyright © 2014, Elsevier Inc.

Radiation has different types and sources. Some types of radiation produce damage in biologic tissue, whereas others do not. Some sources of radiation are considered natural sources because they are always present in the environment. However, other sources are created by humans for specific purposes. The radiation dose to the global population from both natural and manmade sources contributes a percentage of the total amount of radiation that humans receive during their lifetime. This chapter presents an overview of the types and sources of radiation and the doses received from ionizing radiation from both environmental and artificial sources.

## RADIATION

### Types of Radiation

In the simplest terms, energy is the ability to do work, that is, to move an object against resistance. **Radiation** refers to kinetic energy that passes from one location to another and can have many manifestations. By this definition, many types of radiation exist. Some examples are presented in Box 2-1.

### The Electromagnetic Spectrum

The full range of frequencies and wavelengths of electromagnetic waves is known as the **electromagnetic spectrum.** Table 2-1 shows the electromagnetic spectrum in terms of *frequency* (given in units of hertz [Hz] i.e., cycles per second), *wavelength* (in meters), and *energy* (specified in electron volts [eV], a unit of energy equal to the quantity of kinetic energy an electron acquires as it moves through a potential difference of 1 volt). Each frequency within the spectrum has a characteristic wavelength and energy. Some of the practical uses of these different frequency ranges are listed. Note that higher frequencies are associated with shorter wavelengths and higher energies; therefore, as the wavelength ranges from largest to smallest, frequencies and energy cover the corresponding smallest to largest ranges. Precise frequency intervals attributed to different

| BOX 2-1 | **Examples of Different Types of Radiation** |
|---|---|

**Example 1. Mechanical Vibrations of Materials**
Such mechanical vibrations can travel through the air or other materials to interact with structures in the human ear and produce the sensation we call *sound. Ultrasound* is the mechanical vibration of a material in which the rate of vibration does not stimulate the human ear sensors and therefore is beyond the range of human hearing.

**Example 2. The Electromagnetic Wave**
*Radio waves, microwaves, visible light,* and *x-rays* are all representative of the **electromagnetic wave.** In these waves, electric and magnetic fields fluctuate rapidly as they travel through space. A limited range of frequencies of this fluctuation is interpreted by its interaction with the human system as visible light. Within this range, small variations in frequency—the number of cycles or wavelengths of a simple harmonic motion per unit of time—are interpreted as different colors. However, frequencies both above and below the visible range exist and have many uses. Electromagnetic waves are also characterized by their wavelength, which is simply the physical distance between successive maximum values of electric and magnetic fields.

At the beginning of the twentieth century, leading scientists first realized that electromagnetic radiation appears to have a dual nature, referred to as *wave-particle duality.* This means that this form of radiation can travel through space in the form of a wave but can interact with matter as a particle of energy. For this reason, x-rays may be described as both waves and particles.

parts of the electromagnetic spectrum may vary in different references, and there is substantial overlap of ranges (note that FM radio falls completely within the television range). Box 2-2 demonstrates the calculation of the wavelength and energy of electromagnetic radiation.

### Ionizing and Nonionizing Radiation

For our purposes in the study of radiation protection, the electromagnetic spectrum (Fig. 2-1) can be divided into two parts:

1. Ionizing radiation
2. Nonionizing radiation

| Use | Frequency | Wavelength | Energy |
|---|---|---|---|
| AM radio | 0.54-1.6 MHz | 0.6-0.2 km | 2-7 neV |
| FM radio | 88-108 MHz | 3.4-3 m | 370-440 neV |
| Television | 54 MHz-0.8 GHz | 5.6-0.4 m | 220 neV-3.3 μeV |
| Microwaves | 0.1-100 GHz | 3 m-3 mm | 0.4 eV-0.4 meV |
| Infrared | 100 GHz-400 THz | 3 mm-0.7 m | 0.4 meV-1.6 eV |
| Visible | 400-700 THz | 0.7-0.4 m | 1.6-2.8 eV |
| Ultraviolet | 1-100 PHz | 300-3 nm | 4-400 eV |
| X-rays | 100 PHz-100 EHz | 3 nm-3 am | 0.4-400 keV |
| Gamma rays | 100 EHz-infinity | 3-0 am | 400 keV-infinity |

**TABLE 2-1   The Electromagnetic Spectrum***

*Frequency (in units of hertz [Hz] or cycles per second), wavelength (in meters), and energy (in electron volts [eV]). Each member of the spectrum has a characteristic wavelength and frequency. Some of the uses of different frequency ranges are listed. Note that higher frequencies are associated with shorter wavelengths and higher energies. The values shown here are typical representations. See Appendix B for an explanation of the abbreviations (M, G, T, P, μ, etc.).

Of the entire span of electromagnetic radiations included in the electromagnetic spectrum, only the following radiations are classified as ionizing radiations[1]:

- X-rays
- Gamma rays
- High-energy ultraviolet radiation (energy higher than 10 eV)

Because they do not have sufficient kinetic energy to eject electrons from the atom, the following radiations are considered to be nonionizing:

- Low-energy ultraviolet radiation
- Visible light
- Infrared rays
- Microwaves
- Radio waves

If **electromagnetic radiation** is of a high enough frequency, it can transfer sufficient energy to some orbital electrons to remove them from the atoms to which they were attached. This process, called **ionization,** is the foundation of the interactions of x-rays with human tissue. It makes them valuable for creating images but has the undesirable result of potentially producing some damage in the biologic material. The amount of energy transferred to electrons by ionizing radiation is

the basis of the concept of **radiation dose.** Thus, a radiation quantity such as equivalent dose (EqD), which correlates the absorbed dose in biologic tissue with the type and energy of the radiation to which a human has been subjected, applies only to ionizing types of radiation. EqD cannot be used to specify the amount of energy imparted to a potato in a microwave oven or to a sunbather on the beach because no ionization is produced by microwaves or sunlight.* Additional information about EqD is found later in the chapter and in Chapter 4.

## Particulate Radiation

In addition to electromagnetic radiation, there is another category of ionizing radiation, called **particulate radiation.** This form of radiation includes the following:

- Alpha particles
- Beta particles

*Actually, a small amount of ionizing radiation is produced by the sun in the form of solar flares. However, this amount is negligible, and the small amount of ionizing radiation is not what produces the sensation of heat or the chemical changes that produce suntan and sunburn. These are the results of nonionizing infrared and ultraviolet radiation.

---

**BOX 2-2 | Calculation of the Wavelength and Energy of Electromagnetic Radiation**

The speed of light (c), wavelength ($\lambda$), and frequency ($\nu$), are related by the following equation:

$$c = \lambda\nu$$

where $c = 3 \times 10^8$ m/sec.

Therefore, if the frequency of an electromagnetic wave is known, the wavelength may be calculated as follows:

$$\lambda = \frac{c}{\nu}$$

**Example:** Find the wavelength of a 0.5-MHz radio wave.

$$\lambda = \frac{3 \times 10^8 \text{ m/sec}}{0.5 \times 10^6 \text{ sec}^{-1}} = 6.0 \times 10^2 \text{ m} = 0.6 \times 10^3 \text{ m} = 0.6 \text{ km}$$

The energy (in electron volts, eV) of an electromagnetic wave may be calculated using the frequency ($\nu$) and Planck's constant (h) as follows:

$$E = h\nu$$

where $h = 4.14 \times 10^{-15}$ eV-sec.

**Example:** Find the energy of an x-ray having a wavelength of 1 picometer (1 pm = $10^{-12}$ m).

**Solution:** The energy is given by the following relation:

$$
\begin{aligned}
E = h\nu &= hc/\text{wavelength} \\
&= (4.14 \times 10^{-15} \text{ eV-sec})(3 \times 10^{10} \text{ m/sec})/(1 \times 10^{-12} \text{ m}) \\
&= 12.42 \times 10^7 \text{ eV} \\
&= 124 \text{ MeV}
\end{aligned}
$$

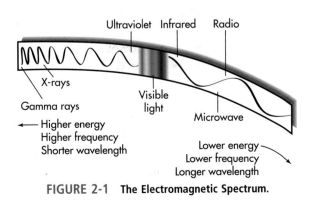

FIGURE 2-1    **The Electromagnetic Spectrum.**

- Neutrons
- Protons

All these are subatomic particles that are ejected from atoms at very high speeds. They possess sufficient kinetic energy to be capable of causing ionization by direct atomic collision. However, no ionization occurs when the subatomic particles are at rest.

*Alpha particles* (also known as alpha rays) are emitted from nuclei of very heavy elements such as uranium and plutonium during the process of radioactive decay. Radioactive decay is a naturally occurring process in which unstable nuclei relieve that instability by various types of nuclear spontaneous emissions, one of which is the emission of charged particles. Alpha particles each contain two protons and two neutrons. They are simply helium nuclei (i.e., helium atoms minus their electrons). Alpha particles have a large mass (approximately four times the mass of a hydrogen atom) and a positive charge twice that of an electron. This permits them to have the potential of transferring very substantial kinetic energy to orbital electrons of other atoms.[2]

Particulate radiations vary in their ability to penetrate matter. Compared with beta particles, which are just fast electrons, alpha particles are less penetrating. Because they lose energy quickly as they travel a short distance in biologic matter (i.e., into the superficial layers of the skin), they are considered virtually harmless as an external source of radiation. A piece of ordinary paper can absorb them or function as a shield. However, as an internal source of radiation, the reverse is true. If emitted from a radioisotope deposited in the body, for example, in the lungs, alpha particles can be absorbed in the relatively radiosensitive epithelial tissue and are very damaging to that tissue. It is in a way analogous to what a bowling ball does to a set of pins.

*Beta particles*, also known as *beta rays*, are identical to high-speed electrons except for their origin. Electrons originate in atomic shells outside of the nucleus, whereas beta particles, like alpha particles, are emitted from within the nuclei of radioactive atoms, but radioactive atoms that relieve their instability in a different fashion. This process of *beta decay,* along with some therapeutic uses of beta radiation, is discussed in Chapter 14. Beta particles are 8000 times lighter than alpha particles and have only one unit of electrical charge (−1) as compared with the alpha's two units of electrical charge (+2). These attributes mean that beta particles will not interact as strongly with their surroundings as alpha particles do. Therefore, they are capable of penetrating biologic matter to a greater depth than alpha particles with far less ionization along their paths. Not all high-speed electrons are beta radiation. Alternate sources of high-speed electrons are produced in a radiation oncology treatment machine called a *linear accelerator.* These electrons are most often used to treat superficial skin lesions in small areas or to deliver radiation boost treatments to breast tumors at tissue depths typically not exceeding 5 to 6 cm. Such very high-energy electrons require either millimeters of lead or multicentimeter thick slabs of wood to absorb them. As previously stated, alpha rays can be absorbed by a piece of ordinary paper because they interact so readily with matter and lose their kinetic energy quite rapidly as a consequence. Beta rays, however, with a lesser probability of interaction, can penetrate matter more deeply and therefore cannot be stopped by an ordinary piece of paper. For energies of less than 2 MeV, either a 1-cm-thick piece of wood or a 1-mm-thick lead shield would be sufficient for absorption.

*Protons* are positively charged components of an atom. An isolated proton, which is simply an ionized hydrogen atom, has a relatively small mass that, however, exceeds the mass of an electron by a factor of 1800. The number of protons in the nucleus of an atom constitutes its atomic number, or "Z" number. The atomic number identifies an element and determines its placement in the periodic table of elements (see Appendix C).

*Neutrons* are the electrically neutral components of an atom and have approximately the same mass as a proton. If two atoms have the same number of protons but a different number of neutrons in their nuclei, they are referred to as *isotopes.* If one of these combinations of Z protons and so many neutrons leads to an unstable nucleus, then that combination is called a "radioisotope."

## Radiation Dose Specification: Equivalent Dose

**Equivalent dose** (EqD) is a radiation *quantity* used for radiation protection purposes when a person receives exposure from various types of ionizing radiation. This quantity attempts to specify numerically the differences in transferred energy and therefore potential biologic harm produced by different types of radiation. EqD enables the calculation of the **effective dose (EfD)**. EfD is essentially a manufactured quantity that takes into account the dose for all types of ionizing radiation (e.g., alpha, beta, gamma, x-ray) to various irradiated organs or tissues in the human body (e.g., skin, gonadal tissue, thyroid). By including specific weighting factors for each of those parts of the body mentioned, EfD takes into account the chance or risk that each of those body parts will develop radiation-induced cancer. In the case of the reproductive organs, the risk of **genetic damage** (radiation damage to generations yet unborn) is considered. Because EfD includes all the organ weighting factors, it represents the uniform whole-body dose that would give an equivalent biologic response or chance of cancer. In the International System of Units (SI), the unit of EqD is the **sievert (Sv)**. Both occupational and nonoccupational dose limits are expressed as EfD and are also stated in sieverts. EfD, EqD, and other units of dosimetry are discussed in substantial detail in Chapter 4.

## Biologic Damage Potential

While penetrating body tissue, ionizing radiation produces **biologic damage** primarily by ejecting electrons from the atoms composing the tissues. Destructive radiation interaction at the atomic level results in molecular change, and this in turn can cause **cellular damage,** leading to abnormal cell function or even entire loss of cell function. If excessive cellular damage occurs, the living organism will have a significant possibility of exhibiting genetic or somatic changes such as the following:

- Mutations
- Cataracts
- Leukemia

*[handwritten: destructive rad @ atomic level - molecular change - cellular damage - organic damage]*

Changes in blood count are classic examples of **organic damage** that results from non-negligible exposure to ionizing radiation. An EqD as low as 0.25 Sv delivered to the whole body may cause a decrease within a few days in the number of lymphocytes (white blood cells that defend the body against foreign invaders by producing antibodies to combat disease) in the blood. Table 2-2 provides some basic information on the known biologic effects that result

| TABLE 2-2 | Radiation Equivalent Dose and Subsequent Biologic Effects Resulting from Acute Whole-Body Exposures* |
|---|---|
| **Radiation EqD** | |
| **Sv** | **Subsequent Biologic Effects** |
| 0.25 | Blood changes (e.g., measurable hematologic depression, decreases in the number of lymphocytes present in the circulating blood) |
| 1.5 | Nausea, diarrhea |
| 2.0 | Erythema (diffuse redness over an area of skin after irradiation) |
| 2.5 | If dose is to gonads, temporary sterility |
| 3.0 | 50% chance of death; lethal dose for 50% of population over 30 days (LD 50/30) |
| 6.0 | Death |

Adapted from *Radiologic health,* unit 4, slide 17, Denver, Multi-Media Publishing (slide program).
*Radiation exposures are delivered to the entire body over a time period of less than a few hours.

when radiation exposures of various EqDs are delivered to the whole body over a time period of less than a few hours (acute exposures). Because of the potential for biologic damage from different radiation EqDs to the whole body, the use of ionizing radiation should be limited whenever possible.

## Sources of Radiation

Human beings are continuously exposed to sources of ionizing radiation. Sources of ionizing radiation may be one of the following:

- Natural
- Manmade (artificial)

Table 2-3 provides a quick, current reference for average annual radiation EqDs for estimated levels of radiation exposure for humans resulting from both natural background and manmade sources of radiation. Since 1987, there has been little change in the amount of natural background radiation to which the U.S. population is exposed. However, significant changes have occurred in the amount of radiation exposure to this population from medical imaging procedures. This increase in exposure results from the increased use of imaging modalities such as computed tomography (CT), cardiac nuclear medicine examinations, and interventional procedures.[3] The number of "repeat" CT scans for patients has especially grown.

To provide greater understanding of the various sources of ionizing radiation to which the U.S. population has been exposed since the publication of the 1987 National Council on Radiation Protection and Measurements (NCRP) report, the NCRP (see Chapter 10 for information on the Radiation Standards Organization) issued another report on March 3, 2009. It is NCRP Report No. 160, *Ionizing Radiation Exposure of the Population of the United States.* This document "estimates the total amount of radiation delivered in 2006 and compares those amounts to the estimates published in 1987."

**Natural Radiation.** Natural sources of ionizing radiation have always been a part of the

| TABLE 2-3 | Average Annual Radiation Equivalent Dose for Estimated Levels of Radiation Exposure for Humans | |
|---|---|---|

| | | Dose |
|---|---|---|
| Category | Type of Radiation | mSv |
| Natural | Radon | 2.0 |
| | Cosmic | 0.3 |
| | Terrestrial | 0.3 |
| | Internal | 0.3 |
| | Total | 3.0 |
| Medical imaging | CT scanning | 1.5 |
| | Radiography | 0.6 |
| | Nuclear medicine | 0.7 |
| | Interventional procedures | 0.4 |
| | Total | 3.2 |
| Other manmade | | 0.1 |
| | Total Annual EqD from All Sources | 6.3 |

Adapted from Bushong SC: *Radiologic science for technologists: physics, biology, and protection,* ed 10, St. Louis, 2013, Mosby.
*CT,* Computed tomography; *EqD,* equivalent dose.

human environment since the formation of the universe. Ionizing radiation from environmental sources is called **natural background radiation** and has the following three components:

- Terrestrial radiation from radioactive materials in the crust of the earth ex. radon, thoron
- Cosmic radiation from the sun (solar) and beyond the solar system (galactic)
- Internal radiation from radioactive atoms (also known as *radionuclides*) that make up a small percentage of the body's tissue

If radiation from any of these natural sources grows larger because of accidental or deliberate human actions such as mining, the sources are termed *enhanced natural sources.*

***Terrestrial Radiation.*** Long-lived radioactive elements such as uranium-238, radium-226, and thorium-232 that emit densely ionizing radiations are present in variable quantities in the crust of the earth. These sources of ionizing radiation are classified as *terrestrial radiation.* The quantity of terrestrial radiation present in any area depends on the composition of the soil or rocks in that geographic region. As of 2006, as reported in NCRP Report No. 160, 37% of natural background radiation exposure comes primarily from the gaseous radionuclide **radon** and from a smaller amount of thoron,* a much less hazardous gas (Fig. 2-2). Both these gases emit alpha radiation. Radon initially does not cling to other particles. Rather, it behaves as a free agent that floats around in the soil and so is referred to as a *noble gas.* As a consequence, the natural flow of air can draw radon gas into the lower levels of homes, and then the gas may permeate upward through such structures as it decays and becomes solid particles.[4,5]

---

*Thoron is a radioactive decay product of an isotope of radon, namely radon-220, with a half-life of 54.5 seconds. It is given the name thoron because radon-220 was itself derived from the radioactive decay of thorium-232, a naturally occurring material.

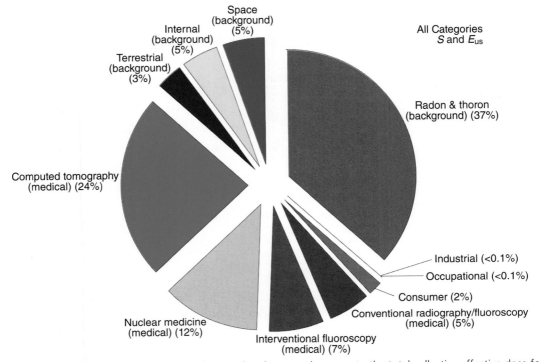

**FIGURE 2-2** Percentage contribution of each natural and manmade source to the total collective effective dose for the population of the United States, 2006.

Geologic formations or soils containing granite, shale, phosphate, and pitchblende produce higher concentrations of radon than other commonly encountered materials. Radon is by far the largest contributor to background radiation. As of 2006, the average U.S. resident received approximately 2.0 mSv per year from indoor and outdoor levels of radon. Radon is the first decay product of radium and is produced as radium decays in soil. It is a colorless, odorless, heavy radioactive gas that, along with its own decay products, polonium-218 ($^{218}$Po) and $^{214}$Po (solid form), is always present to some degree in the air. Because radon has a half-life of 3.825 days,[5] it can gradually percolate up through the soil. Radon enters buildings through cracks or holes in their frameworks. In homes, it may gain access through the following areas (Fig. 2-3):

- Crawl spaces under the living areas
- Floor drains
- Sump pumps
- Porous cement block foundations

In many cases, a pressure gradient exists between a house and the soil on which it rests so that the house draws on the ground like a vacuum cleaner. Commonly used building materials such as bricks, concrete, and gypsum wallboard contain radon. These construction materials are classified as earth-based materials.[2]

Radon concentrations in a particular structure vary across days and seasons. In the cooler months, when homes and buildings are tightly closed, radon levels are usually higher. This is the best time to perform tests for radon.*

---

*Detection kits are relatively easy to use and may be purchased at retail stores or obtained at minimal cost from the National Safety Council in Washington, DC, by calling 1-800-SOS-RADON.

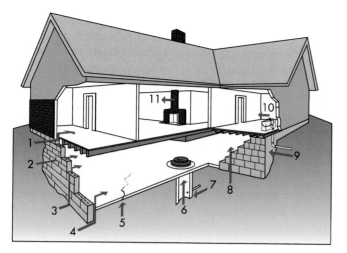

**FIGURE 2-3**   Radon gas can percolate up through soil and enter a home through holes or cracks in its framework, crawl spaces under the living areas, floor drains, sump pumps, and porous cement block foundations. *1,* Spaces behind brick veneer on top of block foundation; *2,* pores and cracks in concrete block foundation; *3,* open top of block foundation walls; *4,* floor to wall joints; *5,* cracks in concrete floor; *6,* exposed soil as in basement sump; *7,* weeping drain tile draining into open sump; *8,* mortar joints; *9,* loose-fitting pipe wall penetration; *10,* well water from some wells; *11,* building materials such as stone.

High indoor concentrations of radon and radon decay products, which are actually solid particles that have attached themselves to dust, have the potential to cause serious health hazards for humans.[4] After being inhaled, these airborne radioactive gases and decay products produce daughter radioactive isotopes that remain for lengthy periods in the epithelial tissue of the lungs. As these secondary isotopes decay, they give off alpha radiation that may injure lung tissues, thereby increasing the risk for lung cancer. The severity of this risk depends on the concentration of the radon and the length of time to which the person is exposed to the gas and solid particles.[6] Smokers exposed to high radon levels face a higher risk of lung cancer than do nonsmokers. One reason for this may be that smokers have already been exposed to higher concentrations of radioactivity from the lead-210 ($^{210}$Pb) and polonium-210 ($^{210}$Po) isotopes contained in tobacco and tobacco smoke. As mentioned earlier, an isotope is an atom that contains a different number of neutrons but the same number of protons in its nucleus as does the reference atom (e.g., helium-3 and helium-4, whose nuclei contain one and two neutrons, respectively). Radioactive isotopes of atoms that make up biologic materials may be used in medical imaging nuclear medicine studies.

The Environmental Protection Agency (EPA) considers radon to be the second leading cause of lung cancer in the United States. Radon is responsible for approximately 20,000 cancer deaths per year. (For more information on the EPA, see Chapter 10). The EPA recommends that action be taken to reduce elevated levels of radon to less than 4 picocuries* per liter (pCi/L) of air (a concentration that specifies the number of radioactive processes per second that occur on average in 1 L of air). A radon concentration of 4 pCi/L results in a yearly EqD to the lung of approximately 0.05 mSv.[7] The presence of this level of radon is considered statistically safe by the EPA. The EPA estimates that 10% of the homes in the United States exceed the recommended limit of 4 pCi/L. Hence, accurate radon testing and appropriate structural repair, if required, are essential to reducing the risk of lung cancer from radon. In actuality, radiation exposure to radon cannot be entirely eliminated, but with suitable structural correction it can be significantly reduced.

***Cosmic Radiation.*** Cosmic rays are of extraterrestrial origin and result from nuclear interactions that have taken place in the sun and other

---

*1 picocurie = $10^{-12}$ curie.

stars. The intensity of cosmic rays varies with altitude relative to the earth's surface. The greatest intensity occurs at high altitudes, and the lowest intensity occurs at sea level. The earth's atmosphere and magnetic field help shield the planet from cosmic rays. The shielding is diminished at higher elevation where less atmosphere separates the earth from cosmic rays. As of 2006, the average U.S. inhabitant received an EqD of approximately 0.3 mSv per year from extraterrestrial radiation (see Table 2-3). Cosmic radiations consist predominantly of high-energy protons; as a result of interactions with molecules in the earth's atmosphere, these protons may be accompanied by alpha particles, atomic nuclei, mesons, gamma rays, and high-energy electrons. These other forms of radiation are collectively referred to as *secondary cosmic radiation*. The gamma rays among them are energetic enough to penetrate several meters of lead.

***Terrestrial and Internal Radiation.*** The tissues of the human body contain many naturally existing radionuclides that have been ingested in minute quantities from various foods or inhaled as particles in the air. A **radionuclide** is an unstable nucleus that emits one or more forms of ionizing radiation to achieve greater stability. These forms of ionizing radiation may include the following:

- Alpha particles (helium nuclei)
- Beta particles (electrons)
- Gamma rays (similar to x-rays, but usually of higher energy, in the range of a million electron volts [MeV])

Certain types of radioactive decay also affect the distribution of electrons around the atom and result in the emission of x-rays. Examples of radioactive nuclides that exist in small quantities in the human body are as follows:

- Potassium-40 ($^{40}$K) (mainly)
- Carbon-14 ($^{14}$C)
- Hydrogen-3 ($^{3}$H; tritium)
- Strontium-90 ($^{90}$Sr)

Radionuclides in the soil and air also add to the human radiation dose burden. As of 2006, the average member of the general population received approximately 0.7 mSv per year from combined exposure to radiations from the earth's surface (terrestrial) and radiation within the human body. In the 2006 total, the radon (2.00 mSv), cosmic ray radiations (0.3 mSv), terrestrial, and internally deposited radionuclides (0.7 mSv) that comprise the natural background radiation in the United States resulted in an estimated average annual individual EqD of approximately 3.0 mSv (see Table 2-3).

**Manmade (Artificial) Radiation.** Ionizing radiation created by humans for various uses is classified as **manmade, or artificial, radiation.** Sources of artificial ionizing radiation include the following:

- Consumer products containing radioactive material
- Air travel
- Nuclear fuel for generation of power
- Atmospheric fallout from nuclear weapons testing
- Nuclear power plant accidents
- Nuclear power plant accidents as a consequence of natural disasters
- Medical radiation

As of 2006, manmade radiation contributed about 3.2 mSv to the average annual radiation exposure of the U.S. population. Of this EqD, 0.6 mSv resulted from medical radiographic procedures, 0.7 mSv resulted from nuclear medicine imaging, 1.5 mSv resulted from CT scanning, 0.4 mSv resulted from interventional procedures and 0.1 mSv resulted from other manmade radiation sources (see Table 2-3). Of course, an individual may or may not have the medical radiation procedures listed above in a given year, but these figures represent an "average share" of dose that would be true, if the total medical radiation dose were shared equally among all individuals. A qualified medical physicist can calculate an individual's actual medical radiation exposure from x-ray examinations, if he or she is provided with the essential technical details (e.g., x-ray tube voltage used, exposure time) pertaining to the studies.

***Consumer Products Containing Radioactive Material.*** Consumer products containing radioactive material include the following:

- Airport surveillance systems
- Early televisions
- Electron microscopes
- Shoe-fitting fluoroscopes used in the early 1920s through approximately 1970
- Ionization-type smoke detector alarms
- Phonograph record static eliminators
- Some timepieces with luminous dials and numbers containing promethium-147, radium-226, $^{90}$Sr, and tritium
- Video display terminals that use cathode-ray tubes

These products contribute a small fraction of the total average EqD to each member of the general population.

When color television monitors were first made available to consumers, radiation exposure levels from these devices was substantial. As a result of technologic advances since the 1970s and strict regulations imposed within the United States by the Food and Drug Administration (FDA) regarding such devices, the radiation exposure of the general public may now be considered negligible.

From 1920 until approximately 1970, shoe-fitting fluoroscopes were used in shoe stores so that customers could see how well a pair of shoes fit before purchase. The shoe-fitting fluoroscopic device was constructed of a wooden cabinet with a lead-shielded base and platform on the base on which the customer could stand with his or her feet in the opening provided. The x-ray tube was housed in the lead-lined cabinet base below the platform, and three separate viewing ports (one each for the parent, child, and sales associate to look through to see the feet inside the shoes, when the x-ray tube was energized) were on top of the cabinet. For example, once the child wearing the new shoes placed his or her feet in the cabinet opening, the exposure button could be pushed to activate the fluoroscope, thus permitting those looking into the viewing ports to see "a fluorescent image of the bones within the outline of the new shoes"[8] (Fig. 2-4). Sales associates assisting customers with the purchase of shoes used the shoe-fitting fluoroscope many times throughout their work day, and some sustained excessive radiation exposure, resulting in radiation burns to their hands from manipulating the shoes on the customer's feet while the x-ray machine was energized. Even though sales associates knew how to operate the shoe-fitting fluoroscope, they lacked knowledge of radiation hazards and radiation protection for self and customers. In an attempt to improve the relatively poor quality of the fluoroscopic image, sales associates sometimes removed the cumbersome lead shielding in the cabinet housing the machine. Many states eventually banned this device for use in fitting shoes.[8]

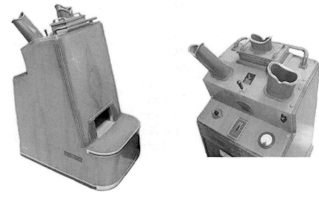

FIGURE 2-4  **Photo of Shoe-Fitting Fluoroscope.**

Porcelain used for making dentures provides a common present-day example of a consumer product that contains radioactive material. Porcelain contains $^{40}K$ and is usually "doped" with uranium to give a more natural color to the denture.[8] Artificial teeth made in the United States are estimated to give the tissues of the oral cavity an average dose of 600 mSv/year, whereas dental porcelain made in Great Britain has been reported to have dose rates 10 times higher.[9]

***Air Travel.*** The normal use of the airplane at high elevations brings many humans in closer contact with high-energy extraterrestrial radiation (e.g., cosmic radiation) and consequently increases exposure. A flight on a typical commercial airliner results in an EqD rate of 0.005 to 0.01 mSv/hour.

Sunspots are dark spots that occasionally appear on the surface of the sun. They indicate regions of increased electromagnetic field activity and are sometimes responsible for ejecting particulate radiation into space. This radiation normally constitutes a small fraction of our dose from cosmic radiation here on earth. However, the solar contribution to the cosmic ray background increases during periods of high sunspot activity.

If a person spends 10 hours flying aboard a commercial aircraft during a period of normal sunspot activity, that individual will receive a radiation EqD that is about equal to the dose received from one chest x-ray examination. During a *solar flare,* "a tremendous explosion on the surface of the sun,"[10] this dose can be 10 to as much as 100 times higher. Awareness of these increases in radiation exposure at high altitudes is important information for pilots and airline crews and the general public. An increase in radiation exposure carries an immeasurably small health risk for those individuals who travel by air infrequently. However, for pilots, flight attendants, and the general public who are "frequent flyers" the possibility exists that they "may unknowingly be exposed to excessively large doses of radiation."[11] With adequate knowledge, a person choosing air travel during periods of high sunspot activity and solar flares can make

an intelligent decision about whether the potential benefit of the air travel outweighs any increased health risk.

If a comparison between workers at a nuclear plant and pilots and flight attendants is made, the "pilots and flight attendants may be more at risk to receive harmful doses of radiation. To prove the harmful effects of this background radiation, data must be collected from various flights by physicians and biologists and submitted for an accurate evaluation of ionization levels."[11]

***Nuclear Fuel for the Generation of Power.*** Nuclear power plants that produce nuclear fuel for the generation of power do not contribute significantly to the annual EqD of the U.S. population. As of 2006, the nuclear fuel cycle, along with other manmade radiations, contributed only a very small portion of 0.1 mSv to the total average annual EqD for persons living in the United States.

***Atmospheric Fallout from Nuclear Weapons Testing.*** An accurate estimate of the total annual EqD from fallout cannot be made because actual radiation measurements do not exist. The *dose commitment* (the dose that may ultimately be delivered from a given intake of radionuclide)[12] may be estimated by using a series of approximations and simplistic models that are subject to considerable speculation. The actual radiation dose to the global population from atmospheric fallout from nuclear weapons testing is not received all at once. It is instead delivered over a period of years at changing dose rates. The changes in the dose rates depend on factors such as characteristics of the fallout field and the elapsed time since the test occurred. No atmospheric nuclear testing has occurred since 1980.

As of 2006, when spread over the inhabitants of the United States, fallout from nuclear weapons tests (Fig. 2-5) and other environmental sources along with other manmade radiations contributed only a small portion of 0.1 mSv to the EqD of each person. This annual EqD is still considered to have a negligible impact on the U.S. population.

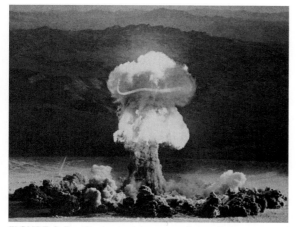

**FIGURE 2-5**   The United States performed aboveground nuclear weapons tests before 1963. During the Priscilla Test, this atomic cloud resulted when a 37-kiloton testing device exploded from a balloon at the Nevada test site on June 24, 1957. The atomic cloud top, which contained manmade ionizing radiation, ascended approximately 43,000 feet.

***Nuclear Power Plant Accidents.*** Although nuclear power benefits humans by creating a needed supply of electricity, unfortunate accidents involving nuclear reactors can occur. This can lead to substantial unplanned radiation exposure for humans and the environment. Examples of two nuclear power plant accidents are addressed in the discussions that follow.

*Three Mile Island Unit 2.* Beginning at approximately 4:00 AM EST on March 28, 1979, the Three Mile Island Unit 2 (TMI-2) pressurized water reactor, situated on an island in the Susquehanna River located about 15 miles southeast of Harrisburg, Pennsylvania (Fig. 2-6, *A*), underwent a loss of coolant that resulted in severe overheating (at a temperature greater than 5000° F) of the radioactive reactor core. Consequently, significant melting of the core occurred. The U.S. Department of Energy estimated that about 40% of the material in the TMI-2 nuclear

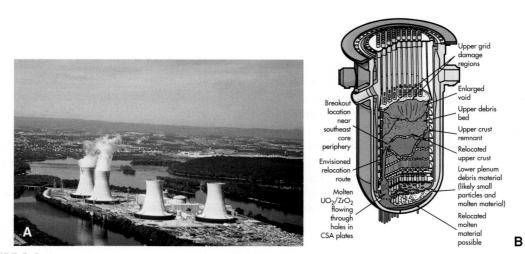

**FIGURE 2-6**   **A,** Nuclear power stations, such as the one located on Three Mile Island (TMI) near Harrisburg, Pennsylvania, house nuclear reactors. The large round containment buildings holding the reactors retain radioactive liquids and gases even in a high-pressure environment. **B,** TMI-2 end-state core conditions illustrating the damage to the radioactive nuclear reactor core after the loss of coolant accident on March 28, 1979. Some of the original core mass formed an upper layer of debris. A hard crust supports this material. Zones of previously molten material and standing fuel rod segments account for some of the core mass lying beneath the upper debris bed. The lower reactor vessel head contains some of the melted core material. Closed-circuit television, mechanical probing, and core-boring operations contributed to assessing the TMI-2 end-state core conditions.

reactor core reached a molten state. Approximately 15% of the melted uranium dioxide fuel of the core actually flowed through the undamaged portions of the core and settled on the bottom of the reactor vessel. This melted material in the nuclear reactor core and bottom of the reactor vessel formed crusts on its outside surfaces and in time cooled to resolidified debris (Fig. 2-6, B). Although significant melting of the core and flowing of the molten radioactive material into intact portions of the reactor vessel occurred, fortunately no "melt-through" of the reactor vessel resulted. The accident did, however, result in the destruction of the reactor.

Even though the potential existed for the release of significant amounts of radioactive material, according to the General Public Utilities Nuclear Corporation (GPU), the quantity of radiation that actually escaped during the accident (approximately 15 curies* of iodine-131 [$^{131}$I][†]) was not sufficient to cause health problems for persons occupationally exposed or for the 2 million people living within 50 miles of the plant. The average dose received by the exposed population living within a 50-mile radius of the TMI nuclear power station was 0.08 mSv. In actuality, this average dose is not above a background radiation level.

According to conventional methods of risk assessment, if 0.08 mGy[‡] is used as an upper limit dose of ionizing radiation, it can be predicted that no more than one additional case of fatal cancer may occur in this population as a result of radiation exposure from this accident.[13]

Therefore, detection of excess cancer deaths in this population as a consequence of the radiation dose it received is not expected.

Additional malignant deaths in the population exposed to radiation during the entire time of the TMI incident can be evaluated in another way. This is by applying the average dose received by the population as the "population dose" for persons living within a 100-mile radius of the nuclear power plant at the time of the accident. During this time, these residents received an average radiation exposure of 15 microgray.[‡] If this dose is used as the population dose, then no more than two additional resulting cancer deaths can be predicted in the exposed inhabitants as a consequence of radiation exposure.[2]

Beginning at the time of the accident and continuing through 1992, the University of Pittsburgh followed more than 32,000 people who lived within 5 miles of TMI and were exposed to the low-level radioactivity released by the accident. Researchers found no link between radiation released (primarily xenon and iodine radioisotopes) during the TMI accident and cancer deaths among persons residing in the area. During the 13-year study of the people who lived within 5 miles of TMI at the time of the accident, only a single death occurred as a consequence of thyroid cancer, and this death was not attributed to radiation exposure.[14]

Because most radiation-induced cancers have a latent period of 15 years or more, continued monitoring of the health of the exposed residents is needed. Studies are expected to continue to obtain the necessary data to evaluate the mortality experience further.

Since the TMI-2 nuclear power plant accident, more than 30 years have passed. There has been no significant increase in cancer-related deaths reported among the population living near the TMI nuclear power station. Psychological stress at the time of the accident and shortly thereafter has been identified as the only detectable effect.[15] The Nuclear Regulatory Commission (NRC) (discussed in Chapter 10) reported that the TMI-2 pressurized water reactor is "permanently shut down and defueled, with the reactor

---

*1 curie represents a quantity of radioactive material that every second produces on average $3.7 \times 10^{10}$ nuclear disintegrations.

[†]$^{131}$I is a radioactive isotope that emits both beta particles (fast electrons) and energetic gamma rays, with the most common beta emissions (89.3%) having 192 keV mean energy and the most common gamma emission (81.2%) having 365 keV energy.

[‡]Gray (Gy) is the SI unit for measuring exposure. A milligray is a subunit of the Gy. It is equal to one thousandth of a Gy. The microgray is also a subunit of the Gy. It is equal to one millionth of a Gy. Radiation quantities and units are covered in Chapter 4.

coolant system drained, the radioactive water decontaminated and evaporated, radioactive waste shipped off-site to an appropriate disposal site, reactor fuel and core debris shipped off-site to a Department of Energy facility, and the remainder of the site being monitored."[16] Long-term monitored storage of TMI-2 is expected to continue "until the operating license for the TMI-1 plant expires at which time both plants will be decommissioned."[16] "In 2009 the TMI-1 operating license was renewed, extending its life by 20 years to 2034."[17]

*Chernobyl.* An explosion at a nuclear power plant in Chernobyl (near Kiev in the Ukraine in the former Soviet Union) (Fig. 2-7) on April 26, 1986, resulted in the release of a number of radioactive nuclides, including 46 megacuries of $^{131}$I, 136 megacuries of xenon radioisotopes, and 2.3 megacuries of cesium-137 ($^{137}$Cs). This is far more than 1 million times the amount of radioactive material released at TMI or "30 to 40 times as much radioactivity as the Hiroshima and Nagasaki atomic bombs combined in 1945."[18] More than 200 people working at the Chernobyl plant received a whole-body EqD exceeding 1 Sv. More than 2 dozen workers died as a result of explosion-related injuries and the effects of receiving doses greater than 4 Sv. The average EqD to the approximately quarter of a million individuals living within 200 miles of the reactor was 0.2 Sv, with thyroid doses (from drinking milk containing radioactive iodine) in some individuals exceeding several sieverts. Adverse health effects from radiation exposure are expected to occur for many years as a consequence of the total collective EqD received by the affected population, and "the number of people who could eventually die as a result of the Chernobyl accident is highly controversial."[19]

*The ETHOS Project.* Beginning in 1996, a 3-year pilot research project called the ETHOS Project[19] was launched in the Republic of Belarus. This project was supported by the radiation project research program of the European Commission (DG XII). In the aftermath of the Chernobyl accident, the local citizens of the contaminated territories were empowered to make

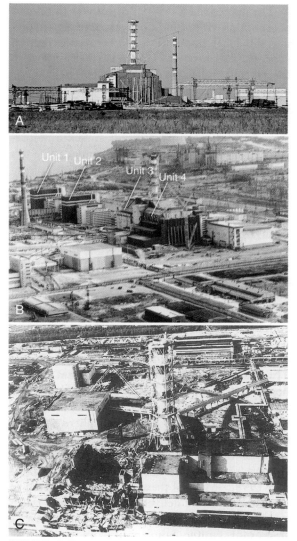

FIGURE 2-7 **A,** Nuclear power plant in Chernobyl, former Soviet Union, site of the 1986 radiation accident. **B,** Aerial view of the four identical units of the Chernobyl nuclear power plant before the accident. Graphics point out each of the reactors. **C,** Chernobyl nuclear power plant after the explosion of unit 4 on April 26, 1986.

their own decisions to facilitate reconstruction of their overall quality of life. They were given the authority to manage their radiologic risk in the same way that the rural communities manage natural risk.[20,21]

The aim of the ETHOS Project was to rebuild acceptable living conditions by actively involving the local population in the reconstruction process. This process encompassed dealing with the aspects of daily living that had been changed or threatened as a consequence of radioactive contamination. One example was the establishment of guidelines for the amount of ash that is allowed to build up in wood stoves and fireplaces before cleaning is recommended. The ash is residue that remains after burning wood from trees that have taken up radioactive materials from the soil. The ash contains radioactive materials and is more compact than the piles of wood from which it came. The elimination of use of wood from the surrounding forests would have posed an unreasonable economic hardship on the population and was unnecessary as long as appropriate guidelines were set. Through this program, local citizens have been engaging in cooperative problem solving as they reconstruct their environment.

*Thyroid Cancer, Leukemia, and Breast Cancer.* Thyroid cancer continues to be the main adverse health effect of the 1986 Chernobyl nuclear power accident. Children and adolescents living in the Ukraine region of Russia, where the dose was heaviest after the disaster, continue to be the focus of the disease. More than 1700 cases of thyroid cancer were diagnosed between 1990 and 1998.[22] Most of these cases are attributed to the radiation dose delivered when [131]I was taken up by the thyroid gland, although previous studies of atomic bomb survivors and Pacific Island inhabitants exposed to fallout predicted only 10 or so extra cases of thyroid cancer.[23] "The 2005 report prepared by the Chernobyl Forum, led by the International Atomic Energy Agency (IAEA) and the World Health Organization (WHO),* attributed 56 direct deaths (47 accident workers, and 9 children with thyroid cancer), and estimated that there may be 4000

extra deaths due to cancer among the approximately 600,000 most highly exposed and 5000 among the 6 million living nearby."[24,25]

Since the time of the Chernobyl accident, there has also been an increase in the incidence of breast cancer directly attributed to the radiation exposure.[26,27] The World Health Organization Expert Group revealed that "reports indicate a small increase in the incidence of pre-menopausal breast cancer in the most contaminated areas, which appear to be related to radiation dose."[28] However, follow-up epidemiologic studies are necessary to confirm these findings. Some early research indicated no other increases in the effects that are generally associated with radiation exposure (leukemia, congenital abnormalities, or adverse pregnancy outcomes).[29] For example, the World Health Organization found no increase in leukemia incidence by 1993 in the population hit hardest by fallout from Chernobyl.[30] Later studies began to show some of the expected effects. It was reported that there has been about a 50% increase in leukemia cases in children and adults in the Gomel region since the Chernobyl disaster.[31,32] Also reported, in June 2001 at the Third International Conference held in Kiev, the Russian liquidators who worked during 1986 and 1987 at the Chernobyl power station complex had a statistically significant rise in the number of leukemia cases.[33,34] The World Health Organization reported that "recent investigations suggest a doubling of the incidence of leukaemia* among the most highly exposed Chernobyl liquidators."[28] Furthermore, this organization also revealed that "no such increase has been clearly demonstrated among children or adults in any of the contaminated areas."[28] Additional time will be required before all the implications of these findings are clearly understood. More information about the Chernobyl catastrophe and its resulting health effects may be found in Chapters 8 and 9.

---

*The World Health organization is the authority that directs and coordinates for health within the United Nations System.

*"Leukaemia" is a variation of the spelling of "leukemia" that is used in some countries and by the World Health Organization. This European spelling can differ from the U.S. spelling, as in, for example, "aluminum" (U.S. spelling) and "aluminium" (British spelling).

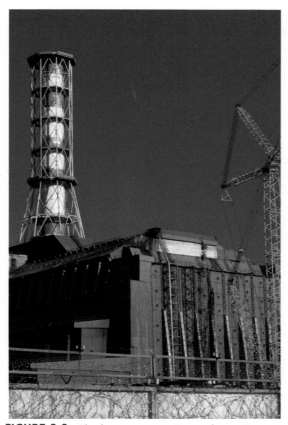

**FIGURE 2-8** The large concrete "sarcophagus," encasing the remains of Chernobyl reactor unit 4. The structure is in danger of collapsing.

During the 6 months after the Chernobyl nuclear power plant disaster, a large concrete shelter known as the "sarcophagus" (Fig. 2-8) was constructed by the Soviets atop the remains of the reactor 4 building so that the other reactors could continue operating to provide nuclear power. Unfortunately, within 10 years after the shelter's construction the walls weakened, leaving the sarcophagus in danger of collapsing. Radiation leaks from the entombed reactor building also became apparent and caused great concern in the scientific community. During 1998 and 1999, some major repair work was carried out on the massive structure to strengthen the roof and structural pillars and stabilize the ventilation stack. In spite of the efforts made to enhance the strength and stability of the sarcophagus, the integrity of the structure remained questionable. Furthermore, lethal radiation levels inside the shelter both complicated and limited opportunities for repair and maintenance.

Plans were made to cover the remains of Chernobyl reactor unit 4 and the concrete sarcophagus that entombs it with a weatherproof, massive steel vault (Fig. 2-9). Construction of this structure began in April 2012, with an estimated completion date of 2016.[35] The arch-shaped steel vault with a 100-year designed lifetime, referred to as the New Safe Confinement structure, is actually being built on site and, when completed, will be moved in place on rails and then slid over the collapsing sarcophagus. After this task has been accomplished, the concrete sarcophagus will be dismantled. The new shelter will provide protection so that highly radioactive fuel and damaged reactor remains can be better confined to protect the environment and the population more effectively.

***Nuclear Power Plant Accidents as a Consequence of Natural Disasters.*** Accidents can occur in nuclear power plants as a consequence of natural disasters such as earthquakes followed by a tsunami (tidal wave). This devastation can result in widespread environmental and health effects on the affected population of the surrounding area.

***Fukushima Daiichi Nuclear Plant Crisis.*** On March 11, 2012, a 9.0-magnitude earthquake that began approximately 60 miles off the northeast coast of Japan triggered a tsunami that slammed into the island's coast and bombarded it with 30-foot-high waves that actually traveled as far as 6 miles inland and devastated everything in their path within minutes.[36]

The Fukushima Daiichi Nuclear Plant, housing six reactors, is located 93 miles southwest of epicenter. As a consequence of the earthquake, the entire Japanese coastline dropped as much as 3 feet, thus leaving the plant much more vulnerable to the seismic waves of the tsunami that was racing toward the shutdown plant in which the reactor cores had been automatically taken offline by sensors. Even though the nuclear plant

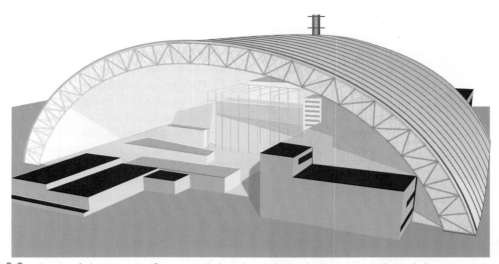

**FIGURE 2-9**   Sketch of the New Confinement Shelter that is being built to cover Chernobyl reactor unit 4 and the concrete sarcophagus that entombs it.

had survived the earthquake, its 18-foot protection walls were not high enough to stop 30-foot waves from flooding the diesel generators cooling the reactor cores. Eventually even the backup batteries that kept the pumps going failed. With the reactors in lockdown and no power being generated to operate the cooling pumps, a critical situation was created as temperatures continued to rise in the reactors. This led to a significant overheating of the fuel rods that resulted in the production of hydrogen gas, which eventually exploded. In desperation, an attempt was made to cool the reactors by dumping seawater on them. Unfortunately, this procedure did not work. Destruction of some reactors and severe damage to others occurred, leading to the release of a considerable amount of radiation (e.g., [137]Cs) in the atmosphere and surrounding area.[36] Because it is extremely difficult to measure the amounts of radiation people received, the long-term effects such as an increased incidence of cancer in the exposed population cannot be accurately determined.[37]

Because humans are unable to control natural background radiation, exposure from artificial sources that can be controlled must be limited to protect the general population from further biologic damage.

***Medical Radiation.*** As mentioned earlier in this chapter, NCRP Report No. 160 was released on March 3, 2009. It reflects data on medical usage patterns through 2006. Data from this report are presented in Table 2-4. The previous report, NCRP Report No. 93 published in 1987, used data on medical usage from 1980 to 1982. The number of medical procedures involving the use of ionizing radiation had increased dramatically since the 1980s. Because of this trend, exposure of the U.S. population from medical sources has increased.

Medical radiation exposure results from the use of diagnostic x-ray machines and radiopharmaceuticals in medicine. Diagnostic medical x-ray radiation (which includes CT scanning, interventional fluoroscopy, and conventional radiography or fluoroscopy) and nuclear medicine procedures are the two largest sources of artificial radiation, and they collectively accounted for 48% of the total collective EfD of the U.S. population as of 2006 (see Fig. 2-2). The main reason for the increase is the enormously expanded use of CT. With the advent of multislice spiral (helical) CT, the utility of this imaging modality in areas such as emergency medicine has increased dramatically. In 1980, the use of CT resulted in a collective dose of 3700

| TABLE 2-4 | Medical Radiation Exposure: 2006 | | | | |
|---|---|---|---|---|---|
| Modalities | Number of Procedures | Percentage (%) | Collective Dose (Person-Sv) | Percentage (%) | Per Capita (mSv) |
| Computed tomography | 67 million | 16 | 440,000 | 49 | 1.50 |
| Nuclear medicine | 18 million | 4 | 231,000 | 26 | 0.80 |
| Radiography and fluoroscopy | 324 million | 76 | 99,000 | 11 | 0.30 |
| Interventional | 17 million | 4 | 129,000 | 14 | 0.40 |
| **Total** | **~426 million** | | **899,000** | | **~3.0** |

person-sieverts. By 2006, that number had risen to 440,000 person-sieverts (see Table 2-4).[3] (See Chapter 4 for a discussion of Radiation Quantities and Units.)

Of course, the use of CT has tremendous medical benefit in the diagnosis of disease and trauma, and the risk-to-benefit ratio is still very small when CT examinations are ordered for appropriate reasons.

According to NCRP Report No. 93, medical radiation was estimated to contribute 0.54 mSv to manmade radiation. As of 2006, medical radiation accounted for approximately 3.2 mSv of the average annual individual EfD of ionizing radiation received (see Table 2-3), an increase of more than a factor of five. The total average annual EfD from manmade and natural radiation, including radon, was 3.6 mSv as of 1987 but increased to 6.3 mSv as a consequence of the greater use of CT scanning, interventional fluoroscopy, and nuclear medicine procedures since that time. Even though it is almost twice as large as the older estimate of 3.6 mSv, it is not associated with any measurable level of harm.[3]

Although the amount of natural background radiation remains fairly constant from year to year at 3.0 mSv, the frequency of exposure to manmade radiation in medical applications continues to increase rapidly among all age groups in the United States for a number of reasons. Because of medicolegal considerations, physicians in general rely more on radiologic diagnoses to assist them in patient care. Greater accuracy in radiologic diagnosis resulting from

educational and technologic improvements makes this increased use understandable. However, to reduce the possibility of genetic damage in future generations, this increase in frequency of radiation exposure in medicine must be counterbalanced by limiting the amount of patient exposure in individual imaging procedures. This can best be accomplished through efficient application of radiation protection measures on the part of the radiographer, radiologist, and physicians performing interventional procedures requiring the use of fluoroscopy. In addition, it is desirable to limit the widespread substitution of unnecessary CT scans by many emergency departments for convenience in place of using other, less costly diagnostic procedures.

Because of the large variety of radiologic equipment and differences in imaging procedures and in individual radiologist and radiographer technical skills, the patient dose for each examination varies according to the facility providing imaging services. The amount of radiation received by a patient from diagnostic x-ray procedures may be indicated in terms of the following:    3 ways

1. Entrance skin exposure (ESE), which includes skin and glandular dose
2. Bone marrow dose
3. Gonadal dose

In pregnant women, fetal dose also may be estimated. A more complete discussion of the amount of radiation received by a patient may be found in Chapter 12. Table 2-5 provides some examples of patient ESEs (skin and glandular),

| TABLE 2-5 | Representative Entrance Skin Exposures, Bone Marrow Dose and Gonadal Dose from Various Diagnostic X-Ray Procedures | | | |
|---|---|---|---|---|
| **Examination** | **Exposure Factors (kVp/mAs)** | **Entrance Skin Dose (mGy$_t$)*** | **Bone Marrow Dose (mGy$_t$)** | **Gonad Dose (mGy$_t$)** |
| Skull | 76/50 | 2.0 | 0.10 | <1 |
| Chest | 110/3 | 0.1 | 0.02 | <1 |
| Cervical spine | 70/40 | 1.5 | 0.10 | <1 |
| Lumbar spine | 72/60 | 3.0 | 0.60 | 2.25 |
| Abdomen | 74/60 | 4.0 | 0.30 | 1.25 |
| Pelvis | 70/50 | 1.5 | 0.20 | 1.50 |
| Extremity | 60/5 | 0.5 | 0.02 | <1 |
| CT (head) | 125/300 | 40.0 | 0.20 | 0.50 |
| CT (pelvis) | 125/400 | 20.0 | 0.50 | 20 |

Adapted from Bushong SC: *Radiologic science for technologists: physics, biology, and protection*, ed 10, St. Louis, 2013, Mosby.
*CT*, Computed tomography.
*Milligray in tissue.

bone marrow, and gonadal doses, whereas Table 2-6 provides some representative entrance exposures and fetal doses for several different radiologic examinations.

## SUMMARY

- Radiation refers to kinetic energy that passes from one location to another.
- For radiation protection purposes, the electromagnetic spectrum can be divided into two categories: ionizing radiation and nonionizing radiation.
- X-rays, gamma rays, and high-energy ultraviolet radiation with energy greater than 10 eV are classified as ionizing radiations.
- Low-energy ultraviolet radiation, visible light, infrared rays, microwaves, and radio waves are classified as nonionizing radiations.
- X-rays are classified as electromagnetic radiation.
- The process of ionization is the foundation of the interaction of x-rays with human tissue. It makes the x-rays valuable for creating images but has the undesirable result of potentially producing some damage in human tissue.
- Alpha particles, beta particles, neutrons, and protons are particulate radiations.

| TABLE 2-6 | Representative Entrance Exposure and Fetal Doses for Radiographic Examinations Frequently Performed With a 400-Speed Image Receptor | |
|---|---|---|
| **Examination** | **Entrance Skin Exposure (mR)** | **Fetal Dose (mrad)** |
| Skull (lateral) | 70 | 0 |
| Cervical spine (AP) | 110 | 0 |
| Shoulder | 90 | 0 |
| Chest (PA) | 10 | 0 |
| Thoracic spine (AP) | 180 | 1 |
| Lumbosacral spine (AP) | 250 | 80 |
| Abdomen (AP) | 220 | 70 |
| Intravenous urogram (IVP) | 210 | 60 |
| Hip* | 220 | 50 |
| Extremity | 5 | 0 |

Adapted from Bushong SC: *Radiologic science for technologists: physics, biology, and protection*, 10 ed, St. Louis, 2013, Mosby.
*AP,* Anteroposterior projection; *IVP,* intravenous urogram; *PA,* posteroanterior projection.
*Gonadal shields should be used if possible.

- Ionizing radiation produces electrically charged particles that can cause biologic damage on molecular, cellular, and organic levels in humans.
- Equivalent dose (EqD) is a radiation quantity used for radiation protection purposes when a person receives exposure from various types of ionizing radiation. This quantity attempts to specify numerically the differences in energy absorption that lead to varying amounts of biologic harm that are produced by different types of radiation. EqD enables the calculation of the effective dose (EfD).
- EfD takes into account the dose for all types of ionizing radiation to irradiated organs or tissues in the human body. By including specific weighting factors for each body part, such as skin, gonadal tissue, and thyroid, EfD takes into account the chance of each of these body parts for developing radiation-induced cancer (or in the case of the reproductive organs, the risk of genetic damage).
- Both occupational and nonoccupational dose limits are expressed as EfD.
- Sievert (Sv) is the metric unit of equivalent dose and effective dose.
- Sources of ionizing radiation may be natural or manmade.
- Natural sources include radioactive materials in the crust of the earth, cosmic rays from the sun and beyond the solar system, internal radiation from radionuclides deposited in humans through natural processes, and terrestrial radiation in the environment.
- Manmade sources include consumer products containing radioactive material, air travel, nuclear fuel, atmospheric fallout from nuclear weapons testing, nuclear power plant accidents, and nuclear power plant accidents as a consequence of natural disaster, and medical radiation from diagnostic x-ray machines and radiopharmaceuticals in nuclear medicine procedures.
- Thyroid cancer continues to be the main adverse health effect of the 1986 Chernobyl nuclear power plant accident.
- Since the 1980s, the number of diagnostic medical imaging procedures using ionizing radiation has increased dramatically.
- CT scanning, interventional fluoroscopy, conventional radiography/fluoroscopy, and nuclear medicine procedures accounted for 48% of the collective EfD of the U.S. population as of 2006.
- As of 2006, medical radiation procedures accounted for approximately 3.2 mSv of the average annual individual EfD of ionizing radiation received.
- The total average annual EfD from natural background and manmade radiations combined is 6.3 mSv.
- The amount of ionizing radiation received by a patient from diagnostic x-ray procedures may be indicated in terms of entrance skin exposure (ESE), bone marrow dose, and gonadal dose. In pregnant women, fetal dose can also be estimated.

## REFERENCES

1. Environmental Protection Agency: *Ionizing and nonionizing radiation.* Available at: http://www.epa.gov/radiation/understand/. Accessed April 7, 2013.
2. Bushong SC: *Radiologic science for technologists: physics, biology, and protection*, ed 10, St. Louis, 2013, Mosby.
3. National Council on Radiation Protection and Measurements (NCRP): *Ionizing radiation exposure of the population of the United States*, Report No. 160, Bethesda, Md, 2009, NCRP.
4. Broadhead B: *The health effects of radon in layman's terms*, 2008, WPB Enterprises Inc.. Available at: www.wpb.radon.com. Accessed October 3, 2012.
5. Broadhead B: *Thoron measurements and health risk*, 2008, WPB Enterprises Inc.. Available at: http://wpb-radon.com/Thoron_measurement.html. Accessed October 3, 2012.
6. Read AB: Radon gas: the invisible threat. *RT Image* 5:12, 1992.
7. National Council on Radiation Protection and Measurements (NCRP): *Exposure of the population in the United States and Canada from natural background radiation*, Report No. 94, Washington, DC, 1987, NCRP.
8. Church EJ: Back then you really did put your foot in it. *ASRT Scanner*, 41:4, 2009.

9. Gollnick DA: *Basic radiation protection technology,* ed 4, Altadena, Calif, 2000, Pacific Radiation Corporation.

10. National Aeronautics and Space Administration (NASA): *Solar flares,* August 14, 2012. Available at: http://solarscience.msfc.nasa.gov/flares.shtml. Accessed October 4, 2012.

11. Pratt L, Strekel A: Prepare for take-off: the risk of cosmic radiation associated with air travel. *RT Image* 20:34, 2007.

12. National Council on Radiation Protection and Measurements (NCRP): *Ionizing radiation exposure of the population of the United States,* Report No. 93, Bethesda, Md, 1987, NCRP.

13. Bushong SC: *Radiologic science for technologists: physics, biology and protection,* ed 8, St. Louis, 2004, Mosby.

14. Talbott EO, Youk AO, McHugh KP, et al: Mortality among the residents of the Three Mile Island accident area: 1979-1992, Research Triangle Park, NC. *Environ Health Perspect* 108:545, 2000.

15. *Three Mile Island: 1979,* March 2001. Available at: www.world-nuclear.org/info/inf36.html. Accessed April 7, 2013.

16. *United States Nuclear Regulatory Commission Fact Sheet on the Three Mile Island Accident.* Available at: www.nrc.gov/reading-rm/doc-collections/fact-sheets/3mile-isle.html. Accessed April 7, 2013.

17. Powell A: Three Mile Island: 25 years later, *About .com pittsburg,* March 2001, minor update January 2012. Available at: http://pbadupws.nrc.gov/docs/ML0929/ML092950481.pdf. Accessed April 11, 2013.

18. *Putting a lid on Chernobyl.* Available at: http://pbadupws.nrc.gov/docs/ML0929/ML092950481.pdf. Accessed April 11, 2013.

19. *The Chernobyl disaster.* Available at: http://news.bbc.co.uk/2/shared/spl/hi/guides/456900/456957/html/nn3page1.stm. Accessed April 7, 2013.

20. Dubreuil GH, Lochard J, Giraard P, et al: Chernobyl post-accident management: the ETHOS project. *Health Phys* 77:361, 1999.

21. Ollagnon H: *Approche patrimoniale de gestion du risque naturel,* Paris, 1992, Etude de CEMAGREFF.

22. United Nations Scientific Committee on the Effects of Atomic Radiation (UNSCEAR): *2000 report to the General Assembly, with Scientific Annexes, UNSCEAR 2000: sources and effects of ionizing radiation,* New York, 2000, United Nations.

23. Lazole E: Thoughts and lessons from the Chernobyl accident. *Health Phys Soc Newsl* 28:10, 2000.

24. *Chernobyl: the true scale of the accident.* Available at: http://www.who.int/mediacentre/news/releases/2005/pr38/en/. Accessed April 11, 2013.

25. International Atomic Energy Agency (IAEA): *Revisiting Chernobyl: 20 years later.* Available at: www.iaea.org/NewsCenter/Focus/Chernobyl/. Accessed April 7, 2013.

26. *Fifteen years after the Chernobyl accident: lessons learned,* Executive Summary, Kiev, April 2001.

27. Swiss Agency for Development and Cooperation: *Chernobyl.info.* Available at: www.chernobyl.info/ Accessed January 2, 2005.

28. World Health Organization: *Health effects of the Chernobyl accident: an overview.* Fact Sheet No. 303, April 2006. Available at: http://www.who.int/ionizing_radiation/chernobyl/backgrounder/en/index.html. Accessed April 7, 2013.

29. Stone R: Living in the shadow of Chernobyl. *Science* 292:420, 2001.

30. Walker SJ: *Permissible dose: a history of radiation protection in the twentieth century,* Berkeley, 2000, University of California Press.

31. Otto Hug Strahleninstit: Information, Ausgabe 9/2001 K, 2001.

32. Chernobyl Children's Project International. Available at: http://www.chernobyl-international.org/documents/chernobylfacts2.pdf. Accessed April 11, 2013.

33. Conclusions of 3rd international conference, health effects of the Chernobyl accident. *Int J Radiation Med* 3:3-4, 2001.

34. *The Ukrainian-American Study of Leukemia and Related Disorders among Chernobyl Cleanup Workers from Ukraine:* 1 study methods. Available at: http://www.ncbi.nlm.nih.gov/pmc/articles/PMC2856482. Accessed April 13, 2013.

35. World Nuclear Association: *Chernobyl accident 1986,* updated December 2012. Available at: http://www.world-nuclear.org/info/Chernobyl/inf07.html. Accessed April 7, 2013.

36. Nova: Japan's killer quake, *An eyewitness account and investigation of the epic earthquake, tsunami, and nuclear crisis.* Aired on February 29, 2012, on PBS, originally aired March 30, 2011. Available at: http://www.pbs.org/wgbh/nova/earth/japan-killer-quake.html. Accessed September 24, 2012.

37. Ritter M: Japan nuclear disaster released higher radiation levels than previously reported, study finds. *Huff Post World,* October 28, 2011. Available at: http://www.huffingtonpost.com/2011/10/27/japan-nuclear-disaster-fukushima-tsunami-earthquake-chernobyl_n_1062605.html. Accessed April 7, 2013.

## GENERAL DISCUSSION QUESTIONS

1. What is radiation?
2. How do electromagnetic and particulate radiations differ?
3. When inhaled into the lungs of a human, why is radon more dangerous than thoron?

4. What is a solar flare?
5. Explain the use of the radiation quantity "equivalent dose" (EqD).
6. What are enhanced natural sources of radiation?
7. How does radon affect the epithelial tissue of the lungs in humans?
8. How can a flight on a typical commercial airliner result in radiation exposure for a passenger?
9. What consumer products contain radioactive materials?
10. What is the main adverse health effect of the 1986 Chernobyl nuclear power plant accident?

## REVIEW QUESTIONS

1. The amount of radiation received by a patient may be indicated in terms of:
   1. Entrance skin exposure (ESE).
   2. Bone marrow dose.
   3. Gonadal dose.
   A. 1 and 2 only
   B. 1 and 3 only
   C. 2 and 3 only
   D. 1, 2, and 3
2. Which of the following processes is the foundation of the interaction of x-rays with human tissue?
   A. Ionization
   B. Linear acceleration
   C. Particle emission
   D. Radioactive decay

3. Why are the long-term effects, such as an increased incidence of cancer in the exposed population living near Japan's Fukushima Daiichi Nuclear Plant, unable to be accurately determined?
   A. Following the tsunami, winds carried all the radiation back out to sea.
   B. It was extremely difficult to measure the amounts of radiation people received.
   C. Radiation from the crippled reactors were negligible.
   D. Radiation levels exceeded the reading scales on the instruments used to measure population exposure.
4. As of 2006, as reported in NCRP Report No. 160, what percentage of natural background comes from radon and thoron?
   A. 10
   B. 29
   C. 37
   D. 48
5. Which of the following are natural sources of ionizing radiation?
   A. Medical x-radiation and cosmic radiation
   B. Radioactive elements in the crust of the earth and in the human body
   C. Radioactive elements in the human body and a diagnostic x-ray machine
   D. Radioactive fallout and environs of atomic energy plants
6. An equivalent dose as low as 0.25 Sv delivered to the whole body may cause which of the following within a few days?
   A. An increase in the number of lymphocytes in the circulating blood
   B. A decrease in the number of lymphocytes in the circulating blood
   C. A drop immediately to zero in the lymphocyte count
   D. A large increase in the number of platelets

7. How is actual radiation dose to the global population from atmospheric fallout from nuclear weapons testing received?
   A. It is received all at once within a short period of time following such a test.
   B. It is received in large quantities within a period of 2 years following such a test.
   C. It is not received all at once but instead is delivered over a period of years at changing dose rates.
   D. No fallout from such testing is ever received.

8. Which of the following was the total average annual radiation exposure from manmade and natural radiation as of 2006?
   A. 1.8 mSv per year
   B. 3.0 mSv per year
   C. 3.2 mSv per year
   D. 6.3 mSv per year

9. The Russian liquidators who worked during 1986 and 1987 at the Chernobyl power complex demonstrated a statistically significant rise in the number of:
   1. Breast cancer cases.
   2. Leukemia cases.
   3. Prostate cancer cases.
   A. 1 only
   B. 2 only
   C. 3 only
   D. 1, 2, and 3

10. Which of the following is recognized as the main adverse health effect from the 1986 Chernobyl nuclear power accident?
    A. Increase in the incidence of leukemia in adults
    B. Increase in the incidence of leukemia in children
    C. Increase in the incidence of thyroid cancer in adults
    D. Increase in the incidence of thyroid cancer in children and adolescents

# Interaction of X-Radiation with Matter

*After completing this chapter, the reader will be able to perform the following:*
- Differentiate between peak kilovoltage (kVp) and milliampere-seconds (mAs) as technical exposure factors.
- Describe the process of absorption, and explain the reason why absorbed dose in atoms of biologic matter should be kept as small as possible.
- Differentiate among the following: primary radiation; exit, or image-formation, radiation; and scattered radiation.
- List two types of x-ray photon transmission, and explain the difference between them.
- Discuss the way x-rays are produced, and explain the range of energies present in the x-ray beam.

- List the events that occur when x-radiation passes through matter.
- Discuss the probability of photon interaction with matter.
- Describe and illustrate by diagram the x-ray photon interactions with matter that are important in diagnostic radiology.
- List the x-ray photon interactions with matter that occur above the energy range used in diagnostic radiology.
- Describe the impact of positive contrast media on photoelectric absorption, and identify its effects regarding absorbed dose in the body structure that contains it.
- Describe the effect of kVp on radiographic image quality and patient absorbed dose.

Copyright © 2014, Elsevier Inc.

---

**KEY TERMS**

absorbed dose (D)
absorption
attenuation
Auger effect
brightness
characteristic photon
characteristic x-ray
coherent scattering
Compton scattered electron,
    or secondary, or recoil,
    electron

Compton scattering
contrast media
effective atomic number (Zeff)
exit, or image-formation,
    photons
fluorescent radiation
fluorescent yield
image receptor (IR) exposure
mass density
milliampere-seconds (mAs)
pair production

peak kilovoltage (kVp)
photodisintegration
photoelectric absorption
photoelectron
primary radiation
radiographic contrast
radiographic density
radiographic fog
radiographic image receptor
small-angle scatter
window level

---

In this chapter, fundamental physics concepts that relate to radiation absorption and scatter are reviewed. The processes of interaction between radiation and matter are emphasized because a basic understanding of the subject is necessary for radiographers to optimally select technical exposure factors such as the following:

- **peak kilovoltage (kVp)**, the highest energy level of photons in the x-ray beam
- **milliampere-seconds (mAs)**, the product of electron tube current and the amount of time in seconds that the x-ray tube is activated

Peak kilovoltage controls the quality, or penetrating power, of the photons in the x-ray beam and to some degree also affects the quantity, or number of photons, in the beam. The product of milliamperes (mA), which is the x-ray tube current, and time (seconds [s] during which the x-ray tube is activated) is the main determinant of how much radiation is directed toward a patient during a selected x-ray exposure. Because the level of energy (beam quality) and the number of x-ray photons are controlled by technique factors selected by the radiographer, the radiographer is actually responsible for the dose the patient receives during an imaging procedure. With a suitable understanding of these factors, radiographers will be able to select appropriate techniques that can minimize the

dose to the patient while producing optimal-quality images.

## SIGNIFICANCE OF X-RAY ABSORPTION IN BIOLOGIC TISSUE

X-rays are carriers of manmade, electromagnetic energy. If x-rays enter a material such as human tissue, they may:

1. Interact with the atoms of the biologic material in the patient.
2. Pass through without interaction.

If an interaction occurs, electromagnetic energy is transferred from the x-rays to the atoms of the patient's biologic material. This process is called **absorption** (Fig. 3-1), and the amount of energy absorbed per unit mass is referred to as the **absorbed dose (D)**. The more electromagnetic energy is received by the atoms of the patient's body, the greater is the possibility of biologic damage in the patient; therefore, the amount of electromagnetic energy transferred should be kept as small as possible. Without absorption and the differences in the absorption properties of various body structures, it would not be possible to produce diagnostically useful images in which different anatomic structures could be perceived and distinguished. The radiographer also benefits when the patient's dose is

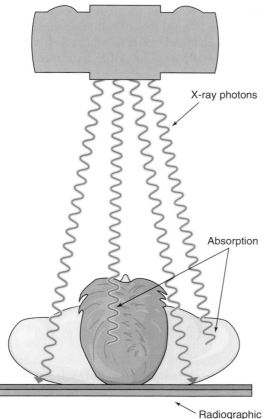

**FIGURE 3-1** X-ray photons can interact with atoms of the patient's body and transfer energy to the tissue. This transference of electromagnetic energy to the atoms of the material is called *absorption*.

X-ray photons

Absorption

Radiographic image receptor

minimal because less radiation is scattered from the patient.

## X-RAY BEAM PRODUCTION AND ENERGY

### Production of Primary Radiation

A diagnostic x-ray beam is produced when a stream of high-speed electrons bombards a positively charged target in a highly evacuated glass tube. In general radiography, this target, also known as the *anode*, is usually made of the metal

tungsten or a metal alloy, tungsten rhenium. These materials have:

- High melting points
- High atomic numbers (tungsten [74] and rhenium [75])

As the electrons interact with the atoms of the target, x-ray photons (particles associated with electromagnetic radiation that have neither mass nor electric charge and travel at the speed of light) emerge from the target with a broad range of energies and leave the x-ray tube through a glass window. The glass window permits passage of all but the lowest-energy components of the x-ray spectrum. It therefore acts as a filter by removing diagnostically useless, very-low-energy x-rays. In addition to this, a certain thickness of added aluminum is placed within the collimator assembly to intercept the emerging x-rays before they reach the patient. This aluminum "hardens" the x-ray beam (i.e., raises its effective energy) by removing low-energy components that would serve only to increase patient dose. The combination of the x-ray tube glass wall and the added aluminum placed within the collimator may be called the *permanent inherent filtration* of the x-ray unit. The emerging x-ray photon beam is collectively referred to as **primary radiation** (Fig. 3-2).

### Energy of Photons in a Diagnostic X-Ray Beam

Although all photons in a diagnostic x-ray beam do not have the same energy, the most energetic photons in the beam can have no more energy than the electrons that bombard the target. The energy of the electrons inside the x-ray tube is expressed in terms of the electrical voltage applied across the tube. In diagnostic radiology, this is expressed in thousands of volts, or kilovolts (kV). Because the voltage across the tube fluctuates, it is usually expressed in kilovolt peak (kVp).

If an electron is drawn across an electrical potential difference of 1 volt, it has acquired

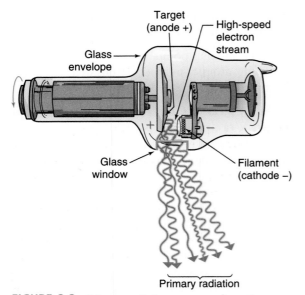

**FIGURE 3-2** Primary radiation emerges from the x-ray tube target and consists of x-ray photons of various energies. It is produced when the positively charged target is bombarded with a stream of high-speed electrons and these electrons interact with the atoms of the target.

energy of 1 electron volt (eV). Therefore, a technique factor of 100 kVp means that the electrons bombarding the target have a maximum energy of 100,000 eV, or 100 keV. X-rays of various energies are produced, but the most energetic x-ray photon can have no more energy than 100 keV. For a typical diagnostic x-ray unit, the energy of the average photon in the x-ray beam is about one third the energy of the most energetic photon. Therefore, a 100-kVp beam contains photons having energies of 100 keV or less, with an average energy of approximately 33 keV.

## ATTENUATION

### Direct and Indirect Transmission X-Ray Photons

When an x-ray beam passes through a patient, it goes through a process called **attenuation**. Attenuation is simply the reduction in the number of primary photons in the x-ray beam through absorption (a total loss of radiation energy) and scatter (a change in direction of travel that may also involve a partial loss of radiation energy) as the beam passes through the patient in its path. Some primary x-ray photons also traverse the patient without interacting. This may be called *direct transmission*. These noninteracting x-ray photons reach the **radiographic image receptor** (**IR**), which may be one of the following:

- Phosphor plate
- Digital radiography receptor
- Radiographic film

Other primary photons can undergo Compton and/or coherent interactions (these processes are discussed later in this chapter) and as a result may be scattered or deflected with a potential loss of energy. Such photons may still traverse the patient and strike the IR. This process is called *indirect transmission*. The optimal x-ray image is formed when only direct transmission x-ray photons reach the IR. In clinical situations, however, scattered photons do reach the IR and degrade image quality (sharpness of the recorded image). Therefore, several methods have been devised to limit the effects of indirectly transmitted x-ray photons. The most common methods include the following:

- Air gap techniques
- Radiographic grids

These methods are described in Chapters 11 and 12. In conventional or digital radiography, the IR covers a broad enough area that x-ray photons scattered from one part of the beam may still strike the IR in another area. Consequently, the resulting radiographic image is formed from both directly transmitted x-ray photons and indirectly transmitted (i.e., scattered) x-ray photons.

### Primary, Exit, and Attenuated Photons

Figure 3-3 illustrates the passage of four x-ray photons through a patient. Before the four photons produced by the x-ray source enter

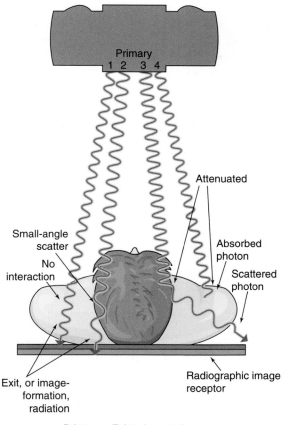

**Primary – Exit 5 Attenuation**

**FIGURE 3-3** Primary, exit, and attenuated photons. Primary photons (photons 1, 2, 3, and 4) are photons that emerge from the x-ray source. Exit, or image-formation, photons (photons 1 and 2) are photons that pass through the patient being radiographed and reach the radiographic image receptor. Attenuated photons (photons 3 and 4) are photons that have interacted with atoms of the patient's biologic tissue and been scattered or absorbed such that they do not reach the radiographic image receptor.

human tissue, they are referred to as *primary photons.* Only two photons emerge from the tissue and strike the radiographic IR below it. They are referred to as **exit,** or **image-formation, photons.** The two that do not strike the IR are attenuated. The term *attenuation* is rather broad; with respect to x-rays, *attenuation* may be used to refer to any process decreasing the intensity of the primary photon beam that was directed toward a destination. The ultimate destination of

the photons in Figure 3-3 is the IR. Therefore, photon 3, which has deviated from its path (i.e., it has been "scattered") to the extent that it will not strike the IR, is said to have been attenuated. Photon 4 seems to disappear. It has transferred all its energy to the atoms of the patient and has therefore been eliminated. Because a photon has no mass, it ceases to exist when it gives up its energy. *Attenuation,* then, refers to both absorption and scatter processes that prevent photons from reaching a predefined destination. Figure 3-3 shows that the path of photon 2 was bent, but not so much that the photon missed its target. Because photon 2 reaches the IR, it is part of the exit, or image-formation, radiation, but the bending of its path represents what is called **small-angle scatter.** Scattered photons in this category have essentially the same energy as the incident photons. Small-angle scatter degrades the appearance of a completed radiographic image by blurring the sharp outlines of dense structures. Because many billions of such scatter events occur, a greater overall exposure of the image receptor (IR) occurs, thus interfering with the radiologist's ability to distinguish different structures in the image. This undesirable, additional exposure is called **radiographic fog.** Reducing the amount of tissue irradiated decreases the amount of fog produced by small-angle scatter. Therefore, adequately collimating the x-ray beam is one way to reduce fog (Fig. 3-4). Other methods used to decrease the image-degrading effects of scatter are discussed later.

## PROBABILITY OF PHOTON INTERACTION WITH MATTER

Because the interaction of photons with biologic matter is random, it is impossible to predict with certainty what will happen to a single photon when it enters human tissue. When dealing with a large number of photons, however, it is possible to predict what will happen on the average, and this is more than adequate to determine the characteristics of the image that results from such numerous interactions (Table 3-1). An example is provided in Box 3-1.

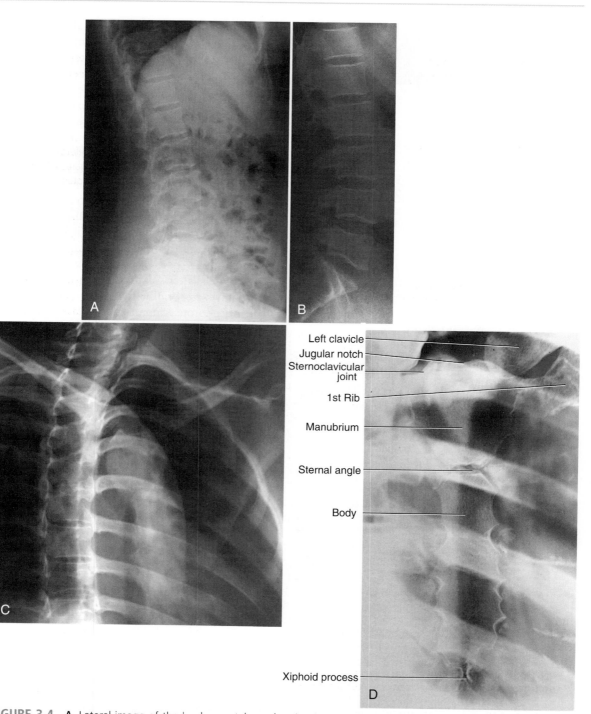

**FIGURE 3-4    A,** Lateral image of the lumbar vertebrae showing improper collimation, which results in the production of radiographic fog and a consequent lack of radiographic clarity. **B,** Lateral image of the lumbar vertebrae showing adequate collimation, which eliminates radiographic fog and consequently increases radiographic clarity. **C,** Posterolateral (PA) oblique projection (right anterior oblique [RAO] position) of the sternum demonstrating poor collimation. **D,** PA oblique projection (RAO position) of the sternum demonstrating good collimation.

| TABLE 3-1 | Interaction of X-Radiation with Soft Tissue: Overview | | | |
|---|---|---|---|---|
| **X-Ray Photon Energy Range** | **Site of Interaction** | **X-Ray Photon** | **Typical Interaction** | **By-Products of Interaction** |
| 1-50 kVp | An atom | Energy: unchanged; direction after interaction: slight change (<20 degrees) | Coherent scattering* | None |
| 1-50 kVp | Inner-shell electron (usually K or L shell) | Energy: absorbed; direction after interaction: not applicable | Photoelectric absorption[†] | Photoelectron (characteristic photon) |
| 60-90 kVp | Outer-shell electron | Energy: reduced; direction after interaction: changed (x-ray photon energy partially absorbed) | Compton scattering[‡] | Compton-scattered electron Compton-scattered photon |
| 200 kVp-2 MeV | Outer-shell electron | Energy: reduced; direction after interaction: changed | Compton scattering[§‖] | Compton-scattered electron Compton-scattered photon |
| Begins at about 1.022 MeV; becomes important at 10 MeV; becomes predominant at 50 MeV and greater | Nucleus of atom | Energy: disappears after interaction with nucleus; transformed into two new particles that annihilate each other; direction after interaction: energy reappears in form of two 0.511-MeV photons moving in opposite directions | Pair production | Positive electron (positron); ordinary electron (negatron); two 0.511-MeV photons |
| Greater than 10 MeV | Nucleus of atom | Energy: absorbed by nucleus after collision with high-energy photon; excess energy in nucleus creates instability that is usually alleviated by emission of a neutron; other emissions possible | Photodisintegration | Neutron; other types of emissions possible if sufficient energy is absorbed by the nucleus: proton or proton-neutron combination (deuteron) or even an alpha particle |

*This scattering occurs mostly in this energy range, but it is still much less probable than photoelectric absorption.
[†]The interaction most responsible for radiation dose in this energy range.
[‡]Both Compton and photoelectric interactions occur in this energy range.
[§]Compton interaction is predominantly responsible for radiation dose in this energy range.
[‖]In this energy range, the scattered particles go on to produce many more Compton and photoelectric interactions on their own.

Table 3-2 shows the factors that influence the probability of interactions in matter. In the remainder of this chapter, the different interactions of photons with individual atoms and the effect of a particular type of interaction on the radiographic image are examined.

## PROCESSES OF INTERACTION

Five types of interactions between x-radiation and matter are possible:

1. Coherent scattering
2. Photoelectric absorption
3. Compton scattering
4. Pair production
5. Photodisintegration

Of these, only two are important in diagnostic radiology:

1. Compton scattering
2. Photoelectric absorption

Box 3-2 presents an overview of the various interactions between x-radiation with matter and where they are important.

## Coherent Scattering

**Coherent scattering** is sometimes called the following terms:

- Classical scattering
- Elastic scattering
- Unmodified scattering

It is basically a relatively simple process that actually results in no loss of energy as x-rays scatter.

| BOX 3-1 | Probability of Photon Interaction with Matter |
|---|---|

In an ordinary beam of x-ray photons (which consists of a vast number of such particles) a 50-keV photon on average has a 66% probability of interaction when it travels through 5 cm of soft tissue (see Appendix D); 34% of the time such photons will be likely to just pass through the tissue. As an illustration of this process, consider that in a randomly chosen group of 1000 50-keV photons traveling through 5 cm of soft tissue, 666 interactions may be expected to occur. Of the 666 interactions, 11% (73 of the 666 interactions) should be of a type called *photoelectric*. In the photoelectric interaction, a photon is completely absorbed by the atoms of the tissue (i.e., removed from the beam). If this were the only interaction possible, irradiating 5 cm of soft tissue with 50-keV photons would create a lighter area on a completed radiographic image, which would be the result of fewer photons' reaching that portion of the image receptor. In reality, the process is much more complicated because several additional effects occur, and a typical x-ray beam is composed of photons with a continuous range of energies.

| BOX 3-2 | Importance of Various Interactions of X-Radiation with Matter |
|---|---|

| Interaction | Where Important |
|---|---|
| Coherent scattering | Not important in any energy range |
| Photoelectric absorption | Diagnostic radiology |
| Compton scattering | Diagnostic radiology and therapeutic radiology |
| Pair production | Therapeutic radiology |
| Photodisintegration | Therapeutic radiology |

| TABLE 3-2 | Factors That Influence the Probability of Interaction of Photons with Energy E in Materials with Density $\rho$ |
|---|---|

| Interaction | Photon Energy | Atomic Number | Electron Density $\rho_e$ (e/g) | Physical Density $\rho$ (g/cm³) |
|---|---|---|---|---|
| Photoelectric | $1/E^3$ | $Z^3$ | Independent | $\rho$ |
| Compton | $1/E$ | Independent | $\rho_e$ | $\rho$ |
| Pair production | $E$ | $Z$ | Independent | $\rho$ |

**Process of Coherent Scattering.** When a low-energy photon (typically less than 10 keV), which may be thought of as a moving electromagnetic wave, interacts with an atom, it may transfer its energy by causing some or all of the electrons of the atom to vibrate momentarily. This is analogous to the behavior of electrons in the antenna of a receiver intercepting a radio signal. Because they are charged particles, each of the atom's vibrating electrons radiates energy in the form of electromagnetic waves. These waves coherently (i.e., cooperatively) combine with one another to form a scattered wave, which represents a scattered photon. Because the wavelengths of both incident and scattered waves are the same, no net energy has been absorbed by the atom (see Appendix E). However, a change in the direction of the emitted photon is very likely. In general, this change in direction, which usually occurs in a forward direction, is less than 20 degrees with respect to the initial direction of the original photon. This is the net effect of coherent, or unmodified, scattering, also known as *Rayleigh scattering* in honor of the scientist who first explained it, before the concept of the photon was known, by using wave analysis alone. Although coherent scattering is most likely to occur at less than 10 keV, some of this unmodified scattering occurs throughout the diagnostic range and may result in small amounts of radiographic fog (Fig. 3-5). This source of fog, however, is not significant in general diagnostic imaging. In mammography, which of necessity involves many low-energy photons, coherent scattering also does not contribute noticeably to radiographic fog because during this imaging procedure, breast tissue is gently but firmly compressed. As a result of this compression, the breast actually becomes relatively thin. This eliminates the production of a large amount of scatter radiation.

In addition to Rayleigh scattering is another kind of coherent scattering, known as *Thompson scattering,* in which the low-energy photon interacts with one or more free (i.e., unbound) electrons. As with Rayleigh scattering, the photon energy is absorbed and then reradiated in a

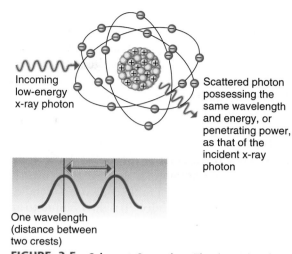

Incoming low-energy x-ray photon

Scattered photon possessing the same wavelength and energy, or penetrating power, as that of the incident x-ray photon

One wavelength (distance between two crests)

**FIGURE 3-5   Coherent Scattering.** The incoming low-energy x-ray photon interacts with an atom and transfers its energy by causing some or all of the electrons of the atom to vibrate momentarily. The electrons then radiate energy in the form of electromagnetic waves. These waves nondestructively combine with one another to form a scattered wave, which represents the scattered photon. Its wavelength and energy, or penetrating power, are the same as those of the incident photon. Generally, the emitted photon may change in direction less than 20 degrees with respect to the direction of the original photon. (Wavelength is the distance from one crest to the next.)

different direction with no change in wavelength of the associated electromagnetic wave. Rayleigh scattering and Thompson scattering play essentially no role in radiography. These types of scattering do not affect x-rays very much, but they do affect visible light. This is why the sky is blue and sunsets are red.[1] Shorter visible wavelengths (e.g., blue light) are more likely to be scattered and to scatter over a greater angle. Therefore, when you look up in the sky in any direction, you tend to see the blue light scattered toward you. At sunset, looking toward the sun, the blue light is mainly scattered away from you, so the sun appears to consist of mostly longer wavelength visible light, that is, mostly red.

A summary of facts about the process of coherent scattering is presented in Box 3-3 for quick reference.

## Photoelectric Absorption

Within the energy range of diagnostic radiology (23 to 150 kVp), which also includes mammography, photoelectric absorption is the most important mode of interaction between x-ray photons and the atoms of the patient's body for producing useful images.

**Process of Photoelectric Absorption. Photoelectric absorption** is an interaction between an x-ray photon and an inner-shell electron (usually in the K or L shells [Table 3-3; for a detailed explanation see Appendix F]) tightly bound to an atom of the absorbing medium (Fig. 3-6). To dislodge an inner-shell electron from its atomic orbit, the incoming x-ray photon must be able to transfer a quantity of energy as large as or larger than the amount of energy that binds the electron in its orbit. On interacting with an inner-shell electron, the x-ray photon surrenders all its energy to the orbital electron and ceases to exist. The electron is ejected from its inner shell, thus creating a vacancy. The ejected orbital electron, called a **photoelectron,** possesses kinetic energy equal to the energy of the incident photon less the binding energy of the electron shell. This photoelectron may interact with other atoms, thereby causing excitation or ionization, until all its kinetic energy has been spent. The photoelectron is usually absorbed within a few micrometers of the medium through which it travels. In the human body, this energy transfer results in increased patient dose and contributes to biologic damage of tissues.

As a result of the photoelectric interaction, a vacancy has been created in an inner shell of the target atom. For the ionized atom, this represents an unstable energy situation. The instability is alleviated by filling the vacancy in the inner shell with an electron from an outer shell, which spontaneously "falls down" into this opening. To do this, the descending electron must lose energy,

| BOX 3-3 | Summary of the Process of Coherent Scattering |
|---------|-----------------------------------------------|

The process of coherent scattering is of no importance in any energy range. When the low-energy x-ray photon interacts with an atom of human tissue, it does not lose kinetic energy. The emitted photon merely changes direction by 20 degrees or less. No ionization of the biologic atom occurs.

| TABLE 3-3 | Electron Shell Occupancies for Some Common Atoms* | | | | | | |
|-----------|--------|------------------|---|---|---|---|---|
| | | | **Shell** | | | | |
| **Atom** | **Symbol** | **Atomic Number** | **K** | **L** | **M** | **N** | **O** | **P** |
| Hydrogen | H | 1 | 1 | | | | | |
| Helium | He | 2 | 2 | | | | | |
| Lithium | Li | 3 | 2 | 1 | | | | |
| Carbon | C | 6 | 2 | 4 | | | | |
| Oxygen | O | 8 | 2 | 6 | | | | |
| Sodium | Na | 11 | 2 | 8 | 1 | | | |
| Aluminum | Al | 13 | 2 | 8 | 3 | | | |
| Calcium | Ca | 20 | 2 | 8 | 8 | 2 | | |
| Copper | Cu | 29 | 2 | 8 | 18 | 1 | | |
| Molybdenum | Mo | 42 | 2 | 8 | 18 | 13 | 1 | |
| Tungsten | W | 74 | 2 | 8 | 18 | 32 | 12 | 2 |
| Lead | Pb | 82 | 2 | 8 | 18 | 32 | 18 | 4 |
| Radon | Rn | 86 | 2 | 8 | 18 | 32 | 18 | 8 |

*For a detailed discussion of electron shell structure, please see Appendix F.

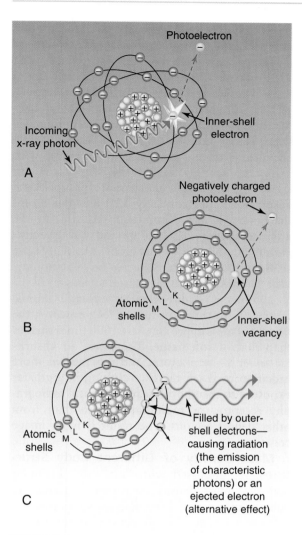

A

B

C

**FIGURE 3-6**  **Photoelectric Absorption. A,** On encountering an inner-shell electron in the K or L shells, the incoming x-ray photon surrenders all its energy to the electron, and the photon ceases to exist. **B,** The atom responds by ejecting the electron, called a *photoelectron,* from its inner shell, thus creating a vacancy in that shell. **C,** To fill the opening, an electron from an outer shell drops down to the vacated inner shell by releasing energy in the form of a characteristic photon. Then, to fill the new vacancy in the outer shell, another electron from the shell next farthest out drops down and another characteristic photon is emitted, and so on until the atom regains electrical equilibrium. There is also some probability that instead of a characteristic photon, an Auger electron will be ejected.

that is, must pass from a less tightly bound atomic state (farther from the nucleus) to a more tightly held status (closer to the nucleus). The amount of energy loss involved is simply equal to the difference in the binding or "holding" energies associated with each electron shell. For a large atom such as those in lead, this energy can be in the kiloelectron volt range, whereas for the small or low atomic number atoms that are associated with the human body, the energy is on the order of 10 eV. The "released" energy is carried off in the form of a photon that is called a **characteristic photon,** or **characteristic x-ray,** because its energy is directly related to the shell structure of the atom from which it was emitted. Characteristic x-rays are also known as **fluorescent radiation.** Those generated from photoelectric interactions within human tissue are low enough in energy that they are predominantly absorbed within the body. In general, ensuing vacancies in other electron shells are successively filled and associated characteristic photons are emitted until the atom achieves an electronic equilibrium.

One additional process can occur as a result of photoelectric interactions. It is called the **Auger effect** (pronounced "awzhay"), named after the French scientist, Pierre Victor Auger, who discovered it in 1925. When an inner electron is removed from an atom in a photoelectric interaction, thus causing an inner-shell vacancy, the energy liberated when this vacancy is filled can be transferred to another electron of the atom, thereby ejecting the electron, instead of emerging from the atom as fluorescent radiation. Such an emitted electron is called an *Auger electron.* Its energy is equal to the difference between that released by an outer electron in filling the initial created vacancy and the binding energy of the emitted or Auger electron. Because this process does not include any x-ray emission, it is called a *radiationless effect.* It reduces the total amount of characteristic radiation produced by photoelectric interactions. **Fluorescent yield** refers to the number of x-rays emitted per inner-shell vacancy. Because the Auger effect is more prevalent in materials with higher atomic number atoms, the fluorescent yield per photoelectron is generally lower in such materials than for substances with low atomic numbers (see Fig. 3-6, C).

In summary, the by-products of photoelectric absorption include the following:

1. Photoelectrons (those induced by interaction with external radiation and the internally generated Auger electrons)
2. Characteristic x-ray photons (fluorescent radiation)

When the energy of these by-products is locally absorbed in human tissue, both the dose to the patient and the potential for biologic damage increase.

A summary of facts about the process of photoelectric absorption is presented in Box 3-4 for quick reference.

**Probability of Occurrence of Photoelectric Absorption.** The probability of occurrence of photoelectric absorption depends on the energy (E) of the incident x-ray photons and the atomic number (Z) of the atoms comprising the irradiated object; it increases markedly as the energy of the incident photon decreases and the atomic number of the irradiated atoms increases. Experimentally, it is observed to vary approximately as $Z^4/E^3$ per atom and $Z^3/E^3$ per electron because there are Z electrons per atom. Thus in the radiographic kilovoltage range, compact bone (effective atomic number 13.8; **effective atomic number [Zeff]** is a composite Z value for when multiple chemical elements comprise a material), with a high content by weight (14.7%) of calcium (Z = 20), undergoes much more photoelectric absorption (approximately 12 times per atom) than an equal mass of soft tissue (effective atomic number approximately 7.4) and air (effective atomic number 7.6). Thus because of the "x-ray shadow" that it casts, bone can be exceptionally well demonstrated in diagnostic images.

Air has a slightly higher effective atomic number (7.6) than soft tissue (7.4); however, the density of air is approximately 1000 times smaller than that of soft tissue. Therefore, air absorbs far fewer x-ray photons, and this permits more radiation to reach the IR, resulting in a greater exposure to the phosphor plate, digital radiography receptor, or radiographic film than from other denser regions. The result is more image contrast.

**Mass Density of Different Body Structures.** As discussed with "air," the dissimilar densities (**mass density** measured in grams per cubic centimeter) of different body structures also influences attenuation. A density increase leads to a corresponding increase in atoms with which x-ray photons can interact and therefore to an increased probability of photon absorption. Thus, in any given sample of biologic material, both density and atomic number are important in determining attenuation. For example, if radiography is performed on an equal thickness of bone and soft tissue, the bone, which is approximately twice as dense as soft tissue, will absorb about nine times as many photons in the diagnostic energy range as will the soft tissue. A factor of 4.5 is caused by the higher atomic number of the bone, and a factor of 2 is caused by the higher density of bone. The total effect is $2 \times 4.5$, for an overall factor of 9 (Fig. 3-7, A).

| BOX 3-4 | Summary of the Process of Photoelectric Absorption |
|---|---|

Photoelectric absorption is the most important mode in the interaction between x-radiation and the atoms of the patient's body in the energy range used in diagnostic radiology because this interaction is responsible for both the patient's dose and contrast in the image. During the process of photoelectric absorption, the kinetic energy of the incident photon is completely absorbed as it interacts with and ejects an inner-shell electron of biologic tissue from its orbit. The newly ejected photoelectron possesses kinetic energy and can ionize other atoms it encounters until its energy is spent. After losing an electron, the original ionized atom is unstable and attempts to restabilize. This occurs as an electron from a higher shell drops down and fills the vacancy in the inner shell by releasing energy as a characteristic photon. This cascading effect of electrons dropping down to fill existing shell vacancies continues until the original atom regains its stability.

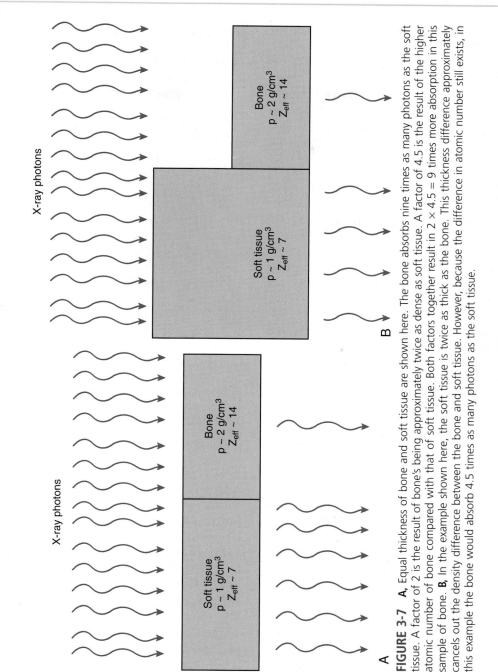

**FIGURE 3-7   A,** Equal thickness of bone and soft tissue are shown here. The bone absorbs nine times as many photons as the soft tissue. A factor of 2 is the result of bone's being approximately twice as dense as soft tissue. A factor of 4.5 is the result of the higher atomic number of bone compared with that of soft tissue. Both factors together result in $2 \times 4.5 = 9$ times more absorption in this sample of bone. **B,** In the example shown here, the soft tissue is twice as thick as the bone. This thickness difference approximately cancels out the density difference between the bone and soft tissue. However, because the difference in atomic number still exists, in this example the bone would absorb 4.5 times as many photons as the soft tissue.

**Body Part Thickness.** Thickness of body parts also plays a role. The thickness factor is approximately linear. If two structures have the same density and atomic number but one is twice as thick as the other, the thicker structure will absorb twice as many photons. Consequently, if a 2-cm-thick bone sample is radiographed next to a 4-cm-thick tissue sample, the density and thickness factors will cancel each other out (Fig. 3-7, *B*). The bone is half as thick in this example, but it is approximately twice as dense. However, the remaining factor, the higher atomic number of bone, causes the bone to absorb approximately 4.5 times as many photons as the soft tissue.

**Difference in Absorption Properties among Different Body Structures.** Such differences in absorption properties among different body structures make diagnostically useful images possible. In other words, the ability to perceive and distinguish among different body structures in an image depends on the presence of differences in the amount of x-radiation these structures permit to pass through them to reach the radiographic IR.

The less a given structure attenuates radiation, the darker its radiographic film image will be (i.e., the greater the **radiographic density,** or degree of overall blackening on a radiographic film), and vice versa. A radiograph must have sufficient density to visualize the anatomic structures of interest. Thus bone, with a higher effective atomic number and greater mass density than either soft tissue or air cavities, absorbs more radiation and appears white on a finished radiographic film image, whereas soft tissue presents a gray image, and air-containing structures (e.g., lungs, stomach) appear black (Fig. 3-8). *Density* is the term that is most commonly used when the IR is film. In the digital environment, the term **image receptor** (**IR**) **exposure** is used because radiographic film is no longer used as the primary IR. "**Brightness** is a monitor function that can change the lightness or darkness of the image on a display monitor,"[2] as controlled by the radiographer. Brightness is the intensity of the display monitor's light emission. It is not

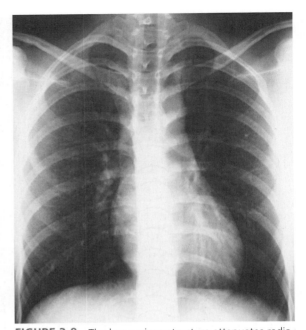

**FIGURE 3-8**   The less a given structure attenuates radiation, the darker its radiographic film image will be (i.e., the greater its radiographic density), and vice versa. Thus, compact bone, with a higher effective atomic number and greater mass density than either soft tissue or air cavities, absorbs more radiation and appears white on a finished radiographic film image, whereas soft tissue presents a gray image, and air-containing structures such as the lungs appear black.

affiliated with the controlling factors of density, which are milliamperage and exposure time (mAs). "Brightness and density are not interchangeable terms."[2] The **window level** sets the midpoint of the range of densities visible on the image. Adjusting the window level, also known as *windowing,* refers to changing the brightness, either to be increased or decreased throughout the entire range of densities. Increasing the window level on the displayed image (increased brightness) decreases the density on the hard copy image, whereas decreasing the window level on the monitor image (decreased brightness) increases density on the hard copy. In both screen-film and digital imaging, the visibility of the image has always been the result of correct exposure to the IR, which is achieved by selecting the appropriate mAs.[2-4]

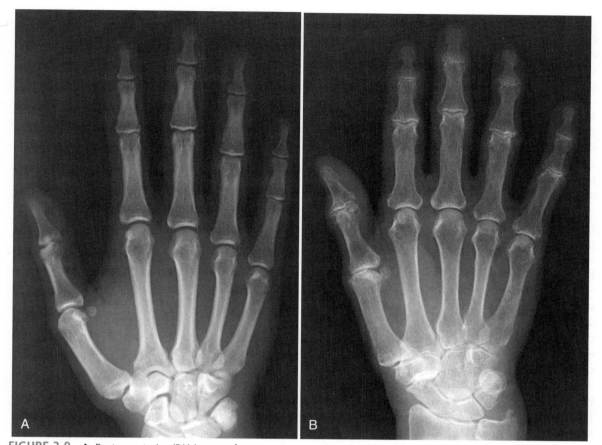

**FIGURE 3-9** **A,** Posteroanterior (PA) image of a young person's hand exhibiting substantial quantities of calcium in the bones. **B,** PA image of an elderly person's hand exhibiting demineralized bone as a consequence of a decrease in bone calcium. This and other degenerative changes account for the almost transparent appearance of the bones.

In Figure 3-9, two posteroanterior (PA) hand projections illustrate age-related changes in bone density resulting from changes in calcium content.

1. Image *A* exhibits substantial quantities of calcium in the bones of a young person.
2. Image *B* exhibits the demineralized bones of an elderly person. The lack of x-ray absorption results from the decrease in bone calcium. Hence the elderly person's bones are almost transparent in radiographic appearance. Pathologic conditions such as degenerative arthritis also contribute to differences in absorption. Technical radiographic exposure factors must be adjusted to compensate for such changes.

**Impact of Photoelectric Absorption on Radiographic Contrast.** Within the energy range of diagnostic radiology, the greater the difference is in the amount of photoelectric absorption, the greater the contrast in the radiographic image will be between adjacent structures of differing atomic numbers. However, as absorption increases, so does the potential for biologic damage. For those regions in which the photoelectric absorption occurs most frequently (e.g., in dense atomic number areas such as cortical bone), the absorbed dose to the patient may be greater by a factor of 6 to 9 than in adjacent low atomic number and less dense regions. Thus, to ensure both radiographic image quality and patient safety, both the radiologist and the radiographer should choose the highest energy x-ray beam that permits adequate **radiographic contrast** for computed radiography, digital radiography, or conventional radiography.

**Use of Contrast Media to Ensure Visualization of Anatomic Structures.** If tissues or structures that are similar in atomic number and mass density must be distinguished, the photoelectric interaction by itself will not be sufficient to produce the contrast needed in that tissue or structure to ensure its visualization in the radiographic image. To resolve the problem, the use of **contrast media** has been adopted. Very simply, positive contrast media consist of solutions containing elements having a higher atomic number than surrounding soft tissue (e.g., barium or iodine based) that are either ingested or injected into the tissues or structures to be visualized. The high atomic number of the contrast media (barium, Z = 56; iodine, Z = 53) significantly enhances the occurrence of photoelectric interaction relative to similar adjacent structures that do not have the contrast media. In addition, the inner-shell electrons of iodine and barium have a binding energy that is in the energy range of the x-ray photons that is most commonly used in general-purpose radiography (30 to 40 keV). This means that photoelectric absorption of the photons in the x-ray beam is greatly increased. In the radiographic image, positive contrast–enhanced structures therefore appear lighter than adjacent structures that did not receive the contrast. Figure 3-10, *A* presents an anteroposterior (AP) projection of the abdomen without the aid of a positive contrast medium to visualize the urinary system, whereas Figure 3-10, *B* presents an AP projection of the abdomen with a positive contrast medium that shows the urinary system, thus permitting each contrast-filled structure to be distinguished.

Caution must be exercised in the use of contrast media because some patients may not be able to tolerate their presence. The use of a positive contrast medium also leads to an increase in absorbed dose in the body structures that contain it. A negative contrast medium such as air or gas is also used for some radiologic examinations. These negative agents result in areas of increased density on the completed image.

## Compton Scattering

**Compton scattering** is also known by the following terms:

- Incoherent scattering
- Inelastic scattering
- Modified scattering

It is responsible for most of the scattered radiation produced during radiologic procedures (Fig. 3-11). This scatter may be directed forward as small-angle scatter, backward as backscatter, and to the side as sidescatter. The intensity of radiation scatter in various directions is a major factor in planning protection for medical imaging personnel during a radiologic examination (Fig. 3-12).

**Process of Compton Scattering.** In the Compton process, an incoming x-ray photon interacts with a loosely bound outer electron of an atom of the irradiated object (Fig. 3-13). On encountering the electron, the incoming x-ray photon surrenders a portion of its kinetic energy to dislodge the electron from its outer-shell orbit, thereby ionizing the biologic atom (see Appendix G for an extended discussion of this type of interaction). The freed electron, called a **Compton scattered electron,** or **secondary,** or **recoil electron,** possesses excess kinetic energy and is capable of ionizing other atoms. It loses its kinetic energy by a series of collisions with nearby atoms and finally recombines with an atom that needs another electron. This usually occurs within a few micrometers of the site of the original Compton interaction.

The incident x-ray photon that surrendered some of its kinetic energy (see Appendix G) to free the loosely bound outer-shell electron from its orbit continues on its way but in a new direction and is now called a *Compton scattered photon*. It has the potential to interact with other atoms either by the process of photoelectric absorption or by subsequent Compton scattering. It also may emerge from the patient, in

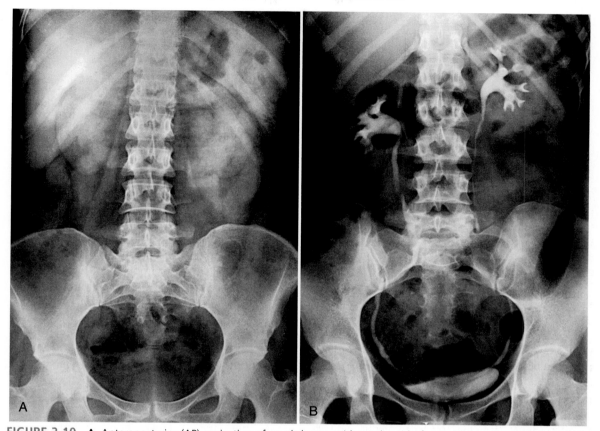

**FIGURE 3-10** **A,** Anteroposterior (AP) projection of an abdomen without the aid of a positive contrast medium. Parts of the urinary system other than the kidneys, which have their own unique density, are not radiographically demonstrated. **B,** AP projection of the abdomen after the intravenous injection of an appropriate positive contrast medium that permits visualization of the entire urinary system, thus allowing each contrast-filled structure to be distinguished.

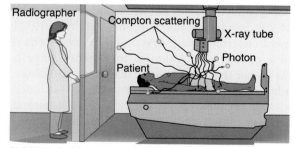

**FIGURE 3-11** Compton scattering is responsible for most of the scattered radiation produced during a radiologic procedure.

which case it may contribute to degradation of the radiographic image by creating an additional, unwanted exposure (radiographic fog) or, in fluoroscopy, it may expose personnel who are present in the room to scattered radiation. The Compton interaction's probability of occurrence has no explicit dependence on atomic number. Instead, it shows something of an energy and density dependence. Density dependence just means that the more targets per unit volume, the greater is the likelihood of an interaction to occur in that volume. With increasing x-ray photon energy, the chance for a billiard ball–like interaction between the photon and an outer atomic electron decreases. What must be emphasized, however,

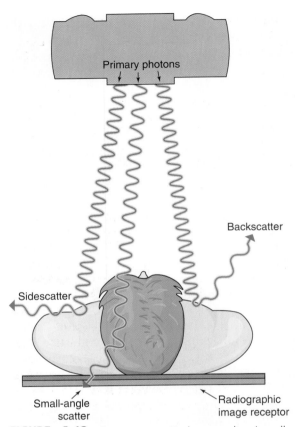

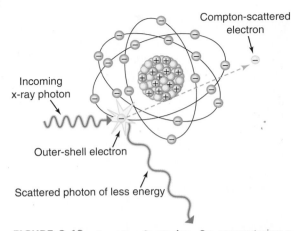

**FIGURE 3-13** **Compton Scattering.** On encountering a loosely bound outer-shell electron, the incoming x-ray photon surrenders a portion of its kinetic energy to dislodge the electron from its orbit. The energy-degraded x-ray photon then continues on its way but in a new direction. The high-speed electron ejected from its orbit is called a *Compton-scattered electron*, or *secondary*, or *"recoil" electron.*

**FIGURE 3-12** Compton scattering results in all-directional scatter. The scatter created may be directed onward as small-angle scatter, backward as backscatter, and to the side as sidescatter. The intensity of radiation scatter in various directions is a major factor in planning the protection for medical imaging personnel during a radiologic examination.

is that the Compton interaction's lack of Z dependence implies that it does not differentiate between equal amounts of bone and soft tissue and thus does not serve as a useful contrast mechanism for radiographic imaging. Fortunately, another type of interaction known as *photoelectric interaction* provides that mechanism.

In diagnostic radiology, the probability of occurrence of Compton scattering relative to that of the photoelectric interaction increases as the energy of the x-ray photon increases. Compton scattering and photoelectric absorption in tissue are equally probable at approximately 35 keV.

Therefore, in a 100-kVp x-ray beam when the photons have an average energy in the range of 30 to 40 keV, significant numbers of Compton events occur.

A summary of facts about the process of Compton scattering is presented in Box 3-5 for quick reference.

## Pair Production

**Pair production** does not occur unless the energy of the incident x-ray photon is at least 1.022 mega electron volts (MeV; a unit of energy equal to 1 million eV). Although this energy range is far higher than that used in diagnostic radiology, a brief description of pair production is included in this chapter to provide the reader with a broader understanding of the basic interactions of x-radiation with matter.

**Process of Pair Production.** In pair production, the incoming x-ray photon strongly interacts with the nucleus of an atom of the irradiated biologic tissue and disappears (Fig. 3-14). In the process, the energy of the photon is transformed into two new particles: a negatron (an ordinary

BOX 3-5 | **Summary of the Process of Compton Scattering**

Compton scattering is important in the energy range used in diagnostic radiology. Because the scattered x-ray photon produced from the interaction of the incoming photon with an outer-shell electron of an atom of human tissue results only in a partial transfer of kinetic energy to that biologic atom, the scattered photon now traveling in a different direction can become a potential health hazard for imaging personnel by increasing their occupational radiation exposure. In the event that Compton scattered photons reach the image receptor, they can decrease contrast of the image by adding an additional, undesirable exposure called *radiographic fog*. Because its energy dependence decreases much more slowly with increasing energy than does the photoelectric interaction, Compton scattering is very important even at therapeutic energies.

BOX 3-6 | **Mass-Energy Equivalent**

$$\text{Mass (electron or positron)} = 9.1 \times 10^{-31}\ \text{kg}$$

$$c = 3 \times 10^8\ \text{m/sec}$$

$$E\,(\text{total}) = E\,(\text{electron}) + E\,(\text{positron})$$
$$= 2mc^2\,(\text{electron or positron}) = 16.38 \times 10^{-14}\ \text{J}$$

$$1\ \text{MeV} = 1.602 \times 10^{-13}\ \text{J}$$

$$\text{Therefore,}\ E = 16.38 \times 10^{-14}\ 1.602 \times 10^{-13} = 1.022\ \text{MeV}$$

electron) and a positron (a positively charged electron). The negatron and the positron have the same mass and magnitude of charge; the only difference is in the "sign" of their electrical charges. The incoming photon must have enough energy to produce the combined rest mass of these two particles. The minimum energy required to produce an electron-positron pair is 1.022 MeV (Box 3-6). For this reason, pair production does not occur at lower energies. The electron loses its kinetic energy by exciting and ionizing atoms in its path. The electron eventually loses enough energy that it may be captured by an atom in need of another electron.

As far as is known, no large quantities of positrons freely exist in the universe. The positron is classified as a form of antimatter. It interacts destructively with a nearby electron. During this interaction, the positron and the electron annihilate each other, a conversion of matter into energy in accordance with Albert Einstein's famous theory of relativity, mathematically expressed as $E = mc^2$ ($c$ is the speed of light in a vacuum). This energy that appears from the annihilation of the negatron and positron is carried off by two 0.511-MeV photons moving in opposite directions. Although pair production does not occur unless the energy of the incoming photon is at least 1.022 MeV, its probability of occurrence starts to become significant (i.e., noticeably greater than zero) at 10-MeV x-ray energies and higher.

**Use of Annihilation Radiation in Positron Emission Tomography.** Annihilation radiation is used in positron emission tomography (PET)

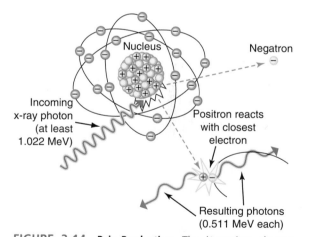

**FIGURE 3-14** **Pair Production.** The incoming photon (equivalent in energy to at least 1.022 MeV) strongly interacts with the nucleus of the atom of the irradiated object and disappears. In the process, the energy of the photon is transformed into two new particles: a negatron (electron) and a positron. The negatron eventually recombines with any atom that needs another electron. The positron interacts destructively with a nearby electron. During the interaction, the positron and the electron annihilate each other, with their rest masses converted into energy, which appears in the form of two 0.511-MeV photons, each moving in the opposite direction.

(see Chapter 14). In PET scanning, the source of the positrons is atomic nuclei that are unstable because they contain too many protons relative to their number of neutrons. To relieve this instability, the surplus proton is converted in the nucleus into a neutron while a positron and another particle called a *neutrino* are ejected from the nucleus. This process is called *positron decay*. Within a very short distance (several micrometers or less), the emitted positron interacts with a local electron, and the two mutually annihilate, yielding a pair of photons emerging in opposite directions from the electron-positron interaction site. These annihilation photons are intercepted by a ring of detectors surrounding the patient and are used to build a cross-sectional image of the radioactivity within the patient. Some examples of unstable nuclei used in PET scanning are as follows:

- Fluorine-18 ($^{18}$F)
- Carbon-11 ($^{11}$C)
- Nitrogen-13 ($^{13}$N)

## Photodisintegration

**Photodisintegration** is an interaction that occurs at more than 10 MeV in high-energy radiation therapy treatment machines. As with pair production, this energy range is also far higher than useful diagnostic energies; therefore, a brief account of this interaction process of radiation with matter is included so the reader will have been introduced to all possible types of radiation and matter encounters.

**Process of Photodisintegration.** In photodisintegration, a high-energy photon collides with the nucleus of an atom, which directly absorbs all the photon's energy. This energy excess in the nucleus creates an instability that in most cases is alleviated by the emission of a neutron by the nucleus. Other types of emissions— a proton or proton-neutron combination (deuteron) or even an alpha particle—are possible if sufficient energy is absorbed by the nucleus. Because emission of charged and/or uncharged particles has occurred from a previously inactive nucleus, we can say that the photodisintegration

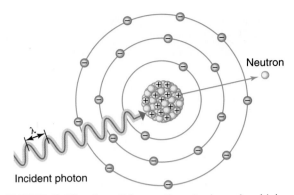

**FIGURE 3-15   Photodisintegration.** An incoming high-energy photon collides with the nucleus of the atom of the irradiated object and absorbs all the photon's energy. This energy excess in the nucleus creates an instability that is usually alleviated by the emission of a neutron. In addition, if sufficient energy is absorbed by the nucleus, other types of emissions will be possible, such as a proton or proton-neutron combination (deuteron), or even an alpha particle.

interaction has made a nucleus radioactive (Fig. 3-15).

## SUMMARY

- Biologic damage in the patient may result from the absorption of x-ray energy.
- Variations in x-ray absorption properties of various body structures make radiographic imaging of human anatomy possible.
- Attenuation results when, through the processes of absorption and scatter, the intensity of the primary photons in an x-ray beam decrease as it passes through matter.
- Scattered radiation can result in decreased contrast of the image by adding additional, undesirable exposure to the IR (radiographic fog) or, in fluoroscopy, Compton-scattered photons may expose personnel who are present in the room to scattered radiation.
- The amount of energy absorbed by the patient per unit mass is called the *absorbed dose*.
- Two interactions of x-radiation are important in diagnostic radiology: photoelectric absorption and Compton scattering. The photoelectric effect is the basis of radiographic imaging, whereas the Compton effect is its bane.

- For each radiographic procedure, an optimal peak kilovoltage (kVp) and milliampere-seconds (mAs) combination exists that minimizes the dose to the patient and produces an acceptable image.
- Within the energy range of diagnostic radiology (23 to 150 kVp), which also includes mammography, when kVp is decreased, the number of photoelectric interactions increases and the number of Compton interactions decreases; however, the patient absorbs more energy, and therefore the dose to the patient increases.
- When kVp is increased, the patient receives a lower dose, but image quality may be compromised.
- kVp selection is usually based on type of procedure and body part imaged.
- Radiographers must balance other variables such as type of image receptor used, patient thickness, and degree of muscle tissue to arrive at technical exposure factors that will provide an acceptable image yet stay within the standards of radiation protection.
- Coherent scattering is most likely to occur at less than 10 keV; pair production and photodisintegration occur far above the range of diagnostic radiology.

# REFERENCES

1. Hendee WR, Ritenour ER: *Medical imaging physics*, ed 4, Chicago, 2002, John Wiley & Sons.
2. Carlton RR, Adler AM: *Principles of radiographic imaging: an art and a science*, ed 5, New York, 2013, Delmar Cengage Learning.
3. Fauber TL: *Radigraphic image and exposure*, ed 4, St. Louis, 2013, Mosby.
4. Johnston JN, Fauber TL: *Essentials of radiographic physics and imaging*, St. Louis, 2012, Mosby.

# GENERAL DISCUSSION QUESTIONS

1. Why is it necessary for radiographers to have a basic understanding of the processes of interaction between radiation and matter?
2. How is an x-ray beam produced?
3. Why is tungsten or tungsten rhenium used in the target of the x-ray tube?
4. Describe the function of filtration in a diagnostic x-ray beam.
5. What is attenuation?
6. Why do human bones appear white in a completed diagnostic image?
7. Describe the interactions between x-radiation and matter that occur within the diagnostic radiology range.
8. In the mathematical expression $E = mc^2$, what does $c$ represent?
9. What type of radiation is used in positron emission tomography?
10. When a high-energy photon collides with the nucleus of an atom during the process of photodisintegration, how much of the photon's energy is directly absorbed by the nucleus?

# REVIEW QUESTIONS

1. Exit, or image-formation, radiation is composed of which of the following?
   A. Primary photons and Compton-scattered photons
   B. Noninteracting and small-angle scattered photons
   C. Attenuated photons
   D. Absorbed photons
2. Which of the following contributes *significantly* to the exposure of the radiographer?
   A. Positrons
   B. Electrons
   C. Compton-scattered photons
   D. Compton-scattered electrons
3. Which of the following defines attenuation?
   A. Absorption and scatter
   B. Absorption only
   C. Scatter only
   D. Weakened only

4. In the radiographic kilovoltage range, which of the following structures undergoes the *most* photoelectric absorption?
   A. Air cavities
   B. Compact bone
   C. Fat
   D. Soft tissue

5. In which of the following x-ray interactions with matter is the energy of the incident photon *partially* absorbed?
   A. Compton
   B. Photoelectric
   C. Coherent
   D. Pair production

6. When a high atomic number solution is either ingested or injected into human tissue or a structure to visualize it during an imaging procedure, which of the following occurs?
   A. Photoelectric interaction becomes greatly decreased, resulting in an increase in the absorbed dose in the body tissues or structures that contain the contrast medium.
   B. Photoelectric interaction becomes significantly enhanced, leading to an increase in the absorbed dose in the body tissues or structures that contain the contrast medium.
   C. Photoelectric interaction becomes greatly decreased, resulting in a decrease in the absorbed dose in the body tissues or structures that contain the contrast medium.
   D. Photoelectric interaction becomes significantly enhanced, leading to a decrease in the absorbed dose in the body tissues or structures that contain the contrast medium.

7. Which of the following characteristics primarily differentiates the probability of occurrence of the various interactions of x-radiation with human tissue?
   A. Energy of the incoming photon
   B. Direction of the incident photon
   C. X-ray beam intensity
   D. Exposure time

8. Which of the following influences attenuation?
   1. Effective atomic number of the absorber
   2. Mass density
   3. Thickness of the absorber
   A. 1 and 2 only
   B. 1 and 3 only
   C. 2 and 3 only
   D. 1, 2, and 3

9. A decrease in contrast of the image by adding an additional, unwanted exposure (radiographic fog) results from which of the following interactions between x-radiation and matter?
   1. Compton scattering
   2. Pair production
   3. Photoelectric absorption
   A. 1 only
   B. 2 only
   C. 3 only
   D. 1, 2, and 3

10. The interactions of x-ray photons with any atoms of biologic matter are:
   A. Able to be preplanned to selective atoms to limit radiation exposure to those atoms.
   B. Important only in therapeutic radiology.
   C. Random, and therefore the effects of such interactions cannot be predicted with certainty.
   D. Unimportant in diagnostic radiology, thus making radiation protection unnecessary.

## CHAPTER 4

# Radiation Quantities and Units

## OBJECTIVES

*After completing this chapter, the reader will be able to perform the following:*

- Explain the concepts of skin erythema dose, tolerance dose, and threshold dose.
- List five examples of early deterministic somatic effects, three examples of late deterministic somatic effects, and two examples of late stochastic effects.
- Differentiate between somatic and genetic (hereditary) effects.
- Differentiate among the radiation quantities exposure, air kerma, absorbed dose, equivalent dose, and effective dose, and identify the appropriate symbol for each quantity.
- List and explain the International System (SI) units for radiation exposure, air kerma, absorbed dose, equivalent dose, and effective dose.
- Define the term *dose area product* (DAP).
- Explain how the quantity surface integral dose is determined.
- Describe the function of a tissue weighting factor.

- Given the numeric value for an absorbed dose of radiation stated in grays, the radiation weighting factor for the type and energy of radiation in question, and the tissue weighting factor, determine the effective dose.
- State the purpose of the radiation quantity collective effective dose, and list its SI unit.
- Explain the importance of linear energy transfer as it applies to biologic damage resulting from irradiation of human tissue.
- State the formula for determining the equivalent dose.
- Determine the equivalent dose in terms of SI units when given the radiation weighting factor and the absorbed dose for different ionizing radiations.
- Explain the concept of effective dose when used for radiation protection purposes.
- State the formula for determining the effective dose.
- State the whole-body total effective dose equivalent (TEDE) for occupationally exposed personnel and for the general public.

Copyright © 2014, Elsevier Inc.

| | | |
|---|---|---|
| Exposure | Equivalence of Radiation- | Effective Dose |
| Air Kerma | Produced Damage from | Collective Effective Dose |
| Absorbed Dose | Different Sources of | Total Effective Dose |
| Surface Integral | Ionizing Radiation | Equivalent |
| Dose | Equivalent Dose | **Summary** |

## KEY TERMS

absorbed dose (D)
air kerma
collective effective dose
   (ColEfD)
committed effective dose
   equivalent (CEDE)
coulomb (C)
coulombs per kilogram (C/kg)
deep dose equivalent (DDE)
dose area product (DAP)
early deterministic somatic
   effects

effective dose (EfD)
equivalent dose (EqD)
exposure (X)
genetic, or heritable, effects
gray (Gy)
International System of Units
   (SI)
linear energy transfer (LET)
late deterministic somatic
   effects

late stochastic effects
occupational exposure
radiation weighting factor
   ($W_R$)
sievert (Sv)
somatic damage
surface integral dose (SID)
total effective dose equivalent
   (TEDE)
tissue weighting factor ($W_T$)

As the potentially harmful effects of ionizing radiation became known, the medical community sought to reduce radiation exposure throughout the world by developing standards for measuring and limiting this exposure. To be able to measure patient and personnel exposure in a consistent and uniform manner, diagnostic imaging personnel should be familiar with the radiation quantities and units discussed in this chapter. Chapter 10 describes the standardized effective dose limits on radiation exposure expressed in these units; the dose limits are designed to minimize the associated risk and the potentially harmful effects of such exposure. Equivalent dose limits for tissues and organs are also described.

## HISTORICAL EVOLUTION OF RADIATION QUANTITIES AND UNITS

### Discovery of X-Rays

On November 8, 1895, while working in a modest laboratory at the University of Wurzburg, in Bavaria, German physics professor Wilhelm Conrad Roentgen (Fig. 4-1) discovered a mysterious ray. While performing an experiment investigating the nature of cathode rays and fluorescent materials, Roentgen passed electricity through a Crookes tube that he had covered with a shield made of black cardboard (Fig. 4-2). As he passed a charge through the pear-shaped, partial vacuum discharge tube, he observed light emanating from a piece of paper coated with barium platino-cyanide that was lying on a bench several feet away. Roentgen hypothesized that some type of radiant energy had been emitted from the Crookes tube that caused the barium platino-cyanide to glow. To determine whether any object had the ability to obstruct the mysterious rays, he held various items between the Crookes tube and the fluorescent-coated paper. He found that most materials would allow some of these new rays to pass through. Roentgen called this momentous discovery "x-ray." Roentgen also found that x-rays could expose photographic film. In late November 1895, he took the world's first x-ray picture on film, which clearly showed the bones of his wife's hand (Fig. 4-3). In December 1895, he announced his scientific findings in

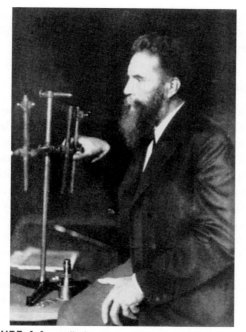

**FIGURE 4-1**   Wilhelm Conrad Roentgen, the discoverer of x-rays.

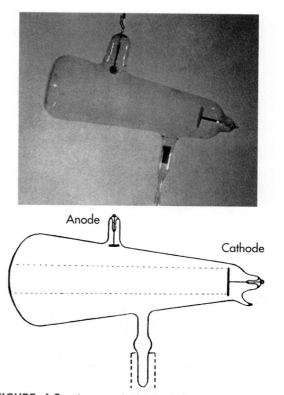

**FIGURE 4-2**   Photograph (**A**) and diagram (**B**) of the original type of x-ray tube. The cathode stream produced x-rays by impinging on the large area of the glass wall of the tube.

an abbreviated manuscript titled, "On a New Kind of Ray, a Preliminary Communication," which was presented to the Physical Medical Society of Würzburg.

## First Reports of Injury

In the months that followed the announcement of Roentgen's discovery, experimentation with the new "wonder rays" resulted in acute biologic damage to some patients and pioneer radiation workers. Cases of **somatic** (from the Greek term *soma*, meaning "of the body") **damage,** biologic damage to the body of the exposed individual caused by exposure to ionizing radiation, were reported in Europe as early as 1896. In the United States, Clarence Madison Dally (Fig. 4-4, *A*), glass-blower, tube maker, assistant, and long-time friend of fluoroscope inventor Thomas A. Edison (Fig. 4-4, *B*), became the first American radiation fatality. Dally died of radiation-induced cancer in October of 1904 at the age of 39 years. Because of Clarence Dally's severe injuries and

death, Thomas Edison discontinued his x-ray research.

Among physicians, cancer deaths attributed to x-ray exposure were reported as early as 1910. As a result of **occupational exposure,** radiation exposure received by radiation workers in the course of exercising their professional responsibilities, many radiologists and dentists developed a reddening of the skin called *radiodermatitis*. Many of these skin lesions on the hands and fingers eventually became cancerous as a consequence of continued exposure to ionizing radiation (Fig. 4-5). Blood disorders such as aplastic anemia, which results from bone marrow failure, and leukemia, an abnormal overproduction of white blood cells, were more common among early radiologists than among nonradiologists.

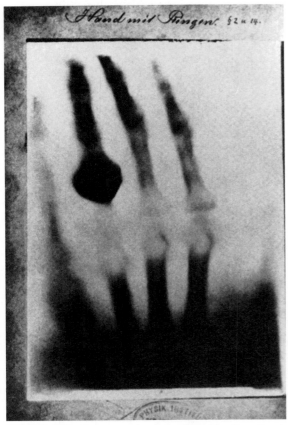

**FIGURE 4-3**   First x-ray picture on film: Mrs. Roentgen's hand.

## Investigation of Methods for Reducing Radiation Exposure

Alarmed by the increasing number of radiation injuries reported, the medical community decided to investigate methods for reducing radiation exposure. In 1921, the British X-Ray and Radium Protection Committee was created to perform this task. The committee planned to formulate guidelines for the manufacture and use of radium and x-ray equipment and devices to eliminate the chance of occupational injury. Even though the committee members recognized the danger of excessive radiation exposure, they were handicapped because they did not have accurate measurement techniques or adequate background knowledge of radiobiology. Unfortunately, because they could not agree on a workable unit of radiation exposure, the members of the committee were unable to fulfill their responsibility.

## Skin Erythema Dose

From 1900 to 1930, the unit in use for measuring radiation exposure was called the *skin erythema dose,* defined as the received quantity of radiation that causes diffuse redness over an area of skin after irradiation. This amount of absorbed radiation corresponds roughly to a modern dose of several grays. The radiation unit, gray (Gy), is discussed later in this chapter. Because the amount of radiation required to produce an erythema reaction varied from one person to another, the skin erythema dose was a crude and inaccurate way to measure radiation exposure. Scientists felt compelled to continue searching for a more reliable unit. The new unit selected was to be based on some exactly measurable effect produced by radiation, such as ionization of atoms or energy absorbed in the irradiated object.

## Early Definition of Quantities and Units

The First International Congress of Radiology was held in London, England, in 1925. This international meeting allowed radiologists from all over the world to collaborate. Unfortunately, no definite decisions for measuring the effects of ionizing radiation were made based on the recommendations presented. The International Commission on Radiation Units and Measurements (ICRU) was also formed in 1925. In 1928, a Second International Congress of Radiology was held in Stockholm, Sweden. Although the "roentgen" was accepted as a unit of exposure, it was not adequately defined. The congress charged the ICRU to define this conventional unit of exposure. The congress also established the International X-Ray and Radium Protection Commission, predecessor of the International Commission on Radiological Protection (ICRP), which is discussed in Chapter 10.

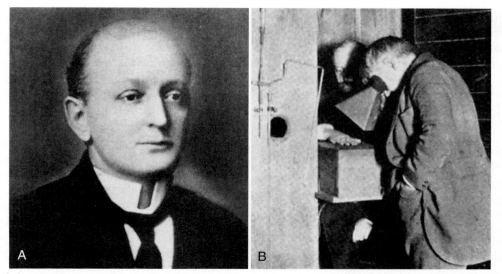

**FIGURE 4-4**   **A,** Clarence Madison Dally (1865-1904), the first American radiation fatality. **B,** Dally, assistant to Thomas A. Edison, is seen holding his hand over a box containing an x-ray tube while Edison examines the hand through a fluoroscope that he invented.

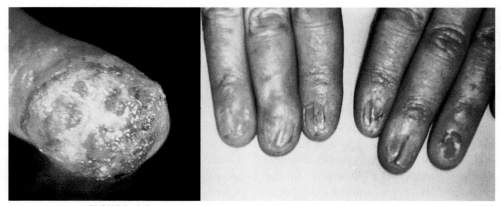

**FIGURE 4-5**   Lesions of the fingers induced by ionizing radiation.

Since the early days of radiology, biologic effects in humans caused by exposure to ionizing radiation were only too apparent. These **early deterministic somatic effects** (Box 4-1), which appeared within minutes, hours, days, or weeks of the time of radiation exposure, were believed to be preventable, if doses to radiation workers were limited and kept lower than a value at which no adverse biologic effects were demonstrated (see Chapters 8 and 10 for additional information on early deterministic somatic effects).

A *tolerance dose* is a radiation dose to which occupationally exposed persons could be continuously subjected without any apparent harmful acute effects, such as erythema of the skin. The general belief was that no adverse effects from radiation exposure would be demonstrated at doses lower than this level. Alternatively, this tolerance exposure level could be regarded as a *threshold dose,* that is, a dose of radiation lower than which an individual has a negligible chance of sustaining specific biologic damage.

---

| BOX 4-1 | Effects of Ionizing Radiation |
| --- | --- |

**Early Deterministic Somatic Effects**
Nausea
Fatigue
Diffuse redness of the skin
Loss of hair
Intestinal disorders
Fever
Blood disorders
Shedding of the outer layer of skin

**Late Deterministic Somatic Effects**
Cataract formation
Fibrosis
Organ atrophy
Loss of parenchymal cells
Reduced fertility
Sterility

**Late Stochastic Effects**
Cancer
Genetic (hereditary) effects

---

The tolerance dose was stated in units of what at that time was an imprecise measure of the quantity called "exposure." This unit, the *roentgen*, was the principal guideline for occupational radiation exposure during the 1930s. Neither tolerance dose nor threshold dose is currently used for the purposes of radiation safety.

In 1934, the International X-Ray and Radium Protection Commission recommended a tolerance dose daily limit of 0.2 roentgen. In the United States, the Advisory Committee on X-Ray and Radium Protection, which was formed in 1931 to formulate recommendations for radiation control, also recommended a tolerance dose equal to 0.2 roentgen per day.

In 1936, the Committee reduced this dose to 0.1 roentgen per day. As scientists began to recognize the **late deterministic somatic effects** and **late stochastic effects** (see Chapters 8, 9, and 10 for additional information) of ionizing radiation that appeared months or years after exposure and the possibility of **genetic,** or **heritable, effects,** they began to focus on finding ways to minimize the risk of sustaining such damage (see Box 4-1).

The search was on for a more reliable unit to replace the tolerance dose.

In 1937, the ICRU finished its assignment from the Second International Congress of Radiology, and, although still not accurately defined, the roentgen became internationally accepted as the unit of measurement for exposure to x-radiation and gamma radiation (short-wavelength, higher-energy electromagnetic waves emitted by the nuclei of radioactive substances). This unit was redefined in 1962 to increase accuracy and acceptability.

In 1946, the U.S. Advisory Committee on X-Ray and Radium Protection became known as the National Committee on Radiation Protection. The name of this radiation standards organization underwent another change in 1956 and again in 1964, when it became the National Council on Radiation Protection and Measurements (NCRP). Functions of the NCRP are discussed in Chapter 10.

The General Conference of Weights and Measures, which was responsible for the development and international unification of the metric system, assigned its International Committee for Weights and Measures the responsibility of developing guidelines for the units of measurement in 1948. To fulfill this responsibility, the committee developed the **International System of Units (SI),** from the French "Système International d'Unités." This system makes possible the interchange of units among all branches of science throughout the world.

## The Modern Era of Radiation Protection

By the early 1950s, maximum permissible dose (MPD) replaced the tolerance dose for radiation protection purposes. MPD basically indicated the largest dose of ionizing radiation that an occupationally exposed person was permitted and that was not anticipated to result in major adverse biologic effects as a consequence of radiation exposure. This meant that absorbed doses of ionizing radiation lower than the established

MPD would not result in any appreciable bodily injury or in injury to the reproductive cells. However, some small risk of damage could exist with radiation doses at the MPD level. MPD was expressed in rem (an acronym for "radiation equivalent man," historically known as "Roentgen equivalent man"), the traditional British unit used for radiation protection purposes at that time.

Eventually the concept of "tolerance dose" was no longer accepted as a means for protecting radiation workers from the acute effects of ionizing radiation. This meant that *no amount* of radiation was considered completely safe. The probability of long-term harm, such as the development of cancer, was expected to decrease as the dose decreased, but it was not expected to become zero at any dose. This raised a dilemma: If no amount of radiation was safe, and if it was impossible to design a work environment where the dose was zero (and still be able to perform procedures such as interventional angiography), then what would determine the maximum allowed occupational exposure? The solution was to compare rates of death and accident among various occupations. Insurance companies had been using this method of comparison for many years to determine insurance rates. Some occupations are very hazardous. Examples of such occupations are:

- Deep sea diving
- Professional mountaineering

Some nonhazardous occupations are:

- Trade
- Government desk work

However, even in nonhazardous occupations, there is still a small risk of fatality or serious injury (approximately 1 chance in 10,000 each year[1]). With this in mind, the decision was made to base recommendations for dose limits on the concept that the probability of harm associated with typical dosimeter readings should be no more than the amount of harm in industries that are generally considered reasonably safe.

By the 1970s, dosimetry and risk analysis had become quite sophisticated. Radiation units were developed that contained factors that accounted for the varied bioeffects of different types of radiation:

- Alpha
- Beta
- Gamma
- X-radiation
- Neutrons

There was also growing recognition that the consequences for the health of the human as a whole organism depended on which organs and organ systems had been irradiated. For example, irradiation of the bone marrow was seen as more significant to the health of an organism than irradiation of the skin. Equal doses of radiation to bone marrow and skin had different consequences. In the late 1970s, dose limits were calculated and established to ensure that the risk from radiation exposure acquired on the job did not exceed risks encountered in "safe" occupations, such as clerical work, in which the risk is approximately $10^{-4}$ (one chance in 10,000) per year.[1]

In 1991, the ICRP revised tissue weighting factors. The revision was based on data from more recent epidemiologic studies of the atomic bomb survivors. The ICRP adopted the term **effective dose (EfD)**. EfD is based on the energy deposited in biologic tissue by ionizing radiation. It takes into account the following:

1. The type of radiation (e.g., x-radiation, gamma, neutron)
2. The variable sensitivity of the tissues exposed to radiation

This quantity, EfD, is actually a measure of the overall risk arising from the irradiation of biologic tissue and organs. It takes into consideration the exposure to the entire body. EfD is expressed in **sieverts (Sv)**, which are SI units, or in millisieverts (mSv), subunits of the sievert. Further discussion of this radiation quantity and its associated units of measure follows.

## Quantities and Units in Use Today

In 1980, the ICRU adopted SI units, a unified system of metric units, for use with ionizing radiation and urged full implementation of the units as soon as possible. Many developed countries, particularly in Europe, have already made the transition to SI units. In the United States, SI units, the gray, and the centigray are now used routinely in therapeutic radiology to specify absorbed dose. Even though the NCRP (see Chapter 10) adopted the internationally accepted SI units for use in 1985, traditional units, older special units associated with radiation protection and dosimetry, such as the roentgen* (with minor exceptions) are becoming obsolete. As previously noted, the roentgen (R) was at one time the internationally accepted unit for the measurement of exposure to x-radiation and gamma radiation. The traditional unit, the rem,[†] was previously used for the radiation quantity equivalent dose, a currently used metric quantity especially in radiation dosimetry reports for occupationally exposed personnel. In the SI system of units, the sievert (Sv) replaced the rem for radiation protection purposes. This unit provides a common scale whereby varying degrees of biologic damage caused by equal absorbed doses of different types of ionizing radiation can be compared with the degree of biologic damage caused by the same amount of x-radiation or gamma radiation. One sievert is equal to 100 rem.

Fluoroscopic entrance dose rates can now be measured in milligray per minute ($mGy_{-a}/min$), but in many facilities they are measured as exposure rates in roentgens per minute (R/min), and essentially all radiation survey instruments continue to provide readings in traditional units. In addition, many regulatory criteria are specified in terms of traditional units. Even though the SI units and their subunits are now predominant, the traditional units and their subunits should be recognized because they are still being used in more than a few situations. For this reason, the current generation of radiation workers must understand both the metric unit systems and the traditional system for the safety of patients and personnel until a complete transition to metric units is made. Although this edition of the textbook focuses on the metric units, the traditional units are presented where appropriate. Traditional units are identified in parentheses after the SI units occasionally. Box 4-2 presents an overview of the important dates in the historical evolution of radiation quantities and units and an overview of terminology used in a given period of time to describe radiation dose limitation.

The SI unit of absorbed dose, the **gray** (**Gy**) (discussed later in this chapter), was named after the English radiobiologist Louis Harold Gray (1901-1965), who was instrumental in developing what is arguably the most important theory in all of radiation dosimetry. The Bragg-Gray theory (1936) relates the ionization produced in a small cavity within an irradiated medium or object to the energy absorbed in that medium as a result of its radiation exposure. With the use of appropriate correction factors, the theory essentially links the determination of the absorbed radiation dose in a medium to a relatively simple measurement of ionization charge.

Rolf Maximilian Sievert (1896-1966), the Swedish physicist for whom the SI unit of equivalent dose was named, is best known for his method (the Sievert integral) for determining the exposure rates at various points near linear radium sources (tubes).

## RADIATION QUANTITIES AND THEIR UNITS OF MEASURE

Diagnostic imaging professionals need to understand the following basic radiation quantities:

---

*One roentgen is the photon exposure that under standard conditions of pressure and temperature produces a total positive or negative ion charge of $2.58 \times 10^{-4}$ coulombs per kilogram of dry air.

[†]Rem stands for "radiation equivalent man." It is defined as the dose that is equivalent to any type of ionizing radiation that produces the same biologic effect as 1 rad (radiation absorbed dose) of x-radiation. One rad corresponds to an energy transfer of 100 ergs per gram to an irradiated object.

| BOX 4-2 | Historical Evolution of Radiation Quantities and Units |
|---|---|

| Year | Event |
|---|---|
| 1895 | X-rays are discovered, and the discovery is announced. |
| 1896 | Initial cases of somatic damage caused by exposure to ionizing radiation are reported in Europe. |
| 1900 | Skin erythema dose becomes the unit for measuring radiation exposure. |
| 1904 | Clarence Madison Dally becomes the first American radiation fatality. |
| 1910 | First cancer deaths among physicians that are attributed to x-ray exposure are reported. |
| 1921 | The British X-Ray and Radium Protection Committee is formed to investigate methods for reducing radiation exposure. |
| 1925 | The First International Congress of Radiology is held in London, England; radiologists from all over the world collaborate, but no definite system for measuring ionizing radiation exposure is identified. The International Commission on Radiation Units and Measurements (ICRU) is formed. |
| 1928 | The ICRU is charged by the Second International Congress of Radiology (Stockholm, Sweden) to define a unit of exposure. The International X-Ray and Radium Protection Commission (predecessor of the ICRP) is established by the Second International Congress of Radiology. |
| 1930s | Tolerance dose is used for radiation protection purposes. |
| 1931 | The U.S. Advisory Committee on X-Ray and Radium Protection is formed to formulate recommendations for radiation control. |
| 1934 | A tolerance dose of 0.2 R per day is recommended. |
| 1936 | The tolerance dose is reduced to 0.1 R per day. |
| | The Bragg-Gray theory is introduced. |
| 1937 | The roentgen (R) becomes internationally accepted as the unit of measurement for exposure to x-radiation and gamma radiation. |
| 1946 | The U.S. Advisory Committee on X-Ray and Radium Protection becomes known as the National Committee on Radiation Protection and Measurements (NCRP). |
| 1948 | The International System of Units (SI) is developed. |
| Early 1950s | Maximum permissible dose (MPD) replaces the tolerance dose for radiation protection purposes. |
| 1962 | The roentgen (R) is redefined to increase accuracy and acceptability. |
| 1963 | The National Committee on Radiation Protection and Measurements becomes the National Council on Radiation Protection (NCRP). |
| 1977 | The International Commission on Radiological Protection (ICRP) recommends that the dose equivalent limit or effective dose equivalent replace the MPD. |
| 1980 | The ICRU adopts SI units for use with ionizing radiation. |
| 1985 | The National Council of Radiation Protection (NCRP) adopts SI units for use. |
| 1991 | The ICRP replaces effective equivalent dose with the term *effective dose (EfD)*. |

**History of Terminology Used to Determine Radiation Dose Limitation**

| | |
|---|---|
| 1900-1930 | Skin erythema dose (SED) |
| 1930-1950 | Tolerance dose (TD) |
| 1950-1977 | Maximum permissible dose (MPD) |
| 1977-1991 | Effective dose equivalent |
| 1991-present | Effective dose (EfD) |

- Exposure (X)
- Air kerma
- Absorbed dose (D)
- Equivalent dose (EqD)
- Effective dose (EfD)

In a simplified sense, exposure may be described as the amount of ionizing radiation that may strike an object such as the human body when in the vicinity of a radiation source. Absorbed dose is the deposition of energy per unit mass in the patient's body tissue from exposure to ionizing radiation. As stated in Chapter 2, EqD is a radiation quantity used for radiation purposes when a person receives exposure from various types of ionizing radiation. Besides serving as a measure of absorbed energy resulting from ionization, this quantity also attempts to take into account the potential variation in biologic harm that is produced by different kinds of radiation. Both the type and the energy of the radiation are considered. EfD is another radiation quantity that is important when discussing radiation protection issues. It begins with EqD, and then by incorporating modifying or weighting factors, which correspond to the relative degrees of radiosensitivity of various organs and tissues, attempts to take into account the different levels of radiation effects on the parts of the body that are being irradiated to arrive at an index of overall harm to a human. EfD, then, is the quantity that summarizes the potential for biologic damage to a human from exposure to ionizing radiation (Box 4-3). Each radiation quantity has its own special unit of measure. These units are discussed in detail in the following section.

## Exposure

When a volume of air is irradiated with x-rays or with gamma rays, the interaction that occurs between the radiation and neutral atoms in the air causes some electrons to be liberated from those air atoms as they are ionized. Consequently, the ionized air can function as a conductor and carry electricity because of the negatively charged free electrons and positively charged ions that have been created. As the intensity of x-ray exposure of the air volume increases, the number of electron-ion pairs produced also increases. Thus the amount of radiation responsible for the ionization of a well-defined volume of air may be determined by measuring the number of electron-ion pairs or charged particles in that volume of air. This radiation ionization in the air is termed *exposure*.

**Exposure (X)** is defined as the total electrical charge of one sign, either all pluses or all minuses, per unit mass that x-ray and gamma ray photons with energies up to 3 million electron volts (MeV) generate in dry (i.e., nonhumid) air at standard temperature and pressure (760 mm Hg or 1 atmosphere at sea level and 22° C). It is a radiation quantity "that expresses the concentration of radiation delivered to a specific area, such as the surface of the human body."[2]

Like other forms of radiation measurement, exposure is based on a response produced when radiation interacts with a medium. It can be quickly evaluated.

For precise measurement of radiation exposure in radiography, however, the total amount of ionization (charge) an x-ray beam produces in a known mass of air must be obtained. This type of direct measurement is accomplished in an accredited calibration laboratory by using a standard, or free-air, ionization chamber (Fig. 4-6). The chamber contains a known quantity of air with precisely measured temperature, pressure, and humidity. If in that specified volume of dry air the total charge of all the ions of one sign (either all pluses or all minuses) produced is collected and measured, the total amount of radiation exposure may be accurately determined. The free-air chamber response is modified to correspond to standard temperature and pressure of dry air.

Such an instrument, however, is not a practical device at locations other than a standardization

---

| BOX 4-3 | **Difference between Equivalent Dose and Effective Dose** |
|---|---|

The quantity, *equivalent dose*, uses radiation weighting factors ($W_R$) to adjust the quantity, *absorbed dose*, to reflect the different capacity for producing biologic harm by various types and energies of ionizing radiation.

The quantity, *effective dose*, uses tissue weighting factors ($W_T$) to adjust the quantity, *equivalent dose*, to reflect the difference in harm to the person as a whole depending on the tissues and organs that have been irradiated. Therefore, effective dose takes into account both the type of radiation and the part of the body irradiated.

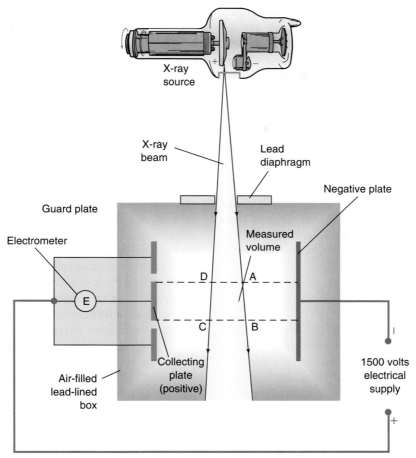

**FIGURE 4-6** This device determines radiation exposure by measuring the amount of ionization (charge) an x-ray beam produces within its air collection volume. The instrument consists of a box containing a known quantity of air, two oppositely charged metal plates, and an electrometer, an instrument that measures the total amount of charge collected on the positively charged metal plate. The chamber measures the total amount of electrical charge of all the electrons produced during the ionization of a specific volume of air at standard atmospheric pressure and temperature. The electrical charge is measured in units called *coulombs* (C) (charge of an electron = $-1.6 \times 10^{-19}$ C). A collected electrical charge of $2.58 \times 10^{-4}$ C/kg of irradiated air constitutes an exposure of 1 roentgen (R).

laboratory. As a result, much smaller and less complicated instruments have been developed for use away from the laboratory. Although very convenient, these instruments must be periodically recalibrated in a standardization laboratory against a free-air chamber.

The **coulomb** (C) is the basic unit of electrical charge. It represents the quantity of electrical charge flowing past a point in a circuit in 1 second when an electrical current of 1 ampere is used. The ampere is the SI unit of electrical current. In the International System, the exposure unit is measured in **coulombs per kilogram (C/kg)**. No special name for this SI quantity has been assigned. This exposure unit is simply equal to an electrical charge of 1 C produced in a kilogram of dry air by ionizing radiation. The roentgen, however, as previously noted, was precisely defined as the photon (either x-ray or gamma ray) exposure, that under standard conditions of pressure and temperature, produces a total positive or negative ion charge of

$2.58 \times 10^{-4}$ C/kg of dry air. An exposure of 1 C/kg equals $(1/2.58 \times 10^{-4})$ R or $3.88 \times 10^3$ R, which represents a very large radiation exposure. Conversion from roentgens to coulombs per kilogram may be accomplished by multiplying the number of roentgens by $2.58 \times 10^{-4}$. In contrast, conversion of coulombs per kilogram (C/kg) to roentgens (R) is achieved by dividing the number of coulombs per kilogram by $2.58 \times 10^{-4}$. Appendix A provides examples of these numeric conversions.

The coulomb per kilogram (roentgen) unit is used for x-ray equipment calibration because x-ray output intensity is measured directly with an ionization chamber. It also is used to calibrate radiation survey instruments (refer to Chapter 5 for further information).

## Air Kerma

**Air kerma** is another SI quantity that can be used to express radiation concentration transferred to a point, which may be at the surface of a patient's or radiographer's body. It is replacing the traditional quantity, exposure. Air kerma actually denotes a calculation of radiation intensity in air. "X-ray tube output and inputs to image receptors are sometimes described in air kerma."[3] A standard or free air ionization chamber is the instrument that can be calibrated to read air kerma.[2] "A conversion factor can also be used to convert between air kerma and exposure values."[2]

"Kinetic energy released in matter," "kinetic energy released in material," and "kinetic energy released per unit mass" all use the word "kerma" as an acronym. In simple terms, air kerma is kinetic energy released in a unit mass (kilogram) of air and is expressed in metric units of joule per kilogram (J/kg).[2] In a similar way one can define *tissue kerma* as the kinetic energy released in a unit mass of tissue. Tissue kerma is also given in units of joules per kilogram. This is in fact the same radiation unit, the gray (Gy), which was previously defined as the SI unit used to measure the radiation quantity absorbed dose. When the Gy is used to indicate kinetic radiation energy deposited or absorbed in a mass of air, it is written as $Gy_a$, where the subscript "$_a$" indicates "air." Conversely, when the Gy is used to indicate the absorbed dose of kinetic radiation energy in tissue, it is written as $Gy_t$, where the subscript "$_t$" indicates "tissue." If air kerma is determined at a specific point within soft tissue of the body, the absorbed dose of radiation in that mass of tissue will be approximately equal to this "tissue" kerma value. With respect to radiographic and fluoroscopic units, however, "air" kerma is the primary concept because in these situations we are concerned with exposure and the patient's entrance dose. Modern radiographic and fluoroscopic units have incorporated an ability to determine the entire amount of energy delivered to the patient by the x-ray beam. This quantity is often referred to as the **dose area product (DAP)**. It is essentially the sum total of air kerma over the exposed area of the patient's surface or, in other words, a measure of the amount of radiant energy that has been thrust into a portion of the patient's body surface. DAP is usually specified in units of mGy-cm$^2$. As an illustration of this concept, consider a patient whose irradiated surface receives an air kerma dose of 0.02 Gy. If the area of the irradiated surface is 100 cm$^2$, then the DAP will be 20 mGy $\times$ 100 cm$^2$ = 2000 mGy-cm$^2$.

## Absorbed Dose

As ionizing radiation passes through an object such as a human body, some of the energy of that radiation is transferred to that biologic material. It is actually absorbed by the body and stays within it. The quantity **absorbed dose (D)** is defined as the amount of energy per unit mass absorbed by an irradiated object. This absorbed energy is responsible for any biologic damage resulting from exposure of the tissues to radiation. For this reason the absorbed dose may be used to indicate the amount of ionizing radiation a patient receives during a diagnostic imaging procedure.

Anatomic structures in the body possess different absorption properties; some structures can absorb more radiant energy than others. The amount of energy absorbed by a structure depends on the atomic number (Z) of the tissues comprising the structure, the mass density of the tissue (measured in kg/m$^3$), and the energy of the incident photon. Absorption increases as atomic number and mass density increase and also as photon energy decreases. Therefore, low-energy photons are more easily absorbed in a material such as biologic tissue than are high-energy photons.

The effective atomic number (Zeff) of a given biologic tissue is a "composite," or weighted average, of the atomic numbers of the many chemical elements comprising the tissue. Bone has a higher effective atomic number (Zeff = 13.8) than does soft tissue (Zeff = 7.4) because bone contains calcium (Z = 20) and phosphorus (Z = 15), whereas soft tissue is composed mostly of fat (Zeff = 5.9) and structures with atomic numbers close to that of water (Zeff = 7.4). Bone absorbs more ionizing radiation than does soft tissue in the diagnostic energy range of 23 to 150 kilovolts peak (kVp), (which includes mammography), because the photoelectric process for bone is the dominant mode of energy absorption within this range. The probability of photoelectric interaction strongly depends on the atomic number of the irradiated material. The higher the atomic number of the material, the greater is the amount of energy absorbed by that material.

In the therapeutic energy range of 100 keV and higher, however, the difference in absorption between bone and soft tissue gradually lessens (Fig. 4-7). This is because the amount of photoelectric absorption decreases and the amount of Compton scattering relative to the photoelectric interaction increases as the energy of the x-ray beam increases. The amount of Compton scattering in a material does not depend on the atomic number of the material. Hence, as energy increases, the difference in the amount of absorption between any two tissues of different atomic number decreases. Because the process of absorption is responsible for biologic damage and absorption properties vary with the quality of the radiation and the type of tissue irradiated, irradiation of tissues in *therapeutic radiology* is

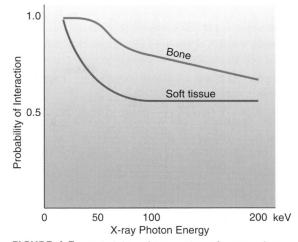

**FIGURE 4-7** Probability of interaction of x-rays when a layer of soft tissue or bone that is 5 cm thick is encountered. The probability is greater at lower energies and is greater for bone than for soft tissue, particularly at low energies.

generally specified in terms of absorbed dose rather than in terms of exposure. It is also important to remember that exposure is only a measure of ionization in air and not in other tissue. However, at all energies, mass density always has an effect on absorption. This effect is linear and directly proportional. Therefore, a material that is twice as dense as another will absorb twice as much energy from the same photon beam.

As stated earlier, the SI unit of absorbed dose is the gray (Gy), previously defined as an energy absorption of 1 joule (J) per kilogram (kg) of matter in the irradiated object. One gray is therefore determined by the following simple equation:

$$1\,Gy = 1\,J/kg$$

A joule may be defined as the work done or energy expended when a force of 1 newton (N) acts on an object along a distance of 1 meter (m). A single joule does not correspond to a large amount of energy. A typical microwave oven, for example, imparts 750 J/sec to the food it is heating.

| BOX 4-4 | Subunits of the Gray |
|---------|----------------------|

Smaller fractions of measured quantities such as the gray (Gy) will have a prefix. Examples follow.

| Prefix | Subunit | Symbol | Fraction | Factor |
|--------|---------|--------|----------|--------|
| centi- | centigray (cGy) | c | $\frac{1}{100}$ | $10^{-2}$ |
| milli- | milligray (mGy) | m | $\frac{1}{1000}$ | $10^{-3}$ |
| micro- | microgray (µGy) | µ | $\frac{1}{1,000,000}$ | $10^{-6}$ |

| BOX 4-5 | How to Convert Grays to Milligrays |
|---------|-------------------------------------|

Rule: Number of grays (Gy) $\times$ 1000 = Number of milligrays (mGy)
Example 1: $0.010 \times 1000 = 10$
Example 2: $0.100 \times 1000 = 100$

Traditionally, the rad* was used as the unit of absorbed dose. One rad is expressed mathematically as follows:

$$1\,\text{rad} = 100\,\text{erg/g}$$

or

$$1\,\text{rad} = 1/100\,\text{J/kg} = 1/100\,\text{Gy}$$

Even though the traditional system of units for radiation quantities is gradually being eliminated in favor of the SI units now used to be consistent with scientific groups, the U.S. government, and many other countries and also current textbooks and scientific journals, some individuals may want to understand how to convert from one system to the other in case they need to do so. As shown earlier, gray and rad units are easily convertible. Appendix A illustrates conversions among the systems of units.

Because many x-ray examinations require relatively small radiation doses, subunits may frequently be used to indicate absorbed dose values. These subunits are only a fraction of a specific unit. Examples of some of these subunits are provided in Box 4-4. In diagnostic radiology

because radiation exposure and absorbed dose are low, a milli-value of $\frac{1}{1000}$ is frequently used for the sake of simplicity. If, for example, a radiation exposure ($Gy_a$), or absorbed dose ($Gy_t$), were stated in grays by using a numeric value with a decimal, it would actually be easier to use a milli-value and convert the number of grays into milligrays (mGy). This can readily be accomplished by multiplying the number of grays by 1000. Examples of this conversion are demonstrated in Box 4-5. It is also easy to convert milligrays to grays. This is just by dividing the number of milligrays by 1000.

SI subunits facilitate conversion from rad to gray and gray to rad (see Appendix A). In therapeutic radiology, for example, the centigray (cGy), which numerically is identical to the rad, is replacing the rad for recording of absorbed dose. Even though SI values and traditional values differ numerically, SI values of dose are all $\frac{1}{100}$ of the older traditional system. For example, 500 rad in the traditional system is now 5 $Gy_t$ in the SI system, and an equivalent dose of 500 rem in the traditional system is now 5 Sv in the new system.[4]

## Surface Integral Dose

The **surface integral dose** (**SID**) is the total amount of radiant energy transferred by ionizing radiation to the body during a radiation exposure. Historically, it has been also known as *exposure area product*. This quantity is determined by the product of the exposure value (in R) and the size of the area ($cm^2$) that receives the total amount of radiation delivered. Thus R-$cm^2$ is the traditional unit for SID.[2] The equivalent SI unit for SID is the Gy-$m^2$.

---

*Rad stands for *radiation absorbed dose*. This unit has been used to indicate the amount of radiant energy transferred to an irradiated object by any type of ionizing radiation. The rad is equivalent to an energy transfer of 100 ergs (another unit of energy and work) per gram of irradiated object.

## Equivalence of Radiation-Produced Damage from Different Sources of Ionizing Radiation

Equal absorbed doses of different types of radiation produce different amounts of biologic damage in body tissue. For example, a 1-Gy absorbed dose of fast neutrons causes more biologic damage than a 1-Gy absorbed dose of x-rays. A 1-Gy dose of neutrons would kill a laboratory rat, but a 1-Gy dose of x-rays would not. The concept of dose equivalence takes this biologic impact into consideration by using a specific modifying, or quality, factor, to adjust the absorbed dose value. Quality factor (Q) is an adjustment multiplier that has been used in the calculation of dose equivalence to specify the ability of a dose of any kind of ionizing radiation to cause biologic damage.

X-rays, beta particles (high-speed electrons), and gamma rays produce virtually the same biologic effect in body tissue for equal absorbed doses. In terms of quality factor, these radiations have been given a numeric adjustment value of 1 and are the basis or standard against which to compare the effectiveness or efficiency of other types of ionizing radiation in producing biologic damage. The quality factors of different kinds of ionizing radiations are listed in Table 4-1. The concept of **linear energy transfer (LET)** helps explain the need for a quality, or modifying, factor. LET (Fig. 4-8) is the amount of energy transferred on average by incident radiation to an object per unit length of track through the object and is expressed in units of keV/μm (see Appendix B).

Radiation with a high LET transfers a large amount of energy into a small area and can therefore do more biologic damage than radiation with a low LET. As a result, a high-LET radiation has a quality factor that is greater than the quality factor for a low-LET radiation. LET and its relationship with biologic damage are discussed again in Chapter 7.

## Equivalent Dose

**Equivalent dose (EqD)** is the product of the average absorbed dose in a tissue or organ in the

| TABLE 4-1 | Quality Factors for Different Types of Ionizing Radiation |
|---|---|
| **Type of Ionizing Radiation** | **Quality Factor** |
| X-ray photons | 1 |
| Beta particles | 1 |
| Gamma photons | 1 |
| Thermal neutrons | 5 |
| Fast neutrons | 20 |
| High-energy external protons | 1 |
| Low-energy internal protons* | 20 |
| Alpha particles | 20 |
| Multiple charged particles of unknown energy | 20 |

Data from National Council of Radiation Protection and Measurements (NCRP): *Limitation of exposure to ionizing radiation,* Report No. 116, Bethesda, Md, 1993, NCRP.
*Protons produced as a result of neutrons interacting with the nuclei of tissue molecules.

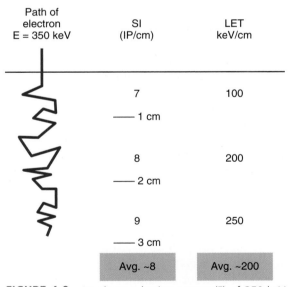

**FIGURE 4-8** An electron having energy (E) of 350 keV interacts in a tissuelike material. Its actual path is tortuous, changing direction a number of times, as the electron interacts with atoms of the material via excitations and ionizations. As interactions reduce the energy of the electron through excitation and ionization, the electron's energy is transferred to the material. The interactions that take place along the path of the particle may be summarized as specific ionization (ion pairs/cm) or as linear energy transfer (LET, keV/cm) along the straight line continuation of the particle's trajectory beyond its point of entry.

human body and its associated **radiation weighting factor** ($W_R$) chosen for the type and energy of the radiation in question. X-radiation and gamma radiation have a $W_R$ of 1, whereby 1 Gy equals 1 Sv. Other types of radiation have different radiation weighting factors.

*Stochastic effects* are nonthreshold, randomly occurring biologic effects of ionizing radiation such as cancer and genetic (hereditary) abnormalities. These effects can result from relatively low radiation exposure, and it can take a long time before they are demonstrated. The probability of occurrence depends on the radiation dose and the type and energy of the radiation. What this means is that some radiations are more biologically efficient for causing damage than others for a given dose (see Chapters 8, 9, and 10 for a more detailed discussion of deterministic and stochastic effects). The radiation weighting factor ($W_R$) takes this into account. The radiation weighting factors are selected by national and international scientific advisory bodies (NCRP, ICRP) and are based on quality factors and LET. The NCRP, in Report No. 116, described the radiation weighting factor as "a dimensionless factor" (a multiplier) that was chosen for radiation protection purposes to account for differences in biologic impact among various types of ionizing radiations.[1] This factor places risks associated with biologic effects on a common scale. Each type and energy of radiation has a specific radiation weighting factor, the numeric value of which may be found in Table 4-2. The radiation weighting factor actually has the same numeric value as the quality factor that was previously used for determining dose equivalence.

EqD is used for radiation protection purposes when a person receives exposure from various types of ionizing radiation. EqD for measuring biologic effects may be determined and expressed in sieverts or in a subunit of the sievert (Box 4-6). The sievert replaces the rem for accounting for differences in biologic effectiveness of various types of ionizing radiations. Equivalent dose is obtained by multiplying the absorbed dose (D) by the radiation weighting factor ($W_R$) as follows:

| TABLE 4-2 | Radiation Weighting Factors for Different Types and Energies of Ionizing Radiation |
|---|---|
| **Radiation Type and Energy Range** | **Radiation Weighting Factor ($W_R$)** |
| X-ray and gamma ray photons and electrons (every energy) | 1 |
| Neutrons, energy <10 keV | 5 |
| 10 keV-100 keV | 10 |
| >100 keV-2 MeV | 20 |
| >2 MeV-20 MeV | 10 |
| >20 MeV | 5 |
| Protons | 2 |
| Alpha particles | 20 |

Data adapted from International Commission on Radiological Protection (ICRP): *Recommendations,* ICRP Publication No. 60, New York, 1991, Pergamon Press.

| BOX 4-6 | Subunits of the Sievert |
|---|---|

Smaller fractions of measured quantities such as the sievert (Sv) will have a prefix. Examples follow.

| Prefix | Subunit | Symbol | Fraction | Factor |
|---|---|---|---|---|
| centi- | centisievert (cSv) | c | $1/100$ | $10^{-2}$ |
| milli- | millisievert (mSv) | m | $1/1000$ | $10^{-3}$ |
| micro- | microsievert (µSv) | µ | $1/1,000,000$ | $10^{-6}$ |

$$EqD = D \times W_R$$

which in terms of units corresponds to:

$$Sv = Gy \times W_R$$

An example of determining and expressing EqD using grays and sieverts is provided in Box 4-7. Appendix A provides an example of using rad and rem for determining and expressing EqD.

Because radiation doses for radiation workers employed in diagnostic radiology are relatively small, they may be specified in terms of millisieverts. To change sieverts to millisieverts,

<table>
<tr><td colspan="2">

**BOX 4-7** | **Determining and Expressing Equivalent Dose Using Grays and Sieverts**

</td></tr>
</table>

Example: An individual received the following absorbed doses: 0.1 $Gy_t$ of x-radiation, 0.05 $Gy_t$ of fast neutrons, and 0.2 $Gy_t$ of alpha particles. What is the total equivalent dose (EqD)?

$$EqD = (D \times W_R)_1 + (D \times W_R)_2 + (D \times W_R)_3$$

(The radiation weighting factor for each radiation in question may be obtained from Table 4-2.)

Answer:

| Radiation Type | D | × | $W_R$ | = | EqD |
|---|---|---|---|---|---|
| X-radiation | 0.1 $Gy_t$ | × | 1 | = | 0.1 Sv |
| Fast neutrons | 0.05 $Gy_t$ | × | 20 | = | 1.0 Sv |
| Alpha particles | 0.2 $Gy_t$ | × | 20 | = | 4.0 Sv |
| | Total EqD | | | = | 5.1 Sv |

---

**BOX 4-8** | **How to Convert Sieverts to Millisieverts**

Rule: Number of sieverts (Sv) × 1000 = Number of millisieverts (mSv)

Example 1: 0.010 × 1000 = 10

Example 2: 0.100 × 1000 = 100

---

**TABLE 4-3** | **Organ or Tissue Weighting Factors**

| Organ or Tissue | Weighting Factor ($W_T$) |
|---|---|
| Gonads | 0.20 |
| Red bone marrow | 0.12 |
| Colon | 0.12 |
| Lung | 0.12 |
| Stomach | 0.12 |
| Bladder | 0.05 |
| Breast | 0.05 |
| Liver | 0.05 |
| Esophagus | 0.05 |
| Thyroid | 0.05 |
| Skin | 0.01 |
| Bone surface | 0.01 |
| Remainder*† | 0.05 |

Data from National Council on Radiation Protection and Measurements (NCRP): *Limitation of exposure to ionizing radiation*, Report No. 116, Bethesda, Md, 1993, NCRP.

*The remainder takes into account the following additional tissues and organs: adrenals, brain, small intestine, large intestine, kidney, muscle, pancreas, spleen, thymus, and uterus.

†In extraordinary circumstances in which one of the remainder tissues or organs receives an equivalent dose in excess of the highest dose in any of the 12 organs for which a weighting factor ($W_T$) is specified, a $W_T$ of 0.025 should be applied to that tissue or organ and a $W_T$ of 0.025 to the average dose in the other remainder tissues or organs.

---

multiply the number of sieverts by 1000, whereas millisieverts can be converted to sieverts by dividing the number of millisieverts by 1000. Examples of these conversions are given in Box 4-8.

## Effective Dose

EfD provides a measure of the overall risk of exposure to humans from ionizing radiation. The NCRP, in Report No. 116, defines it as "the sum of the weighted equivalent doses for all irradiated tissues or organs."[1] EfD incorporates both the effect of the type of radiation used (e.g., x-radiation, gamma, neutron) and the variability in radiosensitivity of the specific organ or body part irradiated through the use of appropriate weighting factors. These factors determine the overall harm to those biologic components and

the risk of developing a radiation-induced cancer or, for the reproductive organs, the risk of genetic damage. The weighting factor that takes into account the relative detriment to each specific organ and tissue is called the **tissue weighting factor** ($W_T$). The tissue weighting factor is a conceptual measure for the relative risk associated with irradiation of different body tissues (see Chapter 10) "to account for the carcinogenic sensitivity of each organ."[5]

The tissue weighting factor (Table 4-3), more precisely, is a value that denotes the percentage of the summed stochastic (cancer plus genetic) risk stemming from irradiation of tissue (T) to the all-inclusive risk, when the entire body is irradiated in a uniform fashion. EfD accounts for the risk to the entire organism brought on by irradiation of individual tissues and organs. The

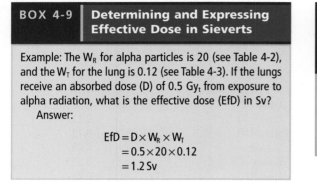

| BOX 4-9 | Determining and Expressing Effective Dose in Sieverts |
|---------|--------------------------------------------------------|

Example: The $W_R$ for alpha particles is 20 (see Table 4-2), and the $W_T$ for the lung is 0.12 (see Table 4-3). If the lungs receive an absorbed dose (D) of 0.5 $Gy_t$ from exposure to alpha radiation, what is the effective dose (EfD) in Sv?
   Answer:

$$EfD = D \times W_R \times W_T$$
$$= 0.5 \times 20 \times 0.12$$
$$= 1.2\,Sv$$

| TABLE 4-4 | Typical Values for Radiation Doses Associated with an Anteroposterior Lumbar Spine Examination |
|-----------|------------------------------------------------------------------------------------------------|

| | |
|---|---|
| Absorbed dose to skin at entrance surface | 6.4 mGy |
| Absorbed dose to bone marrow | 0.6 mGy |
| Absorbed dose to a fetus | 3.5 mGy |
| Equivalent dose to a fetus | 3.5 mSv |
| Effective dose | 3.3 mSv |

ICRP originally introduced the tissue weighting factor concept because uniform, whole-body irradiation seldom occurs, and some organs and body tissues vary considerably in the absorbed dose received and their sensitivity to random radiation-induced responses.

To determine EfD, an absorbed dose (D) is multiplied by a radiation weighting factor ($W_R$) to obtain EqD and that product is multiplied by a tissue weighting factor ($W_T$) to give:

$$EfD = D \times W_R \times W_T$$

EfD is expressed in sieverts or millisieverts. An example of determining and expressing EfD in sieverts is provided in Box 4-9. Appendix A provides an example of expressing EfD in rem.

EfD can be used to compare the average amount of radiation received by the entire body from a specific radiologic examination with that from natural background radiation (see Table 1-1). By using the background equivalent radiation time (BERT) method as discussed in Chapter 1, it is possible to describe the examination radiation dose in terms of the length of time it would take to acquire a comparable EfD from environmental sources.

Table 4-4 gives some typical values for radiation doses that are associated with a radiographic examination of the lumbar spine, and it illustrates some of the principles of the different ways to specify radiation dose. The dose to the patient is highest at the "entrance skin surface," the surface of the patient that is toward the x-ray

tube. This surface will be exposed to the unattenuated primary beam of x-rays. Absorbed doses to various organs may be calculated from standard tables. Two organ absorbed doses are given in Table 4-4, namely, bone marrow and fetus. The EqD to the fetus is also given and is the same as the absorbed dose to the fetus because the radiation weighting factor is 1. Finally, the EfD is given. It was calculated from the various tissue weighting factors and organ absorbed doses for organs in the field of view of this examination.

## Collective Effective Dose

In addition to EqD and EfD, another dosimetric quantity has been derived and implemented for use in radiation protection to describe internal and external dose measurements. The quantity, **collective effective dose** (ColEfD), is used to describe radiation exposure of a population or group from low doses of different sources of ionizing radiation. It is determined as the product of the average EfD for an individual belonging to the exposed population or group and the number of persons exposed. The radiation unit for this quantity is *person-sievert* (previously referred to as *man-rem*). An example using this unit is provided in Box 4-10.

## Total Effective Dose Equivalent

**Total effective dose equivalent** (**TEDE**) is a radiation dosimetry quantity that was defined by the

| BOX 4-10 | Determining Collective Effective Dose Using the Radiation Unit Person-Sievert |
|---|---|

Example: If 200 people receive an average effective dose of 0.25 Sv, the collective effective dose (ColEfD) is 200 × 0.25 = 50 person-sieverts.

Nuclear Regulatory Commission (NRC) to monitor and control human exposure to ionizing radiation. Essentially, as described by NRC regulations, it is the sum of effective dose equivalent from external radiation exposures and a quantity called **committed effective dose equivalent (CEDE)**\* from internal radiation exposures. Thus TEDE is designed to take into account all possible sources of radiation exposure. It is a particularly useful dose monitor for occupationally exposed personnel such as nuclear medicine technologists and interventional radiologists, who are likely to receive possibly significant radiation exposure during the course of a year. Traditionally, for occupationally exposed personnel, the whole-body TEDE regulatory limit is 0.05 Sv and 0.001 Sv for the general public. Radiation monitoring services such as Landauer, Inc. and Global Dosimetry Solutions can provide annual TEDE values for individuals.

Tables 4-5 and 4-6 summarize radiation quantities, units, and equivalents. An additional table emphasizing traditional units and SI units is also found in Appendix A.

---

\*The "committed dose" in radiation protection is a measure of the probabilistic health effect on an individual as a result of an intake of radioactive material into the body. A "committed dose" from an internal source is intended to carry the same effective risk as the same amount of equivalent dose applied uniformly to the whole body from an external source of radiation. This is the origin of the name "committed effective dose equivalent." For nuclear medicine technologists who, through certain procedures (e.g., thyroid ablations using iodine-131), have a possibility of radioisotope absorption and consequent internal radiation exposure, committed dose is certainly an appropriate measure.

| TABLE 4-5 | SI and Traditional Unit Equivalents |
|---|---|
| 1 SI exposure unit equals | 1. $C/kg = \dfrac{1}{(2.58 \times 10^{-4})}R$ |
| 1 coulomb equals | 1. 1 ampere-second |
| 1 coulomb per kilogram of air equals | 1. 1 SI unit of exposure |
| | 2. $\dfrac{1}{(2.58 \times 10^{-4})}R$ |
| 1 gray equals | 1. 1 J/kg |
| | 2. 100 rad |
| | 3. 100 cGy |
| | 4. 1000 mGy |
| 1 sievert equals | 1. 1 J/kg (for x-radiation, Q = 1) |
| | 2. 100 rem |
| | 3. 100 centisievert (cSv) |
| | 4. 1000 mSv |
| 1 erg equals | 1. $10^{-7}$ J |
| 1 joule equals | 1. $10^7$ erg |
| | 2. 1 newton-meter |
| | 3. $6.24 \times 10^{18}$ eV |

## SUMMARY

- Radiation units are now expressed in the International System (SI) because the traditional system of units does not fit into the metric system that provides "one unified system of units for all physical quantities."[2]
- Coulomb per kilogram (C/kg) is used for exposure in air only.
- Air kerma is an SI quantity that can be used for radiation concentration transferred to a point that may be at the surface of a patient's or radiographer's body.
- Dose area product (DAP) is essentially the sum total of air kerma over the exposed area of the patient's surface.
- The gray (Gy) is used for measuring absorbed dose in air ($Gy_a$) or for measuring absorbed dose in tissue $Gy_t$).
- Surface integral dose is determined by the product of the exposure value (in R) and the size of the area $cm^2$ that receives the total amount of radiation delivered.

| TABLE 4-6 | **Summary of Radiation Quantities and Units** | | | |
|---|---|---|---|---|
| **Type of Radiation** | **Quantity** | **SI Unit** | **Measuring Medium** | **Radiation Effect Measured** |
| X-radiation or gamma radiation | Exposure (X) | Coulombs per kilogram (C/kg) | Air | Ionization of air |
| | Air kerma | Gray ($Gy_a$) | | |
| All ionizing radiations | Absorbed dose (D) | Gray ($Gy_t$) | Any object | Amount of energy per unit mass absorbed by object |
| | Air kerma | Gray ($Gy_t$) | | |
| All ionizing radiations | Equivalent dose (EqD) | Sievert (Sv) | Body tissue | Biologic effects |
| All ionizing radiations | Effective dose (EfD) | Sievert (Sv) | Body tissue | Biologic effects |

- Equivalent dose (EqD) and effective dose (EfD) are the quantities of choice for measuring biologic effects when all types of radiation must be considered.
- EqD specifies how the potential for biologic damage from different types and doses of radiation will be equivalent, if correct weighting factors are included.
- EfD describes the way the same effective amount of damage can be attained by giving different equivalent doses to different organs.
- Sievert (Sv) is the SI unit of EqD and EfD.
- Occupational radiation exposure is measured in sieverts or in the subunit, millisieverts.
- Collective effective dose (ColEfD) is used when calculating group or population radiation exposure from low doses of different sources of ionizing radiation.
- Person-sievert is the unit used to calculate the radiation quantity ColEfD.
- To calculate equivalent dose: $EqD = D \times W_R$.
- To calculate effective dose: $EfD = D \times W_R \times W_T$.
- Total effective dose equivalent (TEDE) is a particularly useful dose monitor for occupationally exposed personnel such as nuclear medicine technologists and interventional radiologists. The whole-body TEDE regulatory limit for exposed personnel is 0.05 sievert and 0.001 sievert for the general public.
- The committed effective dose equivalent (CEDE) in radiation protection is a measure of the probabilistic health effect on an individual resulting from an intake of radioactive material into the body.

## REFERENCES

1. National Council on Radiation Protection and Measurements (NCRP): *Limitation of exposure to ionizing radiation*, Report No. 116, Bethesda, Md, 1993, NCRP.
2. Sprawls P: Radiation quantities and units, Sprawls Educational Foundation. *The physical principles of medical imaging online*. Available at: http://www.sprawls.org/ppmi2/RADQU/. Accessed April 8, 2013.
3. Carlton RR, Adler AM: *Principles of radiographic imaging: an art and a science*, ed 5, New York, 2013, Delmar, Cengage Learning.
4. Long BW, Frank ED, Ehrlich RA: *Radiography essentials for limited practice*, ed 4, St. Louis, 2013, Saunders.
5. Nickoloff EL, Lu ZF, Dutta AK, So JC: Radiation dose descriptors: BERT, COD, DAP, and other strange creatures. *Radiographics* 28:1439, 2008. Available at: http://radiographics.highwire.org/content/28/5/1439.full. Accessed September 8, 2012.

## GENERAL DISCUSSION QUESTIONS

1. Why should diagnostic imaging personnel be familiar with standardized radiation quantities and units?
2. When, where, and how did Wilhelm Conrad Roentgen discover x-rays?
3. What types of medical problems did early radiation workers develop as a

consequence of their occupational exposure?

4. What is the benefit of using the International System of Units of measurement for ionizing radiation?

5. What is a threshold dose?

6. In 1991 the International Commission on Radiological Protection (ICRP) revised tissue weighting factors. On what data was this revision based?

7. What radiation quantities are currently in use, and what SI units are used to relate these quantities?

8. What instrument can be calibrated to read air kerma?

9. What factors determine the amount of x-ray energy absorbed by a human anatomic structure?

10. When a person receives exposure from various types of ionizing radiation, what radiation quantity and what SI unit can be used for radiation protection purposes?

## REVIEW QUESTIONS

1. Which of the following was used as the *first* measure of exposure for ionizing radiation?
   A. Air kerma
   B. Skin erythema
   C. Sievert
   D. Roentgen

2. A radiation weighting factor ($W_R$) has been established for each of the following ionizing radiations: x-rays ($W_R$ = 1), fast neutrons ($W_R$ = 20), and alpha particles ($W_R$ = 20). What is the *total* equivalent dose (EqD) in sieverts for a person who has received the following exposures: 0.2 $Gy_t$ of x-rays, 0.07 $Gy_t$ of fast neutrons, and 0.3 $Gy_t$ of alpha particles?
   A. 9.4 Sv
   B. 7.6 Sv
   C. 4.3 Sv
   D. 1.9 Sv

3. Which of the following is the unit of collective effective dose (ColEfD)?
   A. Coulombs per kilogram-sievert
   B. Gray-sievert
   C. Person-sievert
   D. Rad-sievert

4. The concept of tissue weighting factor ($W_T$) is used to do which of the following?
   A. Account for the risk to the entire organism brought on by irradiation of individual tissues and organs
   B. Eliminate the need for determining effective dose
   C. Measure absorbed dose from all different types of ionizing radiations
   D. Modify the radiation weighting factor for different types of ionizing radiation

5. To convert the number of grays into milligrays, the number of grays must be:
   A. Divided by 100.
   B. Divided by 1000.
   C. Multiplied by 100.
   D. Multiplied by 1000.

6. What does the SI radiation unit coulomb per kilogram measure?
   A. Equivalent dose
   B. Absorbed dose in biologic tissue
   C. Radiation exposure in air only
   D. Speed at which x-ray photons travel

7. Which of the following radiation quantities accounts for some biologic tissues' being *more* sensitive to radiation damage than other tissues?
   A. Absorbed dose
   B. Exposure
   C. Equivalent dose
   D. Effective dose

8. The radiation weighting factor for alpha particles is 20, and the tissue weighting factor for the lungs is 0.12. If the lungs receive an absorbed dose of 0.2 $Gy_t$ from exposure to alpha particles, what is the effective dose in sieverts?
   A. 0.48 Sv
   B. 4.8 Sv
   C. 48.0 Sv
   D. 480.0 Sv

9. If 100 people received an average effective dose of 0.35 Sv, what is the collective effective dose?
   A. 17.5 person-sieverts
   B. 35 person-sieverts
   C. 70 person-sieverts
   D. 285 person-sieverts

10. What is the SI unit for surface integral dose?
    A. Coulomb
    B. Erg
    C. Gy-m$^2$
    D. Sievert

# Radiation Monitoring

## OBJECTIVES

*After completing this chapter, the reader will be able to perform the following:*

- State the reason why a radiation worker should wear a personnel dosimeter, and explain the function and characteristics of such devices.
- Identify the appropriate location on the body where the personnel dosimeter(s) should be worn during the following procedures or conditions: (1) routine computed radiography, digital radiography, or conventional radiographic procedures; (2) fluoroscopic procedures; (3) special radiographic procedures; and (4) pregnancy.
- Describe the various components of the optically stimulated luminescence (OSL) dosimeter, thermoluminescent dosimeter (TLD), film badge, and pocket ionization chamber, and explain the use of each of these devices as personnel monitors.
- Explain the function of radiation survey instruments.
- List three gas-filled radiation survey instruments.
- Explain the requirements for radiation survey instruments.
- Explain the purpose of the following instruments: (1) ionization chamber–type survey meter (cutie pie), (2) proportional counter, and (3) Geiger-Müller (GM) detector.
- Identify the radiation survey instrument that can be used to calibrate radiographic and fluoroscopic x-ray equipment.

## CHAPTER OUTLINE

## KEY TERMS

characteristic curve
control badge
control monitor
densitometer
extremity dosimeter
film badge
Geiger-Müller (GM) detector
glow curve
ionization chamber–type
  survey meter (cutie pie)

optical density
optically stimulated
  luminescence (OSL)
  dosimeter
personnel dosimeter
personnel dosimetry
personnel monitoring report
pocket ionization chamber
  (pocket dosimeter)

proportional counter
radiation-dosimetry film
radiation survey instruments
thermoluminescent dosimeter
  (TLD)
TLD analyzer

To ensure that occupational radiation exposure levels are kept well below the annual effective dose (EfD) limit, some means of monitoring personnel exposure must be employed. The radiographer and other occupationally exposed persons should be aware of the various radiation exposure monitoring devices and their functions. This chapter provides an overview of both personnel and area monitoring. In addition, because radiation dosimetry reports still report radiation exposure for workers in traditional units and subunits, the traditional units are identified in parentheses following SI units.

## PERSONNEL MONITORING

### Requirement for Personnel Monitoring

Personnel dosimetry—the monitoring of radiation exposure to any person occupationally exposed on a regular basis to ionizing radiation—is recommended. Exposure monitoring of personnel is *required* whenever radiation workers are likely to risk receiving 10% or more of the annual occupational EfD limit of 50 mSv (5 rem) in any single year as a consequence of their work-related activities. In keeping with the ALARA (as low as reasonably achievable) concept, most health care facilities issue dosimetry devices when personnel could receive approximately 1%

of the annual occupational EfD limit in any month, or approximately 0.04 mSv (4 mrem). Exposure monitoring is accomplished by wearing personnel dosimeters.

## Purpose of Personnel Dosimeter

The **personnel dosimeter:**

- Provides an indication of the working habits and working conditions of diagnostic imaging personnel.
- Determines occupational exposure by detecting and measuring the quantity of ionizing radiation to which the dosimeter has been exposed over a period of time.
- Does not protect the wearer from exposure because the instrument is just meant to detect and measure the amount of ionizing radiation to which it has been exposed.

## Placement of Personnel Dosimeter

**During Routine Radiographic Procedures.** A personnel monitoring device records only the exposure received in the area where the device is worn. During routine computed radiography, digital radiography, or conventional radiographic procedures, when a protective apron is not being used, the primary personnel dosimeter should be attached to the clothing on the front of the body at collar level to approximate the location

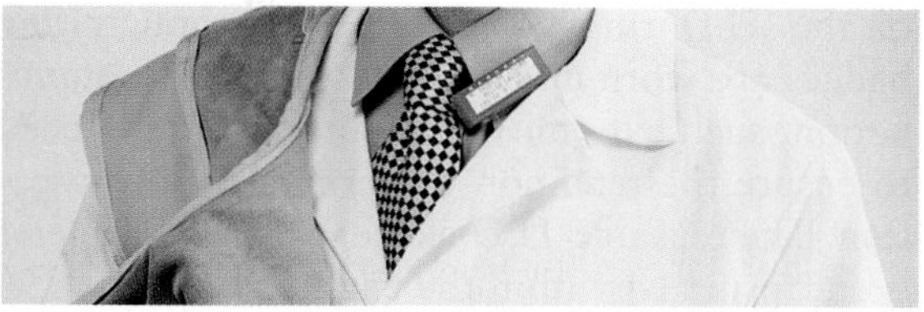

FIGURE 5-1  To approximate the maximum radiation dose to the thyroid and the head and neck during routine computed radiography, digital radiography, or conventional radiographic procedures, the primary personnel monitor should be attached to the clothing on the front of the body at collar level.

| BOX 5-1 | Personnel Monitoring Devices Currently Available |
|---|---|

1. Optically stimulated luminescence (OSL) dosimeter
2. Extremity dosimeter (thermoluminescent dosimeter [TLD] ring)
3. Film badge
4. Thermoluminescent dosimeter (TLD)
5. Pocket ionization chamber (pocket dosimeter)

of maximal radiation dose to the following (Fig. 5-1):

• Thyroid
• Head
• Neck

Consistency of location in wearing the dosimeter is necessary and is the responsibility of the individual wearing the device. A list of the types of personnel monitors available to diagnostic imaging personnel is found in Box 5-1. Discussion of each of the personnel monitoring devices follows.

**When a Protective Apron Is Worn.** Fluoroscopy, surgery, and special radiographic procedures produce the highest occupational radiation exposure for diagnostic imaging personnel. When a protective lead apron is used during such procedures, the dosimeter should be worn outside the apron at collar level on the anterior surface of the body (see Fig. 13-10) because the unprotected head, neck, and lenses of the eye receive 10 to 20 times more exposure than the protected

body trunk. When the dosimeter is located at collar level, it also provides a reading of the approximate equivalent dose to the thyroid gland and eyes of the occupationally exposed person. If the lead apron's shielding integrity is not compromised, a dosimeter reading that is within acceptable limits outside of the apron ensures a minimal reading under the apron.

**As a Second Monitor When a Protective Apron Is Worn.** During lengthy interventional fluoroscopy procedures (e.g., cardiac catheterization), some health care facilities may prefer to have diagnostic imaging personnel wear two separate monitoring devices. As mentioned previously, the first, or primary, dosimeter is to be worn outside the protective apparel at collar level, whereas the second dosimeter should be worn beneath a wraparound-style lead apron at waist level to monitor the approximate equivalent dose to the lower body trunk. Commercially available lead aprons typically have either 0.5-mm lead equivalent shielding over all or in a less heavy version 0.35-mm lead equivalent in the front and 0.25-mm shielding in the back. For those occupationally exposed personnel who use two radiation dosimeters as described earlier, it is useful to have some knowledge of what the difference in equivalent dose readings between those dosimeters could be. From information posted in August 2003 to the "Ask the Experts" section of the Health Physics Society by a certified medical physicist, for a primary beam at 100 kVp and 250 mAs incident at a distance of 100 cm (40 in.) on a 0.5-mm lead apron, the transmission through the apron was on average approximately 3.2%. So the disparity between the outer and inner dosimeter readings was approximately a factor of 30. For a similar situation with the lighter apron in the front, the transmission was approximately 8.5% (factor of 12) and in the rear approximately 10.5% (a factor of 9.5).

**As a Monitor for the Embryo-Fetus.** In addition to a primary dosimeter worn at collar level, pregnant diagnostic imaging personnel should be issued a second monitoring device to record the radiation dose to the abdomen during gestation. This monitor provides an estimate of the equivalent dose to the embryo-fetus.

## Extremity Dosimeter

It is recommended that an **extremity dosimeter,** or **thermoluminescent dosimeter (TLD)** ring (Fig. 5-2), be worn by an imaging professional as a second monitor when performing fluoroscopic procedures that require the hands to be near the primary x-ray beam. The badge cover contains information such as the account number, participant's name and number, wear date, indication of hand (right or left), size, and reference number

of the TLD ring dosimeter. Even though ring badges are worn under gloves to avoid contamination, such extremity monitors are laser-etched to ensure the retention of permanent identification. The reusable TLD element of the dosimeter is encapsulated within the engraved cover.

## Record of Radiation Exposure

A record of exposure should be part of the employment record of all radiation workers. Table 5-1 gives occupational exposure values (gathered from personnel dosimeter readings) for a typical year. The values represent the average annual EfD to the whole body.

## PERSONNEL DOSIMETERS

### Characteristics

A personnel dosimeter should be lightweight and easy to carry and be made of materials durable enough to tolerate normal daily use. The dosimeter must be able to detect and record both small and large exposures in a consistent and reliable manner. Outside influences such as very warm weather, humidity, and ordinary mechanical shock should not affect the performance of

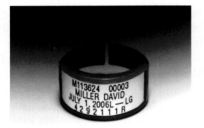

**FIGURE 5-2** An extremity dosimeter (thermoluminescent dosimeter [TLD] ring badge) can be used to monitor the equivalent dose to the hands.

| TABLE 5-1 | Occupational Exposure Values for a Typical Year | | | | |
|---|---|---|---|---|---|
| | Number of Workers (Thousands) | | Average Annual Effective Dose (mSv) | | Collective Effective Dose (Person-Sv)* |
| Category | All | Exposed | All | Exposed | |
| Medicine | 584 | 277 | 0.7 | 1.5 | 416 |
| Industry | 350 | 156 | 1.2 | 2.4 | 380 |
| Nuclear power | 151 | 91 | 3.6 | 5.6 | 550 |
| Flight crews, flight attendants | 97 | 97 | 1.7 | 1.7 | 165 |
| Other† | | | | | 789 |
| | | | | Total | 2300 |

Data from National Council on Radiation Protection and Measurements (NCRP): *Exposure of the U.S. population from occupational radiation,* Report No. 101, Bethesda, Md, 1989, NCRP, pp 65-70.
*See NCRP Report No. 101, p 60.
†Includes workers in the U.S. government (Department of Energy, U.S. Public Health Service), uranium mining, well logging, miscellaneous workers, visitors to facilities, and so forth.

the instrument. Because many employees in a health care facility may be assigned to wear radiation monitors, the monitors are required to be reasonably inexpensive to purchase and maintain. This permits health care facilities to use large numbers of monitors in a cost-effective manner.

## Types

Four types of personnel dosimeters are used to measure individual exposure of the body to ionizing radiation:

- Optically stimulated luminescence (OSL) dosimeters
- Film badges
- Thermoluminescent dosimeters (TLDs)
- Pocket ionization chambers

Extremity dosimeters (TLD ring badges), previously discussed, are used for monitoring of the hands only.

**Optically Stimulated Luminescence (OSL) Dosimeter.** The **optically stimulated luminescence (OSL) dosimeter** for personnel monitoring provides the best features of traditional film badges and TLDs (discussed later in this chapter) while eliminating some of their disadvantages (Fig. 5-3). This radiation monitor is the most common type of device used for monitoring of occupational exposure in diagnostic imaging. It has largely replaced its predecessor, the film badge, for personnel monitoring in many health care facilities.

The OSL dosimeter shown in Figure 5-3 contains an aluminum oxide ($Al_2O_3$) detector (thin layer). The dosimeter is "read out" by using laser light at selected frequencies. When such laser light is incident on the sensing material, it becomes luminescent in proportion to the amount of radiation exposure received. The OSL technology is actually similar to the way in which a luminous dial watch displays information.[1]

Although the OSL dosimeter can be worn for up to 1 year, it is common practice to wear it for a period of 1 to 3 months. Like traditional film badge monitors, OSL dosimeters are usually shipped to the monitoring company for reading

and exposure determination, a task that takes time for the result of a reading to be known. A company such as Landauer Inc (Glenwood, Ill) manufactures and sells an inhouse reader called "microStar" that may be purchased. In this way, occupational exposure can be determined on the day of occurrence.

*Energy Discrimination.* As can be seen in Figure 5-3, three different filters are incorporated into the detector packet of the OSL dosimeter. The filters are, respectively, made of:

- Aluminum (Al)
- Tin
- Copper (Cu)

Each filter blocks a portion of the radiation-sensitive aluminum oxide and causes a different degree of attenuation for any radiation striking the dosimeter, depending on its energy. The aluminum filter offers the least absorption, whereas the copper filter attenuates the most. What this means is that when the exposed aluminum oxide layer is read out by a laser, the degree of luminescence detected in the areas from beneath the filters is a measure of radiation dose occurring within different energy ranges. Thus a situation in which high-energy radiation strikes the dosimeter would show a similar reading through all the filters. Conversely, if the dosimeter had been subjected to only very low-energy radiation, then the laser readout, also known as a **glow curve,**\* would be much more pronounced in the region covered by the aluminum filter than in the other filter-blocked portions. Somewhat more energetic radiation would also enhance the glow curve of the region beneath the tin filter. This is the way that radiation energy discrimination is achieved by the OSL dosimeters. The different energy ranges are typically classified as "deep," "eye," and "shallow" and physically correlate

---

\*Glow curve: A graphical plot that demonstrates the relationship of light output, or emitted thermoluminescence intensity, to temperature variation. The curve represents a unique signature of the exposure received by the TLD dosimeter.

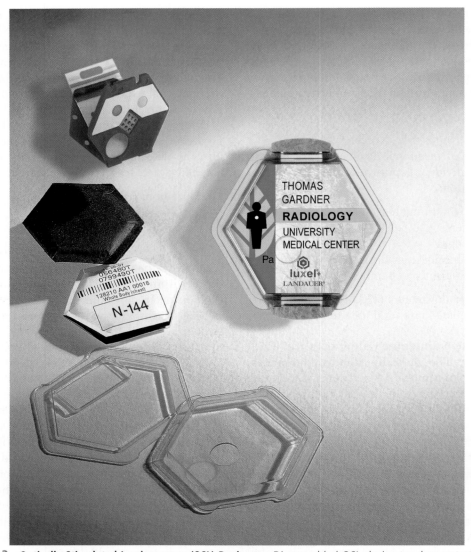

**FIGURE 5-3    Optically Stimulated Luminescence (OSL) Dosimeter.** Disassembled OSL dosimeter demonstrating components of the monitor: sensing material holder, preloaded packet incorporating an $Al_2O_3$ strip sandwiched within a three-element filter pack that is heat sealed within a light-tight black paper wrapper that has been laminated to the white paper label. The front of the white paper packet may also be color-coded to facilitate correct usage and placement of the dosimeter on the body of occupationally exposed personnel. (All components are sealed inside a tamperproof plastic blister pack.)

with different penetration depths and therefore different effective radiation energies, with "deep" being the most penetrating. In the latest type of OSL dosimeter from one manufacturer,[2] a "bare" or unfiltered portion of the aluminum oxide is used to detect dynamic exposures, that is, those received during rapid motion between the source of radiation and the enhanced dosimeter. Examination of the glow curves from this bare region demonstrates a shift or spread in their light frequency that can be correlated with motion (technically classifiable as a Doppler shift*).

***Optically Stimulated Luminescence Dosimeter Sensitivity.*** The OSL dosimeter provides a new degree of sensitivity by giving an accurate reading as low as 1 mrem for x-ray and gamma ray photons with energies ranging from 5 keV to greater than 40 MeV. Because the OSL dosimeter can provide an accurate reading as low as 10 $\mu$Sv (1 mrem), it is actually more sensitive than a TLD, discussed later in this chapter. The OSL dosimeter's maximum equivalent dose measurement for x-ray and gamma ray photons is 10 Sv (1000 rem). For beta particles with energies from 150 keV to in excess of 10 MeV, dose measurement ranges from 100 $\mu$Sv to 10 Sv (10 mrem to 1000 rem). For neutron radiation with energies of 40 keV to greater than 35 MeV, the OSL has a dose measurement range from 200 microsieverts to 250 microsieverts (20 mrem to 25 mrem). In diagnostic imaging, the increased sensitivity of the OSL dosimeter makes it ideal for monitoring employees working in low-radiation environments and for pregnant workers.

***Function of Control Monitor.*** The monitoring company that supplies a health care facility with OSLs provides a **control monitor** with each batch of dosimeters. This control serves as a basis for comparison with the remaining OSL dosimeters after they have been returned to the company for processing. Because the control monitor is supposed to be kept in a radiation-free area within an imaging facility, its optical density reading should be zero. After processing, if a control monitor reading greater than zero is indicated, then the batch of OSLs may have been exposed to radiation while in transit. To ensure that false readings are not recorded, the control

monitor reading is reported to the health care facility. This reading, if different from zero, must be subtracted from each of the remaining OSLs in the batch to ensure accuracy in exposure reporting.

***Advantages of the OSL Dosimeter.*** The OSL is lightweight, durable, and easy to carry. It contains an integrated, self-contained, preloaded packet. Color-coding, graphic formats, and body location icons provide easy identification. Unlike its film badge predecessor, the OSL's tamperproof blister packet is not affected by heat, moisture, and pressure. This device offers complete reanalysis in the event a health care facility believes that an error in reading the dosimeter has occurred. As mentioned previously, in diagnostic imaging the OSL dosimeter has increased sensitivity, providing accurate readings as low as 10 $\mu$Sv (1 mrem) for x-ray and gamma ray photons with energies from 5 keV to 40 MeV. This makes it an excellent, practical monitoring device for employees working in low-radiation environments and for pregnant workers. In addition, when compared with the film badge and the thermoluminescent dosimeter (TLD), described later, the OSL can be worn for longer periods of time (up to 1 year) to record occupational exposure.

***Disadvantages of the OSL Dosimeter.*** As is true with other personnel monitoring devices, occupational radiation exposure is recorded only in the body area where the device is worn. In addition, if the facility does not have an inhouse reader, exposure cannot be determined on the day of occurrence. The OSL dosimeter is not an efficient monitoring device if it is not worn.

**Film Badges.** Although optically stimulated luminescence (OSL) dosimeters are the most common personnel monitoring device in use at the time of this printing, **film badges** are still used for monitoring occupationally exposed imaging personnel in some health care facilities (Fig. 5-4). Film badges are economical and can be used to monitor large numbers of personnel in a cost-effective manner. They record whole-body radiation exposure accumulated at a low rate over a long period of time.

---

*Doppler shift* refers to the apparent change in the frequency of a light wave as observer and light source move toward or away from each other. This is similar to the increase in pitch of a train whistle experienced by a pedestrian as the locomotive moves toward him or her and its decrease in pitch noted by the pedestrian as the train moves away from him or her.

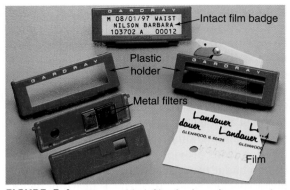

Intact film badge

Plastic holder

Metal filters

Film

**FIGURE 5-4** Disassembled film badge, demonstrating badge components: plastic holder, metal filters, and film packet.

The film badge is composed of three parts:

- A durable, lightweight plastic film holder
- An assortment of metal filters
- A film packet

The film holder should be made of a plastic material of a low atomic number to filter low-energy x-radiation, gamma radiation, and beta radiation. Inside the plastic holder are metal filters of aluminum or copper that are secured in a permanent position. These filters allow the measurement of the approximate energy of the radiation reaching the dosimeter. Penetrating radiations cast a faint shadow of the filters on the processed dosimetry film, whereas soft radiations cast a more pronounced image of the filters. The density of the image cast by each of the filters permits estimation of the energy of the radiation. From these data, the radiation dose can be evaluated as deep (penetrating) or shallow (nonpenetrating). In addition, the direction from which the radiation reached the film (from front to back or from back to front) can be estimated from the appearance of the filter shadows imaged on the processed dosimetry film. The filter images may also be used to determine whether the exposure was the result of excessive amounts of scattered radiation or a single exposure from a primary beam. Excessive exposure to scatter, such as that produced by poor working habits (e.g., radiographer standing too close to a patient during an exposure) or poor facility design, results in a relatively fuzzy image of the filters because the film badge was irradiated from many different angles. A single exposure from a primary beam, such as would result if a radiographer inadvertently left the film badge on a table during an exposure (the badge may have fallen off while the radiographer was positioning the patient and gone unnoticed), results in a sharply defined image.

***Radiation-Dosimetry Film inside the Film Badge.*** The **radiation-dosimetry film** contained in the radiographic film packet is similar to dental film. This film is sensitive to doses ranging from as low as 0.1 mSv (10 mrem) to as high as 5000 mSv (500 rem). Doses less than 0.1 mSv (10 mrem) are not usually detected and are reported as minimal (M) on a personnel monitoring report. The outside of the film packet forms a light-free envelope for the dosimetry film. Inside the envelope, a sheet of lead foil backs the film to absorb scatter radiation coming from behind the dosimeter. Radiation interacting with the film in the badge causes the film to darken once it is developed. After processing, the density, or degree of blackening, of the image of the filters recorded on the dosimeter film is proportional to the amount of radiation received and the energy of the radiation. An instrument called a **densitometer** is used to measure this density (Fig. 5-5). It measures **optical density,** the intensity of light transmitted through a given area of the dosimetry film, and compares it with the intensity of light incident on the anterior side of the film. The amount of radiation to which the film was exposed is determined by locating the exposure value of a control film of a similar optical density on a **characteristic curve.** For example, in the characteristic curve shown in Figure 5-6, if the optical density of the dosimeter film is determined to be 0.5, the film badge has received slightly more than 0.1 mSv (10 mrem).

***Function of a Control Badge.*** The monitoring company that supplies a health care facility with film badges also provides a **control badge** with each batch of badges. As with OSL dosimeters, this control badge serves as a basis for

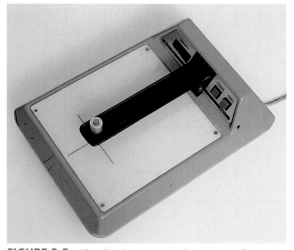

**FIGURE 5-5** The densitometer, an instrument that measures occupational exposure by comparing optical densities of exposed film badge (dosimetry) films.

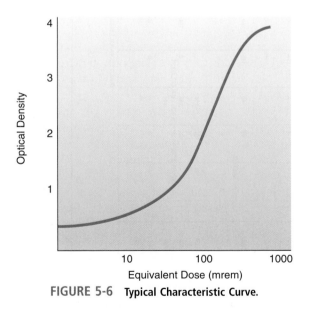

**FIGURE 5-6** **Typical Characteristic Curve.**

radiation while in transit. To ensure that false readings are not recorded, the control badge reading is reported to the health care facility. This reading, if different from zero, must be subtracted from each of the remaining film badges in the batch to ensure accuracy in exposure reporting.

***Personnel Monitoring Reports.*** Results from personnel monitoring programs must be recorded accurately and maintained for review to meet state and federal regulations. To comply with such requirements, health care facilities use established dosimetry services. These monitoring services process film badges and other types of personnel dosimeters, such as the OSL dosimeter (described previously) and the TLD (to be discussed later) and then supply written **personnel monitoring reports** to the health care facility (Fig. 5-7, *A*). These reports, typically one for each hospital department that is being monitored, list the deep, eye, and shallow occupational exposure of each covered person on a monthly (if applicable), quarterly, year to date, and lifetime equivalent basis. In addition, if requested, the total effective dose equivalent (TEDE) for persons of interest can be supplied at year's end. Information on the report is arranged in a series of columns. These columns include the items listed in Box 5-2.

The cumulative columns shown in Figure 5-7, *A* provide a continuous audit of actual absorbed radiation equivalent dose. These totals can be compared with allowable values established by regulatory agencies. Whenever the letter *M* appears under the current monitoring period or in the cumulative columns, it signifies that an equivalent dose below the minimum measurable radiation quantity was recorded during that time. The minimal reporting levels vary according to the dosimeter type and radiation quality as follows:

| | |
|---|---|
| X-ray, gamma | 10 μSv (1 mrem) |
| Beta | 100 μSv (10 mrem) |
| Neutron | 200 μSv (20 mrem) fast, |
| | 100 μSv (10 mrem) thermal |
| Fetal | 10 μSv (1 mrem) |
| Rings | 300 μSv (30 mrem) |

comparison with the remaining film badges after they have been returned to the monitoring company for processing. Because it is supposed to be kept in a radiation-free area within an imaging facility, its optical density reading should be zero. After processing, if a control badge reading greater than zero is indicated, then the batch of badges may have been exposed to

SAMPLE ORGANIZATION
RADIATION SAFETY OFFICER
1000 HIGH TECH AVENUE
GLENWOOD, IL 60425

**LANDAUER®**

Landauer, Inc. 2 Science Road Glenwood, Illinois 60425-1586
Telephone: (708) 755-7000 Facsimile: (708) 755-7016
www.landauerinc.com

luxel®

## RADIATION DOSIMETRY REPORT

| ACCOUNT NO. | SERIES CODE | ANALYTICAL WORK ORDER | REPORT DATE | DOSIMETER RECEIVED | REPORT TIME IN WORK DAYS | PAGE NO. |
|---|---|---|---|---|---|---|
| 103702 | RAD | 9920800151 | 06/11/04 | 06/07/04 | 4 | 1 |

| PARTICIPANT NUMBER | NAME: ID NUMBER / BIRTH DATE | SEX | DOSIMETER | USE | RADIATION QUALITY | DOSE EQUIVALENT (MREM) FOR PERIODS SHOWN BELOW: DEEP DDE | EYE LDE | SHALLOW SDE | QUARTERLY ACCUMULATED DOSE EQUIVALENT (MREM): DEEP DDE | EYE LDE | SHALLOW SDE | YEAR TO DATE DOSE EQUIVALENT (MREM): DEEP DDE | EYE LDE | SHALLOW SDE | LIFETIME DOSE EQUIVALENT (MREM): DEEP DDE | EYE LDE | SHALLOW SDE | RECORDS FOR YEAR | INCEPTION DATE (MM/YY) |
|---|---|---|---|---|---|---|---|---|---|---|---|---|---|---|---|---|---|---|---|
| FOR MONITORING PERIOD: | | | | | | 05/01/04 - 05/31/04 | | | QTR 2 | | | 2004 | | | | | | | |
| 0000H | CONTROL<br>CONTROL<br>CONTROL | | Ja<br>Pa<br>U | CNTRL<br>CNTRL<br>CNTRL | | M<br>M | M<br>M | M<br>M<br>M | | | | | | | | | | 5 | 07/97<br>07/97<br>07/97 |
| 00191 | ADDISON, JOHN | M | Ja | WHBODY | PN<br>P<br>NF | 90<br>60<br>30 | 90<br>60<br>30 | 90<br>60<br>30 | 90<br>60<br>30 | 90<br>60<br>30 | 90<br>60<br>30 | 100<br>70<br>30 | 100<br>70<br>30 | 100<br>70<br>30 | 200<br>170<br>30 | 200<br>170<br>30 | 200<br>170<br>30 | 5 | 07/97 |
| 00192 | JORGENSON, MIKE | M | Pa<br>U | WHBODY<br>RFINGR | | M | M | M<br>M | M | M | M<br>M | M | M | M<br>70 | M | M | M<br>100 | 5 | 07/97<br>07/97 |
| 00193 | THOMAS, LEE | M | Pa<br>U | WHBODY<br>RFINGR | | ABSENT<br>ABSENT | | | M | M | M<br>M | M | M | M<br>M | M | M | M<br>M | 5 | 07/97<br>07/97 |
| 00196 | WALKER, JANE | F | Pa | WHBODY | | 3 | 3 | 3 | 12 | 11 | 11 | 12 | 11 | 11 | 22 | 21 | 21 | 5 | 11/97 |
| 00197 | EDWARD, CHRIS | M | Pa | WHBODY | | M | M | M | M | M | M | M | M | M | M | M | M | 5 | 01/98 |
| 00198 | ZERR, ROBERT | M | Pa | WHBODY<br>NOTE | | 40<br>CALCULATED | 40 | 40 | 160 | 160 | 160 | 200 | 200 | 200 | 240 | 240 | 240 | 5 | 07/98 |
| 00199 | ADAMS, JANE | F | Pa | WHBODY | | M | M | M | M | M | M | 9 | 10 | 12 | 9 | 10 | 12 | 5 | 07/98 |
| 00200 | MEYER, STEVE | M | Pa<br>Pa<br><br><br>U | COLLAR<br>WAIST<br>ASSIGN<br>NOTE<br>RFINGR | PL | 105<br>M<br>4<br>ASSIGNED DOSE BASED ON EDE 1 CALCULATION | 105<br>M<br>105 | 105<br>M<br>105<br><br>140 | 6 | 162 | 165<br>400 | 11 | 327 | 334<br>690 | 51 | 1247 | 1284<br>2180 | 5 | 08/98<br>08/98<br><br><br>08/98 |
| 00202 | HARRIS, KATHY | F | Pa<br>U | WHBODY<br>RFINGR | | M | M | M<br>M | M | M | M<br>M | M | M | M<br>30 | M | M | M<br>30 | 4 | 02/99<br>02/99 |

**M: MINIMAL REPORTING SERVICE OF 1 MREM**
**ELECTRONIC MEDIA TO FOLLOW THIS REPORT**

QUALITY CONTROL RELEASE: VS

20 - PR 6774 - RPT130 - N1 - 02013

NVLAP®

NVLAP LAB CODE 100518-0**

A

FIGURE 5-7 **A,** The personnel monitoring report must include the items of information shown here.

**OCCUPATIONAL DOSE RECORD FOR A MONITORING PERIOD**

This form is for use in place of certain reports required by NRC licensees, OSHA and state regulations. It reflects data provided to or by your account and contains information for NRC Form 5 and other equivalent forms.

Prepared by

**LANDAUER** ®

Landauer, Inc.   2 Science Road   Glenwood, Illinois 60425-1586
Telephone: (708) 755-7000     Facsimile: (708) 755-7016

| ACCOUNT NUMBER | SERIES CODE | PARTICIPANT NUMBER |
|---|---|---|
| 103702 | A | 00010 |

1. NAME (LAST, FIRST, MIDDLE INITIAL)

SAMPLE

| 2. IDENTIFICATION NUMBER | 3. ID TYPE | 4. SEX | 5. DATE OF BIRTH |
|---|---|---|---|
| XXX-XX-XXXX | SSN | [X] MALE  [ ] FEMALE | 06/18/56 |

| 6. MONITORING PERIOD | 7. LICENSEE NAME | 8. LICENSE NUMBER(S) | 9A. [X] RECORD  [ ] ESTIMATE | 9B. [X] ROUTINE  [ ] PSE |
|---|---|---|---|---|
| 01/01/09 - 12/31/09 | | | | |

**INTAKES**

| 10A. RADIONUCLIDE | 10B. CLASS | 10C. MODE | 10D. INTAKE IN µCi |
|---|---|---|---|
| | | | |

**DOSES (in rem)**

| | | |
|---|---|---|
| DEEP DOSE EQUIVALENT (DDE) | 11. | 0.410 |
| EYE DOSE EQUIVALENT TO THE LENS OF THE EYE (LDE) | 12. | 0.410 |
| SHALLOW DOSE EQUIVALENT, WHOLE BODY (SDE, WB) | 13. | 0.410 |
| SHALLOW DOSE EQUIVALENT, MAX EXTREMITY (SDE, ME) | 14. | ND |
| COMMITTED EFFECTIVE DOSE EQUIVALENT (CEDE) | 15. | |
| COMMITTED DOSE EQUIVALENT, MAXIMALLY EXPOSED ORGAN (CDE) | 16. | |
| **TOTAL EFFECTIVE DOSE EQUIVALENT,** *(BLOCKS 11 + 15)* *(TEDE)* | 17. | 0.410 |
| **TOTAL ORGAN DOSE EQUIVALENT, MAX ORGAN** *(BLOCKS 11 + 16)* *(TODE)* | 18. | 0.410 |

19. COMMENTS

PERMANENT TO DATE (IN REM)

DDE : 5.060
LDE : 5.390
SDE, WB : 5.160
SDE, ME : 4.960
TEDE : 5.060

| 20. SIGNATURE - LICENSEE | DATE SIGNED | 21. DATE PREPARED |
|---|---|---|
| | | 03/24/09 |

B   - FORM 5 A NI L 1 17 M INCEPTION DATE: 01/01/87

**FIGURE 5-7, cont'd   B,** Modified report showing a summary of occupational exposure.

| BOX 5-2 | Information Found on a Personnel Monitoring Report |
|---|---|

1. Personal data: participant's identification number, name, birth date, and sex.
2. Type of dosimeter: *P* represents Luxel optically stimulated luminescence (OSL) dosimeter* for x-ray, beta, and gamma radiation; *J* represents Luxel OSL dosimeter for x-ray, beta, gamma, and fast neutron radiation; *U* represents a finger badge used to monitor x-radiation and gamma and beta radiation; *G* represents a film badge reading.
3. Radiation quality (e.g., x-rays, beta particles, neutrons, combined radiation exposure).
4. Equivalent dose data, including current deep, eye, and shallow recorded dose equivalents (millirem) for the time indicated on the report (e.g., from the first day of a given month to the last day of that month).
5. Cumulative equivalent doses for deep, eye, and shallow radiation exposures for specific time period, the year to date, and lifetime radiation.
6. Inception date (month and year) that the monitoring company began keeping dosimeter records for a given dosimeter for an individual listed on the account who is wearing a monitoring device.

*Luxel OSL dosimeter is manufactured by Landauer, Inc, Glenwood, Ill.

***Change in Employment by Radiation Worker.*** When changing employment, the radiation worker must convey the data pertinent to accumulated permanent equivalent dose to the new employer so that this information can be placed on file. Figure 5-7, *B* is an example of an appropriate summary of an occupational exposure report. A copy of such a report should be given to the radiation worker on termination of employment.

***Main Advantage of the Film Badge.*** The main advantage of the film badge is that the radiographic film itself, which is maintained by the monitoring company, constitutes a permanent legal record of personnel exposure. In health care facilities that have a well-structured radiation safety program, personnel monitoring reports are received and reviewed by the radiation safety officer (RSO). Film badge readings that exceed a trigger level set by the health care

facility are investigated to ascertain the cause of that reading. Such a process should be an integral component of the facility's radiation safety program. This practice is compatible with the ALARA policy.

***Other Advantages of the Film Badge.*** The film badge is reasonably economical, costing only a few dollars per unit per month. It can be used to record exposure to x-radiation, gamma radiation, and all but very low-energy beta radiation in a reliable manner. Moreover, the film badge can discriminate among the types of radiation and the energies of each of these radiations. Another advantage is its mechanical integrity. For example, the dosimeter will not be damaged if the badge is accidentally dropped.

***Objectionable Characteristics of the Film Badge.*** The film badge does have some objectionable characteristics. Temperature and humidity extremes or wetting can cause fogging of the dosimetry film over long periods of time. This effect increases with the length of time that the badge is worn and can result in a substantially inaccurate high exposure reading. Film badge dosimetry film must be shipped to the monitoring company for processing and exposure determination. Because this task takes time, a radiation worker's exposure cannot be determined on the day of occurrence. Manufacturers usually recommend 1 month as the period of time that a film badge should be worn for personnel monitoring before it is read. However, for those groups of workers who will be monitored even though their likelihood and history of any significant radiation exposure are low and nonexistent, quarterly badge monitoring is available.

***Film Badge Dosimeter Sensitivity.*** Other types of personnel dosimeters are more sensitive to ionizing radiation and are therefore more effective monitors in some situations. The film badge dosimeter is most sensitive to photons having an energy level of 50 keV; for values above and below this energy range, dosimetry film sensitivity decreases.

**Thermoluminescent Dosimeter.** The exterior of a **thermoluminescent dosimeter** (TLD) may resemble that of a film badge (Fig. 5-8).

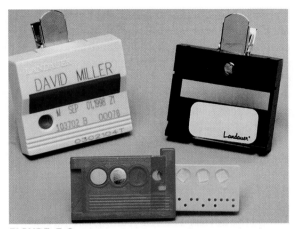

**FIGURE 5-8** Thermoluminescent dosimeter (TLD) containing the sensing material lithium fluoride (LiF).

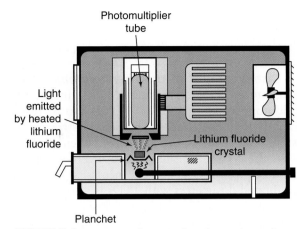

**FIGURE 5-9**  **Diagram of a Typical Analyzer.** The analyzer measures the amount of ionizing radiation to which a badge has been exposed by heating the irradiated lithium fluoride (LiF) crystals of the exposed badge with linearly rising temperatures produced by hot gas. This represents a departure from the previously used heating method, which relied on physical contact between the crystals and a heated plate. The newer method is a technical improvement because it eliminates any need for contact readjustments.

However, the interior of this monitoring mechanism differs completely. This light-free device usually contains a crystalline form (powder or, more frequently, small chips) of lithium fluoride (LiF), which functions as the sensing material of the TLD.

Ionizing radiation causes the LiF crystals in the TLD to undergo changes in some of their physical properties. When irradiated, some of the electrons in the crystalline lattice structure of the LiF molecule absorb energy and are "excited" to higher energy levels or bands. The presence of impurities in the crystal causes electrons to become trapped within these bands. When the LiF crystals are passed through a special heating process, however, these trapped electrons receive enough energy to rise above their present locations into a region called the *conduction band*. From there, the electrons can return to their original or normal state with the emission of energy in the form of visible light. The energy emitted is equal to the difference between the electron-binding energy of the two orbital levels. The intensity of the light is proportional to the amount of radiation that interacted with the crystals.

A device called a **TLD analyzer** measures the amount of ionizing radiation to which a TLD badge has been exposed by first heating the crystals to free the trapped, highly energized electrons and then recording the amount of light

emitted by the crystals (which is proportional to the TLD badge exposure) (Fig. 5-9). Plotting this light intensity versus the crystal heating temperature generates the glow curve.

***Advantages of the Thermoluminescent Dosimeter over the Film Badge.*** The TLD has several advantages over the film badge. The LiF crystals interact with ionizing radiation as human tissue does[*]; hence this monitor determines dose more accurately. Exposures as low as $1.3 \times 10^{-6}$ C/kg (5 mR)[†] can be measured precisely. Humidity, pressure, and normal temperature changes do not affect the TLD. Unlike the film in a monthly film badge, which could possibly fog if it is worn for more than 1 month, the TLD may be worn for up to 3 months. After the TLD reading has been obtained, the crystals can be

---

[*]The effective atomic number of LiF is equal to 8.2, which is similar to that of soft tissue (Z = 7.4).
[†]1 R = $2.58 \times (10)^{-4}$ C/kg by definition.
5 mR = 0.005 R = $5 \times (10)^{-3}$ R $\times 2.58 \times (10)^{-4}$ C/kg per R = $1.3 \times (10)^{-6}$ C/kg.

reused. This makes the device somewhat cost-effective, even though the initial cost is high (approximately twice the cost of a film badge service).

***Disadvantages of the Thermoluminescent Dosimeter.*** TLDs have some disadvantages in addition to their high cost. A TLD can be read only once. The readout process destroys the stored information; the TLD may be reused, but once the crystal is heated, the record of any previous exposure is gone. The necessity of using calibrated dosimeters with TLDs is also a disadvantage because the calibrated dosimeters must be prepared and read with each group, or batch, of TLDs when they are processed.

**Pocket Ionization Chamber.** The **pocket ionization chamber (pocket dosimeter)** is the most sensitive type of personnel dosimeter (Fig. 5-10). However, the use of these monitors in diagnostic imaging is uncommon. Externally, the pocket dosimeter resembles an ordinary fountain pen, but it contains a slender cylindrical (thimble) ionization chamber that measures radiation exposure. A clip on the eyepiece end allows the dosimeter to be attached to an individual's apparel (e.g., like a pen in a laboratory coat pocket).

***Types.*** Two types of pocket ionization chambers exist: the self-reading type, which contains a built-in electrometer (a device that measures electrical charge); and the non–self-reading type, which requires a special accessory electrometer to read the device. The self-reading pocket dosimeter has largely replaced the non–self-reading type for most operations. The operating principle of both types is similar to that of the gold leaf electroscope, which detects the presence and sign of an electric charge.

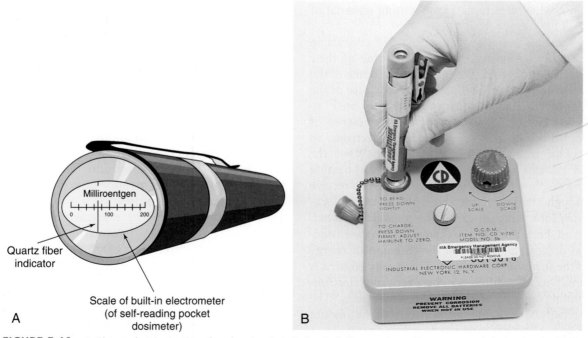

**FIGURE 5-10** **A**, The pocket ionization chamber (pocket dosimeter), the most sensitive personnel dosimeter, looks like a fountain pen on the outside but contains an ionization chamber that measures radiation exposure. Viewed through an eyepiece, the quartz fiber indicator of the built-in electrometer of the self-reading pocket dosimeter generally used in radiology indicates exposures of 0 to $5.2 \times 10^{-5}$ C/kg (0 to 200 mR). Before being used, each pocket dosimeter should be charged to a predetermined voltage by a special charging unit (**B**) so that the charges of the positive and negative electrodes are balanced and the quartz fiber indicator reads zero (0).

**Components.** The pocket ionization chamber contains two electrodes, one positively charged (the central electrode) and one negatively charged (the outer electrode). A quartz fiber may form part of the positive electrode and also function as the indicator on the transparent reading scale; in such a system, the quartz fiber casts a shadow onto a scale so that the quantity of charge on the positively charged electrode determines the position of the shadow along the scale and is equivalent to the scale reading at that position. When the charged electrodes in the device are exposed to gamma or x-radiation, the air surrounding the central electrode (+) becomes ionized and discharges the mechanism in direct proportion to the amount of radiation to which it has been exposed.

*Special Charging Unit.* A special charging unit is required for pocket ionization chambers. Each dosimeter must be charged to a predetermined voltage before use so that the quartz fiber indicator shows a zero (0) reading. As the dosimeter is exposed to ionizing radiation, it discharges, and the fiber indicator advances along the scale in a linear fashion, thereby showing the net exposure in milliroentgens. Pocket chambers generally used in medical imaging are sensitive to exposures ranging from 0 to $5.2 \times 10^{-5}$ C/kg (0 to 200 mR).

**Advantages.** Historically, the pocket ionization chamber was used to provide immediate exposure readouts for radiation workers who worked in high-exposure areas (e.g., a cardiac catheterization laboratory). Such individuals could read the dosimeter on site to determine the dose received at the completion of a given assignment and, if necessary, alter their working habits. Furthermore, pocket ionization chambers were compact, easy to carry, and convenient to use. Reasonably accurate and sensitive, they were useful monitoring devices for procedures of relatively short duration. Currently, however, in many institutions a device such as the Landauer-manufactured microStar system has been substituted.

**Disadvantages.** Pocket ionization chambers are fairly expensive, costing $150 or more per unit. If not read each day, the dosimeter may give an inaccurate reading because the electric charge tends to escape (i.e., the fiber indicator drifts with time; thus a false high reading may be obtained from a dosimeter read too late). In addition, pocket ionization chambers can discharge if they are subjected to mechanical shock, which again would result in a false high reading. Because these devices provide no permanent legal record of exposure, health care facilities that use this method to record personnel exposure must delegate someone to keep such a record. This task is generally the responsibility of the radiation safety officer (RSO), an individual such as a medical physicist or radiologist, qualified through training and experience, who is designated by a health care facility and approved by the Nuclear Regulatory Commission (NRC) (see Chapter 10) and state to ensure that internationally accepted guidelines for radiation protection are followed in the facility.

**Summary of Advantages and Disadvantages of Personnel Monitoring Devices.** Table 5-2 provides a summary of the advantages and disadvantages of the personnel monitoring devices discussed in this chapter.

# RADIATION SURVEY INSTRUMENTS FOR AREA MONITORING

## Radiation Detection and Measurement

**Radiation survey instruments** fall into several categories. The most common of these have as their detector a Geiger-Müller (GM) tube, the operation of which is described later in this chapter. Such instruments can be used in multiple ways, depending on their level of calibration ("the adjustment of an instrument to accurately read the radiation level from a reference source"[3]) and associated components. The simplest version, lacking any readout scale but possibly having adjustable sensitivity levels, is used to just indicate the presence of any radiation above background. It can do this by emitting a repetitive

| TABLE 5-2 | Advantages and Disadvantages of Personnel Dosimeters | |
|---|---|---|
| **Monitoring Device** | **Advantages** | **Disadvantages** |
| Optically stimulated luminescence dosimeter (OSL) | Lightweight, durable, easy to carry<br>Contains an integrated, self-contained, preloaded packet<br>Color-coding, graphic formats, and body location icons provide easy identification<br>Heat, moisture, and pressure will not affect the tamperproof blister packet<br>Has extended wear frequencies<br>Offers complete reanalysis<br>Has increased sensitivity<br>Gives accurate readings as low as 10 μSv (1 mrem) for x-ray and gamma ray photons with energies from 5 keV to 40 MeV<br>Can be used for up to 1 year<br>Excellent monitoring device for employees working in low-radiation environments and for pregnant workers<br>Reasonably inexpensive to purchase and maintain<br>Control monitor indicates whether group dosimeters were exposed in transit | Records occupational exposure only in the body area where the device is worn<br>If the facility does not have an "inhouse reader," exposure is not determinable on day of occurrence<br>Not effective as a monitoring device if not worn |
| Film badge | Lightweight, durable, easy to carry<br>Cost-efficient monitoring for large numbers of people<br>Records radiation exposure accumulated at a low rate over a long period of time<br>Provides permanent, legal record of personnel exposure<br>Detects and records small and large exposure in a consistent, reliable manner<br>Performance not affected by heat, humidity, and nonextreme mechanical shock<br>Possible to estimate direction from which radiation came<br>Filters can indicate whether exposure was the result of excessive amounts of scattered radiation or a single exposure from the primary beam<br>Control monitor indicates whether group badges were exposed in transit<br>Monitors x-radiation and gamma and all but very-low-energy beta radiation<br>Discriminates among types of radiation and energy of x-radiation and gamma and beta radiation | Records only exposure received in the body area where it is worn<br>High temperatures and excess humidity can cause film in the badge to fog over long periods of time, thus producing inaccurate exposure readings<br>Film sensitivity decreased at energy levels greater than or less than 50 keV<br>Exposure not determinable on day of occurrence<br>Accuracy limited to ±20%<br>Not effective as a monitoring device if not worn |

| TABLE 5-2 | Advantages and Disadvantages of Personnel Dosimeters—cont'd | | |
|---|---|---|---|
| **Monitoring Device** | **Advantages** | | **Disadvantages** |
| Thermoluminescent dosimeter (TLD) | Not affected by humidity, pressure, or normal temperature changes<br>Can be worn up to 3 months<br>After a reading has been obtained, TLD crystals can be reused, making the device somewhat cost-effective | | Readings may be lost if not carefully recorded<br>Readout process destroys information stored in TLD; thus preventing the "read" TLD from serving as a permanent legal record of exposure<br>Calibrated dosimeters must be prepared and read with each group of TLDs as they are processed |
| Pocket ionization chamber | Small, compact, easy to carry and use<br>Reasonably accurate and sensitive<br>Can be used for procedures that last a short time<br>Immediate exposure readout | | Not cost-effective for large numbers of personnel<br>Readings may be lost if not carefully recorded<br>Dosimeter must be calibrated to zero or its initial reading must be noted each day it is used<br>Mechanical shock can cause false high readings<br>No permanent, legal record of exposure<br>Records only exposure received in body area where worn<br>Initial cost is greater than film badge service |

sound whose loudness or repetitive frequency is directly associated with the intensity of radiation. Other versions, more fully equipped, have calibrated readout scales as well as audible indicators and are typically used either as area or room monitors or as portable survey instruments for measuring exposure rates at any location or object of interest. These instruments do not directly supply a cumulative radiation exposure reading. Finally, there are ionization chamber–based instruments, which are described in more detail later in this chapter. The most common type of survey meter that incorporates an ionization chamber as its radiation detector is called the "cutie pie" (Fig. 5-11). It acquired this nickname sometime during 1943 or 1944 "due to its diminutive size."[4] This instrument, when

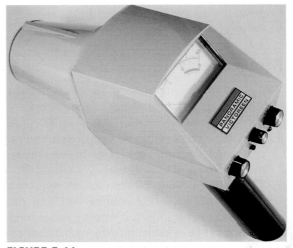

**FIGURE 5-11**  Ionization chamber-type survey meter, or "cutie pie."

properly calibrated, is capable not only of measuring radiation exposure rates over a very wide range but also of determining cumulative radiation exposure for whatever period of time the instrument is irradiated. In this regard, it can be considered a dosimeter, as are all properly calibrated ionization chamber–based devices.

## Types of Instruments

When in contact with ionizing radiation, survey instruments respond because of the charged particles that are produced by the radiation interacting with and subsequently ionizing the gas (usually air) in the detector. These instruments measure either the total quantity of electrical charge resulting from the ionization of the gas or the rate at which the electrical charge is produced.

Three different gas-filled radiation detectors serve as field instruments:

- Ionization chamber–type survey meter ("cutie pie")
- Proportional counter
- GM detector

All three detect the presence of radiation and, when properly calibrated, give a reasonably accurate measurement of the exposure. Each of these instruments has its own special use, and they are not all equally sensitive in the detection of ionizing radiation.

## Requirements

Radiation survey instruments for area monitoring should meet the following requirements:

1. They must be portable, so that one person can carry and operate the device in an efficient manner for a period of time.
2. They must be durable enough to withstand normal use, including routine handling that occurs during standard operating procedures.
3. They must be reliable; only in such a case can radiation exposure or exposure rate in a given area be accurately assessed.

4. They should interact with ionizing radiation similarly to the way human tissue reacts. This permits dose to be determined more accurately.
5. They should be able to detect all common types of ionizing radiation. Such a capability increases their usefulness.
6. The energy of the radiation should not significantly affect the response of the detector, and the direction of the incident radiation should not affect the performance of the unit. Such characteristics ensure consistency in unit operation among individual users.
7. They should be cost-effective. The initial cost and subsequent maintenance charges should be as low as possible.
8. They should be calibrated annually to ensure accurate operation.

## Gas-Filled Radiation Survey Instruments

As mentioned, three types of gas-filled radiation survey instruments exist: the ionization chamber–type survey meter (cutie pie), the proportional counter, and the GM detector.

**Ionization Chamber–Type Survey Meter (Cutie Pie).** The **ionization chamber survey meter (cutie pie)** is both a rate meter device (for exposure rate) used for area surveys and an accurate integrating or cumulative exposure instrument (see Fig. 5-11). It measures x-radiation and gamma radiation, and, if equipped with a suitable window, it can also record beta radiation.

***Sensitivity Ranges and Uses.*** In the rate mode, the cutie pie can measure radiation intensities ranging from 10 to several thousand micrograys per hour (1 mR/hr to several thousand milliroentgens per hour); and in the integrate mode, it can sum exposures from as little as 10 $\mu Gy_{-a}$ to several $Gy_{-a}$ (1 mR to several R). This device is useful for monitoring radiographic x-ray installations when exposure times of a second or more are chosen and for measuring fluoroscopic scatter radiation exposure rates. It is usually the instrument of choice when determining exposure rates from patients containing therapeutic doses of radioactive materials and when assessing the exposure rates in radioisotope storage facilities, and it is especially valuable when quantifying the cumulative exposures received outside of protective barriers.

***Advantages and Disadvantages.*** Among the advantages of the cutie pie is its ability to measure a wide range of radiation exposures within a few seconds while over a broad expanse of radiation energies, exhibiting essentially the same response or sensitivity. The delicate detector of the unit, however, may be considered a disadvantage. Another caveat is that without adequate warm-up time, its meter drifts and produces an inaccurate reading. This device cannot be used to measure exposures produced by typical diagnostic procedures because the exposure times are too short to permit the meter to respond appropriately.

**Proportional Counter.** The **proportional counter** serves no useful purpose in diagnostic imaging. It is generally used in a laboratory setting to detect alpha and beta radiation and small amounts of other types of low-level radioactive contamination. The proportional counter can discriminate between alpha and beta particles. Because alpha radiation travels only a short distance in air, the operator of the proportional counter must hold the unit's probe close to the surface of the object being surveyed to obtain an accurate reading of the alpha radiation emitted by the object.

### Geiger-Müller Detector

***Sensitivity and Use.*** The **Geiger-Müller (GM) detector** serves as the primary portable radiation survey instrument for area monitoring in nuclear medicine facilities (Fig. 5-12). With the exception of alpha particle emission, the unit is sensitive enough to detect individual particles (e.g., electrons emitted from certain radioactive nuclei) or photons. Hence it can easily detect any area contaminated by radioactive material. Because the GM detector allows rapid monitoring, it can be used to locate a lost radioactive source or low-level radioactive contamination. By using its audio mode, the GM detector may also be

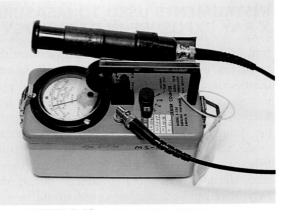

**FIGURE 5-12** Geiger-Müller (GM) Detector.

employed to scan radiation barriers for any shielding defects.

***Components.*** The GM detector has an audible sound system (an audio amplifier and speaker) that alerts the operator to the presence of ionizing radiation. Metal encloses the counter's gas-filled tube or probe, which is the unit's sensitive ionization chamber. When the shield covering the probe's sensitive chamber is open, very low-energy x-radiation and beta and gamma radiation can be detected. Meter readings are usually obtained in milliroentgens per hour. Because GM tubes tend to lose their calibration over time, the instrument generally has a "check source" of a weak, long-lived radioisotope located on one side of its external surface to verify its constancy daily.

***Disadvantages.*** The meter reading of a GM detector is not independent of the energy of the incident photons. This means that photons of widely different energies cause the instrument to respond quite differently, which is a disadvantage in diagnostic imaging. The cutie pie (ionization chamber–type survey meter), as mentioned previously, exhibits a much flatter, or more constant, response, with varying photon energies. In addition, the GM detector is likely to saturate or jam when it is placed in a very high-intensity radiation area (e.g., that associated with a linear accelerator used in radiation therapy), thereby giving a false reading.

## INSTRUMENTS USED TO MEASURE X-RAY EXPOSURE IN RADIOLOGY

Ionization chambers can be used to measure the radiation output from both radiographic and fluoroscopic x-ray equipment. As described previously, a cutie pie ionization chamber is also used for radiation protection surveys. If a cutie pie ionization chamber, operating in "rate" mode, were to be placed in the beam emanating from an x-ray tube during a radiographic exposure, the electrical signal produced during the very brief radiographic exposure would be too small to be recorded and measured reliably. An ionization chamber specifically designed for such measurement purposes is connected to an electrometer, a device that can measure tiny electrical currents with high precision and accuracy. Such a combination is shown in Figure 5-11. Both the ionization chamber and the electrometer system must be calibrated periodically to meet state and federal requirements for patient dose evaluation. Several regional calibration laboratories offer this service. A current listing of calibration laboratories is available from the American Association of Physicists in Medicine.*

Medical physicists use ionization chambers connected to electrometers to perform the standard measurements required by state, federal, and health care accreditation organizations for radiographic and fluoroscopic devices. These measurements include x-ray output in mR/mAs, reproducibility and linearity (i.e., proportionality) of output, timer accuracy, half-value layer, or beam quality, and entrance exposure rates for fluoroscopy units. Furthermore, such a device equipped with a specially calibrated parallel plate chamber may be used for similar measurements for mammography x-ray units.

## SUMMARY

- Personnel monitoring ensures that occupational radiation exposure levels are kept well below the annual effective dose (EfD) limit.

---

* One Physics Ellipse, College Park, Md, or www.aapm.org.

- Personnel monitoring is required whenever radiation workers are likely to risk receiving 10% or more of the annual occupational EfD limit of 50 mSv (5 rem) in any 1 year as a consequence of their work-related activities.
- To keep radiation exposure as low as reasonably achievable (ALARA), most health care facilities issue dosimeter devices when personnel could receive approximately 1% of the annual occupational EfD limit in any month, or approximately 0.04 mSv (4 mrem).
- The working habits and conditions of diagnostic imaging personnel can be assessed over a designated period of time through the use of the personnel dosimeter.
- A radiation worker should wear a personnel monitoring device at collar level during routine computed radiography, digital radiography, or conventional radiographic procedures to approximate the maximum radiation dose to the thyroid and the head and neck.
- During high-level radiation procedures, imaging professionals should wear both a thyroid shield and a protective lead apron, with the dosimeter worn outside the garment at collar level, to provide a reading of the approximate equivalent dose to the thyroid and eyes.
- Pregnant radiation workers should wear a second dosimeter beneath a lead apron to monitor the abdomen during gestation to provide an estimate of the equivalent dose to the embryo-fetus.
- Thermoluminescent dosimeter (TLD) rings are worn under certain conditions (e.g., by interventional radiologists who must insert catheters with fluoroscopic guidance) to monitor and determine equivalent dose to the hands when they are near the primary beam.
- Health care facilities must maintain a record of exposure recorded by personnel dosimeters as part of each radiation worker's employment record.
- In general, personnel dosimeters must be portable, durable, and cost-efficient.
- Four types of personnel monitoring devices exist: optically stimulated luminescence (OSL) dosimeters, TLDs (both extremity and for the

full body), film badges, and pocket ionization chambers.

- Results from personnel monitoring programs must be recorded accurately and maintained by each health care facility to meet state and federal regulations.
- The radiation safety officer (RSO) in a health care facility receives and reviews personnel monitoring reports to assess compliance with ALARA guidelines.
- Monitoring reports list the deep, eye, and shallow occupational exposure of each person wearing a monitoring device in the facility as measured by the exposed monitor.
- Area monitoring can be accomplished through the use of radiation survey instruments.
- A simple detection system (e.g., just a Geiger-Müller [GM] tube with no quantitative readout device) indicates only the presence or absence of radiation, whereas a dosimeter system (i.e., a detector plus a readout device) can quantitatively indicate both cumulative radiation intensity and radiation intensity rates.
- Radiation survey instruments for area monitoring must be durable and easy to carry, be able to detect all common types of ionizing radiation, and not be substantially affected by the energy of the radiation or the direction of the incident radiation.
- Types of gas-filled radiation survey instruments include the ionization chamber–type survey meter (cutie pie), the proportional counter, and the GM detector.
- Radiographic and fluoroscopic units can be calibrated with ionization chambers. When used for this purpose, the ionization chamber is connected to an electrometer that can measure tiny electrical currents with high precision and accuracy.

# REFERENCES

1. Gillman M: Shining a light on dosimetry. *RT Image* 13:22, 27, 2000.
2. Landauer, Inc, 2 Science Road, Glenwood, Ill. Available at: www.landauer.com.
3. Gollnick DA: *Basic radiation protection technology*, ed 4, Altadena, Calif, 2000, Pacific Radiation Corporation.
4. Frame P: *The nicknames of early survey meters*, Oak Ridge, Tenn, 1999, Oak Ridge Associated Universities. Available at: http://www.orau.org/ptp/collection/surveymeters/nicknamessurveymeters.htm. Accessed April 9, 2013.

# GENERAL DISCUSSION QUESTIONS

1. How is exposure monitoring accomplished?
2. Why should a personnel dosimeter be worn outside a protective apron at collar level on the anterior surface of the body during a fluoroscopic procedure?
3. What must personnel dosimeters be able to detect and record from day to day?
4. Why does a monitoring company supply a control monitor with every new batch of dosimeters?
5. What must be done with results from personnel monitoring programs to meet state and federal regulations?
6. When changing employment, what responsibility does a radiation worker have for personal data pertinent to accumulated permanent equivalent dose?
7. How sensitive to x-radiation and gamma radiation is an OSL dosimeter?
8. What are some of the requirements that radiation survey instruments must meet if they are to be used for area monitoring?
9. How does a GM detector alert the operator to the presence of ionizing radiation?
10. What type of diagnostic x-ray equipment would ionization chambers be used to calibrate?

# REVIEW QUESTIONS

1. When laser light is incident on the sensing material in an OSL dosimeter, the material:
   A. Becomes luminescent in proportion to the amount of radiation exposure received.

B. Fluoresces in proportion to the amount of radiation exposure received and then emits beta particles.

C. Phosphoresces in proportion to the amount of radiation exposure received and then darkens.

D. Turns ice blue and fluoresces in proportion to the amount of radiation exposure received.

2. Which of the following chemicals functions as the sensing material in a thermoluminescent dosimeter?
   A. Barium sulfate
   B. Calcium tungstate
   C. Lithium fluoride
   D. Sodium iodide

3. During routine radiographic procedures, when a protective apron is *not* being worn, the primary personnel dosimeter should be attached to the clothing on the front of the body at:
   A. Collar level to approximate the maximum radiation dose to the thyroid and the head and neck.
   B. Chest level to approximate the maximum radiation dose to the heart and lungs.
   C. Hip level to approximate the maximum radiation dose to the reproductive organs.
   D. Waist level to approximate the maximum radiation dose to the small intestine.

4. Which of the following requirements should radiation survey instruments fulfill?
   1. Instruments must be reliable by accurately recording exposure or exposure rate.
   2. Instruments must be durable enough to withstand normal use.
   3. Instruments should interact with ionizing radiation in a manner similar to the way in which human tissue interacts.
   A. 1 only
   B. 2 only
   C. 3 only
   D. 1, 2, and 3

5. During diagnostic imaging procedures, how should the radiation dose to the abdomen of a pregnant radiographer be monitored during gestation?
   A. It should be estimated from the radiation dose recorded by the primary monitor worn at collar level.
   B. It should be obtained from the primary radiation monitor worn at the abdominal level.
   C. It should be obtained from a second radiation monitor worn at the abdominal level.
   D. It is not necessary to monitor the radiation dose to the embryo-fetus that results from occupational exposure of a pregnant radiographer during gestation.

6. When a radiologic procedure requires the hands of a radiation worker to be near the primary beam, the equivalent dose to the hands of that individual may be determined through the use of:
   A. The primary personnel monitor worn at collar level.
   B. A pocket ionization chamber attached to the wristwatch of the radiation worker.
   C. A TLD ring worn on the hand of the radiation worker.
   D. A cutie pie.

7. Which of the following instruments is used to calibrate radiographic and fluoroscopic x-ray equipment?
   A. Proportional counter
   B. GM detector
   C. Ionization chamber with electrometer
   D. Pocket ionization chamber

8. For x-ray and gamma ray photons with energies from 5 keV to in excess of 40 MeV, the _____ gives an accurate reading as low as 1 mrem.
   A. Film badge
   B. OSL dosimeter
   C. Pocket ionization chamber
   D. TLD

9. Which of the following instruments should be used to locate a lost radioactive source or detect low-level radioactive contamination?
   A. GM detector
   B. Proportional counter
   C. Ionization chamber–type survey meter (cutie pie)
   D. TLD analyzer

10. Which of the following instruments should be used in an x-ray installation to assess the fluoroscopic scatter radiation exposure rate?
    A. GM detector
    B. Ionization chamber with electrometer
    C. Proportional counter
    D. TLD

## CHAPTER 6

# Overview of Cell Biology

## OBJECTIVES

*After completing this chapter, the reader will be able to perform the following:*

- State the purpose for acquiring a basic knowledge of cell structure, composition, and function as a foundation for radiation biology.
- Identify and describe some important functions of the major classes of organic and inorganic compounds that exist in the cell.
- List the essential functions of water in the human body.

- Name and describe a landmark event pertaining to the human genome that occurred in 2001.
- Describe the molecular structure of deoxyribonucleic acid, and explain the way it functions in the cell.
- List the various cellular components, and identify their physical characteristics and functions.
- Distinguish between the two types of cell divisions, mitosis and meiosis, and describe each process.

## CHAPTER OUTLINE

## KEY TERMS

amino acids
anaphase
carbohydrates
cell division
cell membrane
chromosomes
cytoplasm
cytoplasmic organelles
deoxyribonucleic acid (DNA)
endoplasmic reticulum (ER)
fats
genes

human genome
inorganic compounds
interphase
lipids
meiosis
messenger RNA (mRNA)
metaphase
mitochondria
mitosis (M)
nucleic acids
nucleus
organic compounds

prophase
proteins
protein synthesis
protoplasm
ribonucleic acid (RNA)
ribosomal RNA (rRNA)
ribosomes
saccharides
telophase
transfer RNA (tRNA)

 Copyright © 2014, Elsevier Inc.

Biology is a science that explores living things and life processes. Cells are the basic units of all living matter and are essential for life. The cell is the fundamental component of structure, development, growth, and life processes in the human body. Before imaging professionals can understand the effects of ionizing radiation on the human body, they must acquire a basic knowledge of cell structure, composition, and function. This chapter provides a foundation for radiation biology.

## THE CELL

The human body is composed of trillions of cells. These cells exist in a multitude of different forms and perform many diverse functions for the body such as the following:

- Conduction of nerve impulses
- Contraction of muscles
- Support of various organs
- Transportation of body fluids such as blood

Some cells are freely moving, independent units (e.g., leukocytes), whereas others remain in one position as part of the tissues of larger organisms throughout their lifetimes (e.g., bone marrow cells). Every mature human cell is highly specialized and has predetermined tasks to perform in support of the body.

Cells:

- Move
- Grow
- React
- Protect themselves
- Repair damage
- Regulate life processes
- Reproduce

To ensure efficient cell operation, the body must provide food as a source of raw material for the release of energy, supply oxygen to help break down the food, and have enough water to transport inorganic substances such as calcium and sodium into and out of the cell. In turn, proper cell function enables the body to maintain homeostasis or equilibrium, which is the ability to function in a normal manner despite any changes the body may undergo because of outside influences such as stress, exercise, injury, or disease.

In summary, cells are engaged in an ongoing process of obtaining energy and converting it to support their vital functions. They absorb molecular nutrients through the cell membrane and use these nutrients to produce energy and synthesize molecules. If exposure to outside influences such as ionizing radiation damages the components involved in molecular synthesis beyond repair, then cells either behave abnormally or die.

## CELL CHEMICAL COMPOSITION

### Protoplasm

Cells are made of **protoplasm**, the chemical building material for all living things. This substance carries on the:

- Complex process of metabolism
- Reception and processing of food and oxygen
- Elimination of waste products

Metabolism enables the cell to perform the vital functions of synthesizing proteins and producing energy.

Protoplasm consists of:

- Organic compounds (those compounds that contain carbon, hydrogen, and oxygen)
- Inorganic materials (compounds that do not contain carbon)

These are either dissolved or suspended in water.

The biomolecules that comprise protoplasm are formed from 24 elements, with the 4 primary elements being the following:

- Carbon
- Hydrogen
- Oxygen
- Nitrogen

When combined with phosphorus and sulfur, they comprise the essential major *organic* compounds:

| BOX 6-1 | Life-Sustaining Role of Water in the Human Body |

- Acts as the medium in which acids, bases, and salts are dissolved
- Functions as a solvent by dissolving chemical substances in the cell
- Functions as a transport vehicle for material the cell uses or eliminates
- Maintains a constant body core temperature of 98.6° F (37° C)
- Provides a cushion for vital organs such as the brain and lungs
- Regulates concentration of dissolved substances
- Lubricates the digestive system
- Lubricates skeletal articulations (joints)

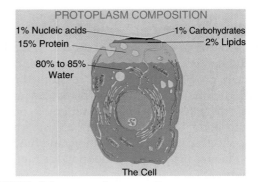

**FIGURE 6-1** Depending on cell type, water normally accounts for 80% to 85% of protoplasm.

| BOX 6-2 | Major Classes of Organic Compounds That Compose the Cell |

| | |
|---|---|
| Proteins | Lipids (fats) |
| Carbohydrates | Nucleic acid |

- Proteins
- Carbohydrates
- Lipids
- Nucleic acids

These compounds are discussed later in this chapter.

The most important *inorganic* substances are:

- Water
- Mineral salts (electrolytes)

Water aids in sustaining life and is the most abundant inorganic compound in the body. The essential functions of water are listed in Box 6-1. These functions are also discussed later in this chapter. Depending on cell type, water normally accounts for 80% to 85% of protoplasm (Fig. 6-1). Mineral salts exist in smaller quantities and are of vital importance in sustaining cell life. They help produce energy and aid in the conduction of nerve impulses. Mineral salts are also responsible for the prevention of muscle cramping.

## Organic Compounds

The four major classes of **organic compounds** (proteins, carbohydrates, lipids [fats], and nucleic acids) all contain carbon (Box 6-2). Carbon is the basic constituent of all organic matter. By combining with:

- Hydrogen
- Nitrogen
- Oxygen

carbon makes life possible. Of all the organic compounds, protein contains the most carbon.

**Proteins.** **Proteins** are the most elementary building blocks of cells, and they constitute approximately 15% of cell content (see Fig. 6-1). They are essential for growth, the construction of new body tissue (including acellular tissue such as hair and nails), and the repair of injured or debilitated tissue. Proteins are formed when organic compounds called **amino acids** combine into long, chainlike molecular complexes. Amino acids are essentially made up of combinations of $NH_2$ (called "amine") and COOH (carboxylic acid) molecules. Thus nitrogen, hydrogen, carbon, and oxygen are the key constituents of amino acids, of which approximately 500 different ones are currently known. An individual amino acid compound is known as a *monomer.*

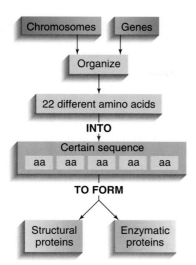

**FIGURE 6-2** Chromosomes and genes organize the 22 different amino acids into certain sequences to form the different structural and enzymatic proteins.

Monomers are molecular units that can chemically combine with other such units in a sequential manner. The resulting combination is called a polymer. Amino acids are examples of natural monomers. When chemical links called *peptide bonds** generate tandem patterns of various amino acids, they form polymers. Such lengthy complexes are what constitute proteins. Protein production, or **protein synthesis,** involves 22 different amino acids. The order of arrangement of these amino acids determines the precise function of each protein molecule, and the types of protein macromolecules (a molecule consisting of a large number of atoms) that any given cell contains determine the characteristics of that cell. Chromosomes and genes organize the amino acids into different orderings to make different types of proteins (Fig. 6-2).

***Structural and Enzymatic Proteins.*** Structural proteins such as those found in muscle provide the body with its shape and form and are a source of heat and energy. Enzymatic

proteins function as organic catalysts, that is, agents that affect the rate or speed of chemical reactions without being altered themselves. Enzymatic proteins (sometimes just called "enzymes") control the cell's various physiologic activities. They cause an increase in cellular activity that in turn causes biochemical reactions to occur more rapidly to meet the needs of the cell. Hence proper cell functioning depends on enzymes.

***Repair Enzymes.*** Many of the proteins produced in the cell are enzymes, initiating vital chemical reactions within the cell at the appropriate time. Some of the enzymes produced, called *repair enzymes,* can mend damaged molecules and are therefore capable of helping the cell to recover from a small amount of radiation-induced damage. Both the catalytic and repair capabilities of enzymes are of vital importance to the survival of the cell.

Repair enzymes work effectively in both the diagnostic and therapeutic energy ranges. However, if the radiation damage is excessive because of the delivered equivalent dose, the damage will be too severe for repair enzymes to have a positive effect. When ionizing radiation is used for therapeutic purposes to destroy malignant cells, a very significant effort using the latest advances in imaging and computer treatment planning algorithms is also made to spare healthy surrounding tissue. In radiation therapy, this concept is referred to as a *therapeutic ratio,* wherein the intent is to deliver enough radiation to kill cancerous cells in a tumor (i.e., damage them sufficiently so that they are irreparable) while delivering a lesser than cell-killing equivalent dose to any surrounding noncancerous tissue structure. This stratagem is the foundation on which successful radiation therapy rests.

***Hormones and Antibodies.*** In addition to providing structure and support for the body, proteins may function as hormones and antibodies. Hormones are chemical secretions manufactured by various endocrine glands and carried by the bloodstream to influence the activities of other parts of the body. For example, hormones produced by the thyroid gland located in the neck control metabolism throughout the body.

---

*Peptide bond: a covalent chemical bond (i.e., the sharing of one or more pairs of electrons between atoms) formed when the carboxyl group of one amino acid combines with the amine group of another amino acid.

Hormones also regulate body functions such as growth and development.

Antibodies are protein molecules produced by specialized cells in the bone marrow called *B lymphocytes*. Lymphocytes are white blood cells involved in the body's immune reactions. Antibodies are produced when other lymphocytes in the body, known as *T lymphocytes*, detect the presence of molecules that do not belong to the body. These foreign objects (e.g., bacteria, flu viruses) are called *antigens*. Although the skin of the body is the initial barrier to any outside invasion by pathogens or the like, once it has been penetrated the body's primary defense mechanism against infection and disease is the antibodies that chemically attack any foreign invaders or antigens.

**Carbohydrates.** Carbohydrates, also referred to as **saccharides,** make up approximately 1% of cell content (see Fig. 6-1). They include starches and various sugars. Carbohydrates range from simple to complex compounds (Box 6-3), even though they are composed of only carbon, hydrogen, and oxygen. Simple sugars such as glucose, fructose, and galactose have six carbon atoms and six molecules of water (e.g., glucose has the chemical formula $C_6H_{12}O_6$). Glucose is the primary energy source for the cell. Because it is a simple sugar, it is called a *monosaccharide*. Other sugars that have two units of a simple sugar linked together are called *disaccharides*. Sucrose (cane sugar) and lactose are examples of disaccharides. Both monosaccharides and disaccharides are relatively small molecules. *Polysaccharides* contain several or many molecules of simple sugar. Plant starches and animal glycogen

are the two most important polysaccharides. Through the process of metabolism, the body breaks these down into simpler sugars for energy.

Carbohydrates, simply described as chains of sugar molecules, function as short-term energy warehouses for the body. Their primary purpose is to provide fuel for cell metabolism. Although carbohydrates are found throughout the human body, they are most abundant in the liver and in muscle tissue. They also are important structural parts of intercellular materials.

**Lipids.** Lipids, also referred to as **fats** or fatlike substances, constitute approximately 2% of cell content (see Fig. 6-1). They are made up of a molecule of glycerin (Box 6-4) and three molecules of fatty acid. When glucose is broken down in the body during respiration, fats are among the generated intermediate products. When some of these fats combine with an acidic group of atoms (e.g., the carboxyl group, COOH), a fatty acid is formed. An example of a fatty acid is $CH_3COOH$, which is commonly known as *acetic acid*. Fatty acids are constituents of amino acids from which proteins are built. Lipids are organic macromolecules, large molecules built from smaller chemical structures. They are the structural parts of cell membranes. Lipids are present in all body tissue. The functions they perform for the body are listed in Box 6-5.

**Nucleic Acids.** Nucleic acids comprise approximately 1% of the cell (see Fig. 6-1). They are very large, complex macromolecules (Fig. 6-3). The much smaller structures that make up nucleic acids are called *nucleotides*. Each nucleotide is a unit formed from a nitrogen-containing

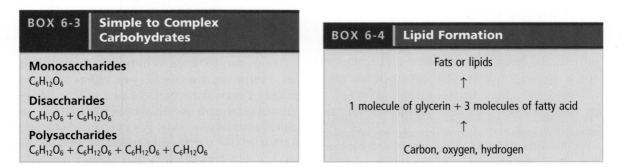

| BOX 6-3 | Simple to Complex Carbohydrates |
| --- | --- |

**Monosaccharides**
$C_6H_{12}O_6$

**Disaccharides**
$C_6H_{12}O_6 + C_6H_{12}O_6$

**Polysaccharides**
$C_6H_{12}O_6 + C_6H_{12}O_6 + C_6H_{12}O_6 + C_6H_{12}O_6$

| BOX 6-4 | Lipid Formation |
| --- | --- |

Fats or lipids

↑

1 molecule of glycerin + 3 molecules of fatty acid

↑

Carbon, oxygen, hydrogen

| BOX 6-5 | **Functions That Lipids Perform for the Body** |

1. Act as reservoirs for the long-term storage of energy
2. Insulate and guard the body against the environment
3. Support and protect organs such as the eyes and kidneys
4. Provide essential substances necessary for growth and development
5. Lubricate the joints
6. Assist in the digestive process

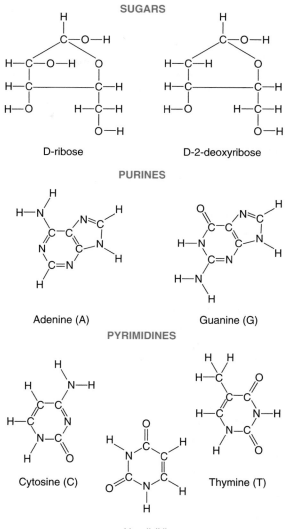

**FIGURE 6-3** The components of nucleic acid (H, hydrogen; C, carbon; N, nitrogen; O, oxygen). Sugars are strung together with phosphate groups, and a base is attached to each sugar. DNA uses D-2-deoxyribose sugar, and RNA uses D-ribose. Both nucleic acids use the same two purines, but thymine (T) in DNA is replaced by uracil (U) in RNA.

organic base, a five-carbon sugar molecule (deoxyribose), and a phosphate molecule.

***Deoxyribonucleic and Ribonucleic Acids.*** Cells contain two types of nucleic acids that are important to human metabolism:

• Deoxyribonucleic acid (DNA)
• Ribonucleic acid (RNA)

The DNA macromolecule is composed of two long sugar-phosphate chains, which twist around each other in a double-helix configuration and are linked by pairs of nitrogenous organic bases at the sugar molecules of the chain to form a tightly coiled structure resembling a twisted ladder or spiral staircase. The sugar-phosphate compounds are the rails, and the pairs of nitrogenous bases, which consist of complementary chemicals, are the steps, or rungs, of the DNA ladderlike structure (Fig. 6-4). Hydrogen bonds attach the bases to each other and join the two side rails of the DNA ladder.

*Nitrogenous Organic Bases in DNA.* The four nitrogenous organic bases in DNA macromolecules are as follows:

• Adenine (A)
• Cytosine (C)
• Guanine (G)
• Thymine (T)

Adenine and guanine are compounds called *purines,* and the compounds cytosine and thymine are classified as *pyrimidines.* A significant characteristic of the organic bases is that purines link with pyrimidines only in certain specific combinations; more precisely, adenine always bonds only with thymine, and cytosine bonds only with guanine. This characteristic is the reason the two strands of DNA are described as complementary.

***DNA: The Master Chemical.*** DNA is sometimes referred to as the master chemical because

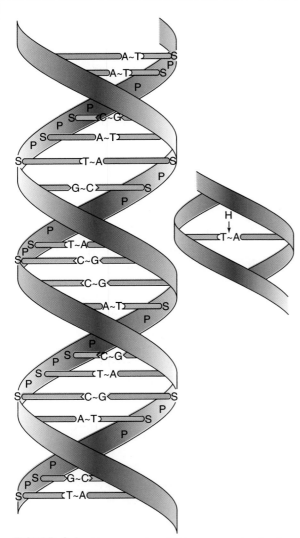

**FIGURE 6-4** Diagram of a DNA macromolecule that illustrates its twisted ladderlike or spiral-staircase–like configuration. Alternating sugar and phosphate molecules form the side rails of the ladder, and the nitrogenous organic bases, which consist of the complementary chemicals adenine (A), thymine (T), guanine (G), and cytosine (C), form the rungs, or steps. A hydrogen bond joins the bases together.

it contains all the information the cell needs to function. It carries the genetic information necessary for cell replication and regulates all cellular activity needed to direct protein synthesis. DNA determines a person's characteristics by

regulating the sequence of amino acids in the person's constituent proteins during the synthesis of these proteins. These sequences of amino acids are determined by the order of adenine-thymine and cytosine-guanine base pairs in the DNA macromolecules. Therefore, the sequence of nitrogenous base pairs in the DNA molecule constitutes the *genetic code*. Different sequences of amino acids produce proteins with different functions. Protein characteristics determine cell characteristics, and cell characteristics ultimately determine the characteristics of the entire individual. All the information necessary to construct and maintain a living organism is written in the "genetic code book" of DNA—the letters, words, and sentences are composed of the nitrogenous organic bases. What makes one person's DNA different from another's? Small differences in base pair arrangements are responsible for variations in human beings. These slightly altered base pair configurations lead to changes in the proteins produced, how much are produced, and when they are produced.

*Structural Differences between DNA and RNA.* The nucleic acid polymer, RNA, plays an essential part in the translation of genetic information from DNA into protein products. RNA functions as a messenger between DNA and the ribosomes, or "protein factories," where synthesis occurs. RNA differs structurally from DNA in several ways, some of which are as follows:

- RNA is a single-strand macromolecular structure, whereas DNA is a double-strand macromolecular structure that exists most frequently in a double-helix configuration.
- RNA contains ribose, whereas DNA contains deoxyribose.
- RNA has uracil with adenine in its base, whereas DNA has thymine paired with adenine in its base.
- RNA performs many different biologic functions (e.g., acts as an enzyme), whereas DNA carries the genetic information.
- RNA has a much shorter chain of nucleotides, whereas DNA has a longer chain of nucleotides.

*Messenger RNA.* Because DNA is found mostly in the cell nucleus, it cannot directly influence cellular activity such as growth and differentiation, which occur in the cytoplasm (the part of the cell that lies outside the nucleus). Instead, DNA regulates cellular activity indirectly, transmitting its genetic information outside the cell nucleus by reproducing itself in the form of **messenger RNA (mRNA)**, which can leave the cell nucleus and, once in the cytoplasm, directs the process of making proteins out of amino acids.

DNA serves as a prototype for mRNA, but mRNA differs from DNA in two important ways:

1. mRNA contains in its backbone the sugar molecule, ribose, which differs only in the presence of an extra O-H bond from the sugar molecule, deoxyribose, found in the backbone of DNA (see Fig. 6-4).
2. In mRNA, a pyrimidine base called *uracil* (U) replaces the thymine that is found in DNA (see Fig. 6-5).

An mRNA macromolecule resembles one half of a DNA macromolecule. It appears as a single strand of the DNA ladderlike configuration, the ladder being severed in half lengthwise (Fig. 6-5).

*Transfer RNA.* Macromolecules of mRNA carry their genetic codes in their sequences of nitrogenous organic bases (e.g., U, U, C, C, A, U, G) from the cell nucleus to the *ribosomes.** Proteins are manufactured in the ribosomes. Within the ribosome, both mRNA and **transfer RNA (tRNA)** macromolecules are present. The mRNA transfers its genetic code to tRNA. This tRNA combines with individual amino acids from different areas of the cell and attaches them to the ribosomes, where the amino acids are arranged in specific orders to form chainlike protein molecules. Each tRNA molecule is coded for a particular amino acid. Because each of the

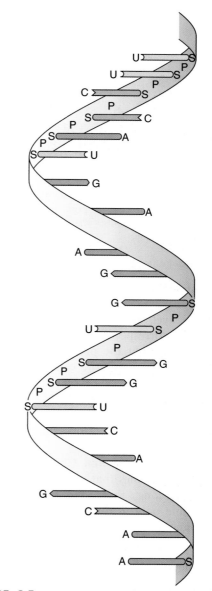

**FIGURE 6-5** Messenger RNA (mRNA) resembles one half of a DNA macromolecule. It appears as a single strand (one side rail) of the DNA ladderlike configuration, the ladder being severed in half lengthwise. Uracil (U) replaces thymine (T) as one of the nitrogenous organic bases in the mRNA molecule.

---

*Ribosomes: small, spherical organelles (subunits of a cell that perform a specific function) that are the assembly sites (similar to an auto assembly line) where mRNA and tRNA combine amino acids into proteins. A further discussion of ribosomes is provided later in this chapter.

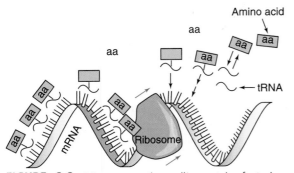

**FIGURE 6-6** Ribosomes, the cell's protein factories, travel along the messenger RNA (mRNA) rails, linking transfer RNA (tRNA) and its corresponding amino acids in the proper sequences to produce the proteins appropriate for the needs of the cell.

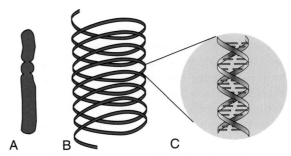

**FIGURE 6-7** A chromosome viewed under a microscope appears rod shaped (**A**); when further magnified, a chromosome appears as a tightly wound spiral structure (**B**) composed of hundreds of genes—a segment of the DNA macromolecule (**C**).

22 different amino acids has an associated tRNA, at least 22 different types of tRNAs exist. The ribosomes travel along the mRNA and link tRNA and its corresponding amino acids in the correct order so that the proteins necessary to provide for the needs of the cell are produced (Fig. 6-6).

*Ribosomal RNA.* Ribosomal RNA (**rRNA**) is another type of RNA. Its function is to assist in the linking of mRNA to the ribosome to facilitate protein synthesis.

*Chromosomes and Genes.* **Chromosomes** are tiny rod-shaped bodies that under a microscope appear to be long, threadlike structures that become visible only in dividing cells (Fig. 6-7). Chromosomes are composed of:

* Protein
* The genetic material DNA

A normal human being has 46 different chromosomes (23 pairs) in each somatic (nonreproductive) cell. Individual male and female reproductive cells, also known as *germ cells*, exist singly. Thus each of these germ cells has only 23 chromosomes, which pair up to form a full set of 46 chromosomes when a sperm fertilizes an egg cell. The DNA, a complex protein that makes up every chromosome, is divided into hundreds of segments called **genes**. Each gene, because of the ordering of its nitrogenous base pairs, contains information responsible for the following:

* Directing cytoplasmic activities
* Controlling growth and development of the cell
* Transmitting hereditary information (e.g., hair color, blood type)

Thus genes are the basic units of heredity. Taken as a whole, they control the formation of proteins in every cell through the intricate process of genetic coding.

*The Human Genome.* The total amount of genetic material (DNA) contained within the chromosomes of a human being is called the **human genome.** The process of locating and identifying the genes in the genome is called *mapping.* A landmark event occurred in 2001, when after years of intense effort two rival groups succeeded in deciphering the human genome. Essentially they uncovered the entire sequence of DNA base pairs (i.e., all of the "rungs" of the DNA ladder structure) on all 46 chromosomes. This major milestone in biology and medicine was accomplished by Celera Genomics, a private company in Rockville, Maryland, and the International Human Genome Sequencing Consortium, a group of academic centers funded mostly by the National Institutes of Health and the Wellcome Trust of London.[1]

The groups found that there are 2.9 billion base pairs in the human genome and that these base pairs are arranged into approximately 30,000 genes. It is estimated that these genes are capable of producing at least 90,000 different proteins.

As amazing as the accomplishment is, it remains only the first step toward a complete understanding of the biochemical processes that occur in health and disease. The challenge in interpreting the map of the human genome is similar to that of a building contractor finding a list of all the things that are needed to build a house but not having a blueprint that shows how often or in what order to do things. Over the next few decades, the great challenge will be to answer questions such as the following:

1. What determines when genes will produce proteins and when genes will not?
2. In what order are various proteins produced during development and throughout life?
3. What genes cause some individuals to be susceptible to a certain disease?
4. Is it possible to learn how to deactivate those genes and turn on other genes that provide resistance?
5. Are there genes that make some people more or less sensitive to the effects of ionizing radiation?
6. Can we use our new insight into the human genome to both detect and properly correct the defective genes that are the root of genetically transmitted disease?

The Human Genome Project has provided data that allow work on problems in molecular biology such as those listed here. It is surprising, then, to realize that the primary stimulus for initiating the project[2] can be traced to an urgency to attack radiobiologic questions that were raised during a scientific conference held in March 1984 at Hiroshima, Japan. At this conference, participants repeatedly stressed the need to use molecular DNA tools to enable direct detection of radiation exposure-induced mutations that could be inherited from the survivors of the atomic bomb blasts. Another conference was held some 9 months later in Alta, Utah. At this meeting, it was concluded that available knowledge was still insufficient to detect such mutations, which could be as few as 30 per individual genome per generation, and that only a massive effort, designed to improve the technology by orders of magnitude, would suffice for unraveling the human genome to the required degree. The intense discussions and ideas put forth at this meeting by the attendees were what ultimately led to the establishment of the Human Genome Project.

## Inorganic Compounds

**Inorganic compounds** are compounds that do not contain carbon. The inorganic compounds found in the body occur in nature independent of living things and are:

- Acids
- Bases
- Salts (electrolytes)

*Acids* are hydrogen-containing compounds such as $HNO_3$ (nitric acid) that can attack and dissolve metal. *Bases* are alkali or alkaline earth OH compounds such as $Mg(OH)_2$ (otherwise known as milk of magnesia) that can neutralize acids. *Salts* are chemical compounds resulting from the action of an acid and a base on each other. Salts are sometimes referred to as *electrolytes*. Chemically, they "are substances that become ions in solution and acquire the capacity to conduct electricity. Electrolytes are present in the human body, and the balance of the electrolytes in our bodies is essential for normal function of our cells and our organs."[3] A list of some of the important electrolytes in the body may be found in Box 6-6.

Water is the primary inorganic substance contained in the human body; it comprises approximately 80% to 85% of the body's weight (Fig. 6-8). The water content in a cell is very important. If water content is insufficient, the cell will collapse, resulting in a lack of ability to continue normal biologic function. Conversely, if water content is excessive, the cell most likely

| BOX 6-6 | **Some of the Important Electrolytes in the Body** |
| --- | --- |

| | |
| --- | --- |
| Sodium ($Na^+$) | Chloride ($Cl^-$) |
| Potassium ($K^+$) | Bicarbonate ($HCO_3^-$) |
| Calcium ($Ca^{++}$) | Phosphate ($HPO_4^-$) |
| Magnesium ($Mg^{++}$) | Sulfate ($SO_4^{-2}$) |

As a transportation system to and from cells

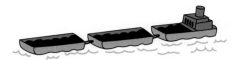

As a medium to dissolve and regulate acids, bases, and salts

As a means of maintaining a constant body temperature

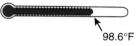

98.6°F

**FIGURE 6-9** Water's Role Outside the Cell.

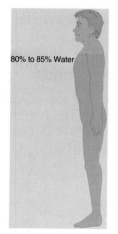

80% to 85% Water

**FIGURE 6-8** Water constitutes approximately 80% to 85% of the body's weight.

will rupture. Therefore, it is imperative that the correct amount of water in a cell be maintained.[4]

**Function of Water within and outside of the Cell.** Within the cell, water is indispensable for metabolic activities because it is the medium in which the chemical reactions that are the basis of these activities occur. It also acts as a solvent, keeping compounds dissolved so that they can more easily interact and their concentration may be regulated. Outside the cell, water functions as a transport vehicle for materials the cell uses or eliminates. In addition, water is responsible for maintaining a constant body core temperature of 98.6° F (37° C) (Fig. 6-9) while at the same time serving to lubricate both the digestive system and skeletal articulations (joints). Organs such as the brain and lungs are also protected by a cushion of compounds comprised primarily of water.

**Function of Mineral Salts within the Cell.** Salts such as sodium (Na) and potassium (K) keep the correct proportion of water in the cell. Mineral salts are necessary for:

- Proper cell performance
- Creation of energy
- Conduction of impulses along nerves

The constituents of salts exist as ions (particles carrying a positive or negative electric charge) in the cell. These ions via chemical reactions cause materials to be altered, broken down, and recombined to form new substances. Potassium (K) contributes most of the positive ions (cations) present in cells, whereas phosphorus (P) contributes the majority of negative ions (anions). Potassium is of primary importance in maintaining adequate amounts of intracellular fluid. Water tends to move across cell surfaces or membranes into areas with a high concentration of ions. This motion is referred to as *osmosis*. Thus, by balancing the concentration of potassium ions (as well as sodium [Na] and chloride [Cl] ions), the cell regulates the amount of fluid it contains. By maintaining the correct proportion of water in the cell, osmotic pressure is maintained. Potassium also aids in maintaining acid-base balance, a state of equilibrium or stability between acids and bases.

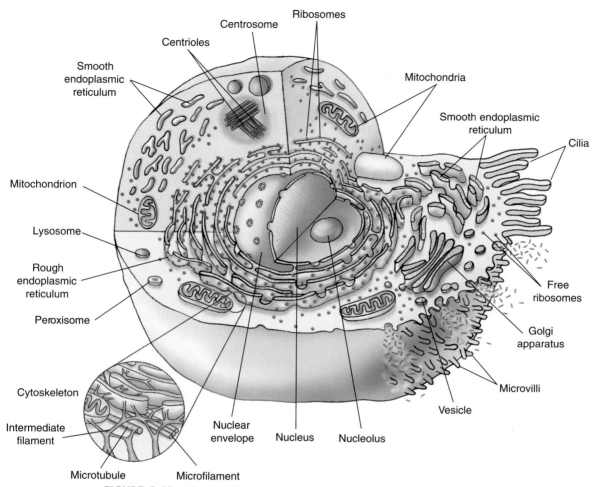

**FIGURE 6-10** Diagram of a typical cell, demonstrating its basic components.

## CELL STRUCTURE

The normal cell has the following components (Fig. 6-10):

1. Cell membrane
2. Cytoplasm
3. Cytoplasmic organelles
   a. Endoplasmic reticulum
   b. Golgi apparatus or complex
   c. Mitochondria
   d. Lysosomes
   e. Ribosomes
   f. Centrosomes
4. Nucleus

## Cell Membrane

The **cell membrane** is a frail, semipermeable, flexible structure encasing and surrounding the human cell.

- It is made up of lipids and proteins.
- It functions as a barricade to protect cellular contents from the outside environment.
- It controls the passage of water and other materials into and out of the cell.

Because the cell membrane allows penetration only by certain types of substances and regulates the speed at which these substances travel within the cell, it plays a primary role in the cell's transport system. When a substance moves through the cell membrane by osmosis, the transport system is classified as passive because the cell uses no energy to maintain the concentration. When the movement of a substance across a cell membrane is controlled more by the properties and powers of the cell membrane than it is by the relative concentrations of particles in fluid, the transport system is classified as active. In active transport, the cell must expend energy to pump substances into and out of it.

## Cytoplasm

**Cytoplasm** is the protoplasm that exists outside the cell's nucleus. It is primarily composed of water but also contains:

- Proteins
- Carbohydrates
- Lipids
- Salts
- Minerals

The cytoplasm makes up the majority of the cell and contains large amounts of all the cell's molecular components with the exception of DNA. All cellular metabolic functions occur in the cytoplasm. The major functions of the cytoplasm are listed in Box 6-7.

---

| BOX 6-7 | Major Tasks of the Cytoplasm |
|---------|------------------------------|

Behaving like a factory, the cytoplasm performs the following major tasks:
1. Accepts and builds up unrefined materials and assembles from these materials new substances such as carbohydrates, lipids, and proteins; the assembly of larger molecules from smaller ones is known as *anabolism*
2. Breaks down organic materials to produce energy (catabolism)
3. Packages substances for distribution to other areas of the cell or to various sites in the body through the circulation
4. Eliminates waste products

---

## Cytoplasmic Organelles

The cytoplasm contains all the miniature cellular components that enable the cell to function in a highly organized manner. These little organs of the cell are collectively referred to as **cytoplasmic organelles.** They consist of the following:

- Tiny tubules (small tubes)
- Vesicles (small cavities or sacs containing liquid)
- Granules (small insoluble nonmembranous particles found in cytoplasm)
- Fibrils (minute fibers or strands that are frequently part of a compound fiber)

Together these structures perform the major functions of the cell in a systematized way. DNA, which is located in the cell nucleus, separated from the cytoplasm, determines the function of each cytoplasmic organelle; mRNA carries the DNA code from the nucleus into the cytoplasm.

**Endoplasmic Reticulum.** The **endoplasmic reticulum (ER)** is a vast, irregular network of tubules and vesicles spreading and interconnecting in all directions throughout the cytoplasm. It enables the cell to communicate with the extracellular environment and transfer food and molecules from one part of the cell to another. Thus the ER functions as the highway system of the cell. For example, mRNA travels from the nucleus to different locations in the cytoplasm through the ER, and lipids and proteins are also routed into and out of the nucleus through the ER tubular network.

Cells have two types of ER:

- Rough surfaced (granular)
- Smooth (agranular)

If numerous ribosomes (the small, spherical organelles that are the sites where mRNA and tRNA assemble amino acids into proteins) are present on the surface of the ER, the surface is rough or granular. If they are not present, the surface is smooth or agranular. The "smooth" or "rough" distinction refers to the ER's appearance when viewed with an electron microscope. The cell type determines the type of ER. For example, cells that actively manufacture proteins for export, such as the pancreatic cells, which produce insulin, need more ribosomes and therefore have extensive rough or granular ER. A lesser amount of rough or granular ER is found in cells that synthesize proteins mainly for their own use.

**Golgi Apparatus or Complex.** The Golgi apparatus, bodies, or complex are minute vesicles that extend from the nucleus to the cell membrane. They consist of tubes and a tiny sac located near the nucleus. This structure unites large carbohydrate molecules and then combines them with proteins to form glycoproteins. When the cell manufactures enzymes and hormones, the Golgi apparatus concentrates, packages, and transports them through the cell membrane so that they can exit the cell, enter the bloodstream, and be carried to the areas of the body where they are required.

**Mitochondria.** The large, double-membranous, oval or bean-shaped structures called **mitochondria** function as the "powerhouses" of the cell because they supply the energy for cells. They contain highly organized enzymes in their inner membranes that produce this energy for cellular activity by breaking down nutrients such as:

- Carbohydrates
- Fats
- Proteins

This breakdown of nutrients occurs through the process of oxidative metabolism. Oxidation is any chemical reaction in which an atom loses electrons. The substance that loses electrons is said to have been oxidized. The oxidation of iron produces iron oxide, commonly known as *rust*. Metabolism is the breaking down of large molecules into smaller ones. Oxidative metabolism is the breaking down of large molecules into smaller ones through the process of oxidation. Some of the enzymes contained within the mitochondria are essential in the production of adenosine triphosphate (ATP), an energy-releasing phosphate compound essential for sustaining life. This compound plays a role in active

transport within the cell. In active transport, molecules are moved through cell membranes regardless of the relative concentrations of particles. This requires energy, which is supplied by ATP. The number of mitochondria in cells varies from a few hundred to several thousand. The greatest number is found in cells exhibiting the greatest activity.

**Lysosomes.** Lysosomes are small, pealike sacs or single-membrane spherical bodies that are of great importance for digestion within the cytoplasm. They contain a group of different digestive enzymes that target proteins, and their primary function appears to be the breaking down of unwanted large molecules that either penetrate into the cell through microscopic channels or are drawn in by the cell membrane itself. If lysosomes fail in their cellular "garbage disposal" tasks, the resulting accumulation of large molecules may ultimately obstruct normal functions in organs. Lysosomes are sometimes referred to as "suicide bags," because the enzymes they contain can break down and digest not only proteins and certain carbohydrates, but also the cell itself should the lysosome's surrounding membrane break. Exposure to radiation may induce such a rupture. When this occurs, the cell is likely to die.

**Ribosomes.** Ribosomes are very small spherical organelles that attach to the ER. They consist of:

- Two thirds RNA
- One third protein

Ribosomes are commonly referred to as the cell's "protein factories" because their job is to manufacture (synthesize) the various proteins that cells require by using the blueprints provided by mRNA. Their role in the assembly of amino acids into proteins is described earlier in this chapter.

**Centrosomes.** Centrosomes are located in the center of the cell near the nucleus. They contain the *centrioles*, which in each centrosome are a pair of small, hollow, cylindrical structures oriented at right angles to each other and embedded in a material mass of more than 100

| TABLE 6-1 | Summary of Cell Components | |
|---|---|---|
| **Title** | **Site** | **Activity** |
| Cell membrane | Cytoplasm | Functions as a barricade to protect cellular contents from their environment and controls the passage of water and other materials into and out of the cell; performs many additional functions such as elimination of wastes and refining of material for energy through breakdown of the materials |
| Endoplasmic reticulum | Cytoplasm | Enables the cell to communicate with the extracellular environment and transfers food from one part of the cell to another |
| Golgi apparatus | Cytoplasm | Unites large carbohydrate molecules and combines them with proteins to form glycoproteins; transports enzymes and hormones through the cell membrane so that they can exit the cell, enter the bloodstream, and be carried to areas of the body in which they are required |
| Mitochondria | Cytoplasm | Produce energy for cellular activity by breaking down nutrients through a process of oxidation |
| Lysosomes | Cytoplasm | Dispose of large particles such as bacteria and food as well as smaller particles; also contain hydrolytic enzymes that can break down and digest proteins, certain carbohydrates, and the cell itself if the lysosome's surrounding membrane breaks |
| Ribosomes | Cytoplasm | Manufacture the various proteins that cells require |
| Centrosomes | Cytoplasm | Believed to play some part in the formation of the mitotic spindle during cell division |
| DNA | Nucleus | Contains the genetic material; controls cell division and multiplication and also biochemical reactions that occur within the living cell |
| Nucleolus | Nucleus | Holds a large amount of RNA |

proteins. The centrioles play a significant role in the formation of the mitotic spindle* by organizing the spindle fibers during cell division. The stages of cell division and the importance of centrosomes in facilitating this process are discussed in detail later in this chapter.

## Nucleus

Separated from the other parts of the cell by a double-walled membrane (nuclear envelope), the **nucleus** forms the heart of the living cell. It is a spherical mass of protoplasm known as *nucleoplasm* that contains the genetic material, DNA, and protein. These two nuclear components are arranged in long threads called *chromatin*. When a cell divides, this gene-containing material contracts into tiny rod-shaped bodies, called *chromosomes*, that carry genes.

The nucleus also contains at least one very small, rounded body, called the *nucleolus*, which manufactures and holds a large amount of RNA and protein inside the ribosomes it contains. When RNA is expelled into the cytoplasm, the nucleolus assists in the manufacturing of protein.

In summary, the nucleus controls cell division and multiplication and the biochemical reactions that occur within the cell. By directing protein synthesis, the nucleus plays an essential role in the following:

- Active transport
- Metabolism
- Growth
- Heredity

A summary of cell components is presented in Table 6-1.

## CELL DIVISION

**Cell division** is the multiplication process whereby one cell divides to form two or more cells

---

*The mitotic spindle is essentially a protein machine that segregates chromosomes to two daughter cells during the cell division process.

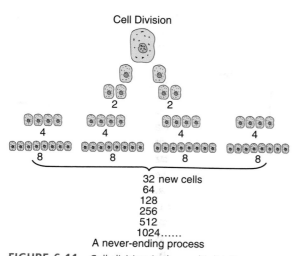

Cell Division

2    2

4    4    4    4

8    8    8    8

32 new cells
64
128
256
512
1024......
A never-ending process

**FIGURE 6-11** Cell division is the multiplication process whereby one cell divides to form two or more cells.

(Fig. 6-11). The two types of cell divisions that occur in the body are:

- Mitosis
- Meiosis

When somatic cells (all cells in the human body except the germ cells) divide, they undergo mitosis, a process in which the nucleus first divides, followed by the division of the cytoplasm. Genetic cells (the oogonium, or female germ cell, and the spermatogonium, or male germ cell) undergo meiosis, a process of reduction division.

## Mitosis

Through the process of **mitosis (M)** (Fig. 6-12), a parent cell divides to form two daughter cells identical to the parent cell. This process results in an approximately equal distribution of all cellular material between the two daughter cells. The cellular life cycle may be pictured as in Figure 6-13. Different phases of cell growth, maturation, and division occur in each cell cycle. Four distinct phases of the cellular life cycle are identifiable:

- M (mitosis phase)
- $G_1$ (pre-DNA synthesis phase)

- S (synthesis phase)
- $G_2$ (post-DNA synthesis phase)

In addition, mitosis (M) can be divided into four subphases:

- Prophase
- Metaphase
- Anaphase
- Telophase

Mitosis is the division phase of the cellular life cycle. It is actually the last phase of the cycle. After it has commenced, it takes only about 1 hour to complete in all cells. Interphase, the period of cell growth that occurs before actual mitosis, consists of three intervals:

1. $G_1$
2. S
3. $G_2$

$G_1$ is the earliest phase among reproductive events. It is the gap in the growth of the cell that occurs between mitosis and DNA synthesis. Depending on the types of cells involved, this interval may take just a few minutes, or it may take several hours. $G_1$ is designated as the pre-DNA synthesis phase. During $G_1$, a form of RNA is synthesized in the cells that are to reproduce. This RNA is needed before actual DNA synthesis can efficiently begin. S is the actual DNA synthesis period. While in S phase, each DNA molecule contained within the chromosome (Fig. 6-14, *A*) is first copied (replicated) and then is divided into two individual sister chromatids,* each containing DNA molecules. Each of these identical sister chromatids is now one half of the replicated chromosome. These chromatids will join together to form another chromosome by the end of the S phase (Fig. 6-14, *B*). Therefore, a chromosome consists of two copies of the DNA that is contained in each chromatid. The region of the chromosome where the two chromatids join together is called the *centromere* (see

---

*A chromatid is a highly coiled strand; one of the two duplicated portions of DNA in a replicated chromosome that appear during cell division.

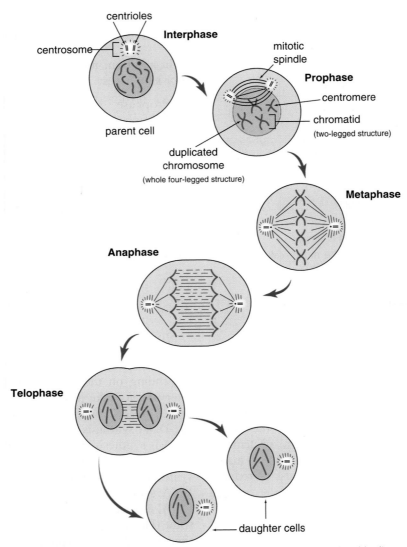

**FIGURE 6-12   Diagram of Mitosis.** An animal cell with four chromosomes first multiplies (duplicates its DNA) and then divides, forming two new daughter cells, each of which contains exactly the same genetic material as the parent cell.

Fig. 6-14, *B*). During the anaphase of mitosis (described later), the paired sister chromatids separate from one another to form individual daughter chromosomes.

When compared with $G_1$ and $G_2$, the S phase is relatively long. It can take up to 15 hours. $G_2$ is the post-DNA manufacturing interval in the cellular life cycle. It is a relatively short period, occupying approximately 1 to 5 hours of the whole cycle. During this phase, cells manufacture

certain proteins and RNA molecules needed to enter and complete the next mitosis. When $G_2$ is complete, cells enter the first phase of mitosis, the prophase, and the process of division commences.

**Interphase.** Interphase is the period of cell growth that occurs before actual mitosis. As previously stated, $G_1$, S, and $G_2$ are the phases of the cell cycle that comprise interphase. Cells are not yet undergoing division during this phase. If

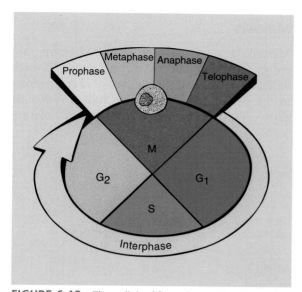

**FIGURE 6-13** The cellular life cycle may be pictured as four distinct, identifiable phases: M, $G_1$, S, and $G_2$. M may be divided into four subphases: prophase, metaphase, anaphase, and telophase.

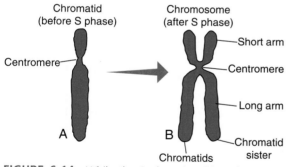

**FIGURE 6-14** While the S phase is taking place, two sister chromatids like the one shown in (**A**) join to become a chromosome (**B**). A centromere links them together.

a cell is viewed through a microscope during interphase, the nucleus looks somewhat odd. DNA may be visualized by using a specific stain designed to make it visible; it appears as clumps of material shaped in different patterns. These patterns are seen throughout the nucleus. Individual chromosomes are not visible during interphase. During the synthesis portion of interphase (S), each chromosome reproduces itself and splits longitudinally, thus forming two sister chromatids attached to each other at the centromere.

Hence, the cell's DNA molecules have duplicated in preparation for cell division. Genetic information also is transcribed into different kinds of RNA molecules such as mRNA and tRNA, which, after passing into the cytoplasm, translate the genetic information by promoting the synthesis of specific proteins.

**Prophase.** During **prophase,** the first phase of cell division, the nucleus enlarges, the DNA complex (the chromatid network of threads) coils up more tightly, and the chromatids become more visible on stained microscopic slides. Chromosomes enlarge, and the DNA begins to take structural form. The nuclear membrane disappears, and the centrioles (small hollow cylindrical structures) migrate to opposite sides of the cell and begin to regulate the formation of the *mitotic spindle,* the delicate fibers that are attached to the centrioles and extend from one side of the cell to the other across the equator of the cell.

**Metaphase.** As **metaphase** begins, the fibers collectively referred to as the mitotic spindle form between the centrioles. Each chromosome, which now consists of two chromatids, lines up in the center or equator of the cell attached by its centromere to the mitotic spindle. This configuration forms the equatorial plate. The centromeres then duplicate, and each chromatid attaches itself individually to the spindle. At the end of metaphase, the chromatids are strung out along the mitotic spindle much like laundry hung on a clothesline. During metaphase, cell division can be stopped, and visible chromosomes can be examined under a microscope. Chromosome damage caused by radiation can then be evaluated.

**Anaphase.** During **anaphase,** the duplicate centromeres migrate in opposite directions along the mitotic spindle and carry the chromatids to opposite sides of the cell. The cell is now ready to begin the last phase of division.

**Telophase.** During **telophase,** the chromatids undergo changes in appearance by uncoiling and becoming long, loosely spiraled threads. Simultaneously, the nuclear membrane forms anew, and two nuclei (one for each new daughter cell) appear. The cytoplasm also divides (cytokinesis) near the equator of the cell to surround each new nucleus. After this cell division completes, each daughter cell has a complete cell membrane and contains exactly the same amount of genetic material (46 chromosomes) as the parent cell.

## Meiosis

**Meiosis** is a special type of cell division that reduces the number of chromosomes in each daughter cell to half the number of chromosomes in the parent cell (Fig. 6-15). Male and female germ cells, or sperm and ova, of sexually mature

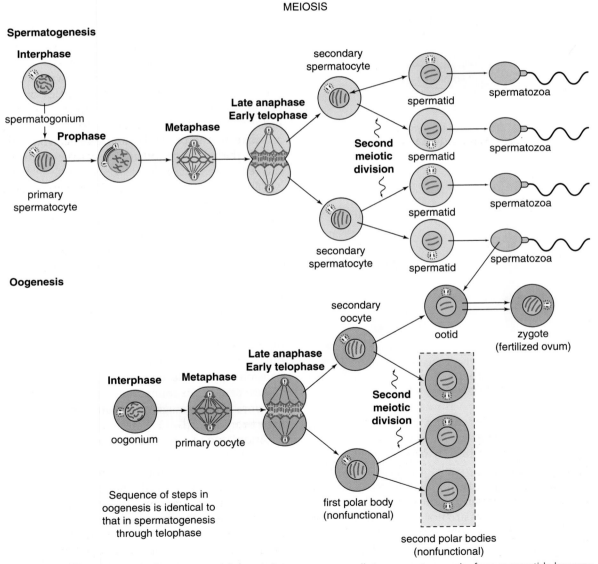

**FIGURE 6-15    Diagram of Meiosis.** Four cells result from one germ cell. In spermatogenesis, four spermatids become mature spermatozoa. In oogenesis, one ootid may be fertilized, and three second polar bodies remain nonfunctional.

individuals each begin meiosis with 46 chromosomes. However, before the male and female germ cells unite to produce a new organism, the number of chromosomes in each must be reduced by one half to ensure that the daughter cells (zygotes) formed when they unite will contain only the normal number of 46 chromosomes. Hence meiosis is really a process of reduction division (Fig. 6-16).

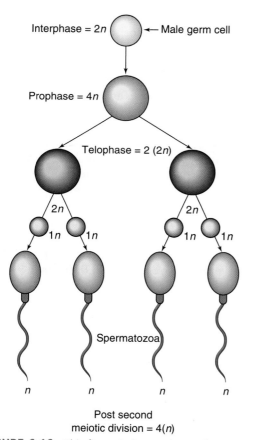

FIGURE 6-16 This figure indicates the total amount of genetic material at different stages of meiosis of a male germ cell. Twenty-three chromosomes, half the amount needed to produce a new human organism, are needed in the spermatozoa. If we refer to 23 chromosomes as an amount of genetic material $n$, then before meiosis (during interphase) the germ cell has $2n$. During prophase, this number doubles to $4n$. There then follows 2 reduction divisions to form the final $1n$ (23 chromosomes) in the spermatozoa. An egg cell undergoes a similar process, but only 1 of the 4 resulting germ cells at the end of the process is functional.

Meiosis begins with a doubling of the amount of genetic material. This doubling of the amount of DNA is called *replication* and occurs during interphase. As a result of DNA replication, each one-chromatid chromosome duplicates, thus forming a two-chromatid chromosome. This means that sperm and egg cells begin meiosis with twice the amount of genetic material as the original parent cell. Thus, at the beginning of meiosis, the number of chromosomes increases from $2n$ to $4n$ ($n = 23$).

The various phases of meiosis are similar to those of mitosis. The major difference between the two types of cell division begins at the end of telophase. In meiosis, after the parent germ cell has formed 2 daughter cells, each of which (in human beings) contains 46 chromosomes, the daughter cells divide without DNA replication; chromosome duplication does not occur at this phase of division. These 2 successive divisions result in the formation of 4 granddaughter cells, each of which contains only 23 chromosomes. This means that the proper number of 46 chromosomes will be produced when a female ovum containing 23 chromosomes is fertilized by a male sperm containing 23 chromosomes.

During meiosis, the sister chromatids exchange some chromosomal material (genes). This process, called *crossover,* results in changes in genetic composition and traits that can be passed on to future generations.

**Multiple Births.** Multiple births can occur during one pregnancy in one of two ways. The first way is if a fertilized ovum (zygote) splits after fertilization and two separate offspring develop. The two offspring would be referred to as *monozygotic* (coming from one zygote) *twins.* Monozygotic twins are also known as *identical twins* because they contain exact replicas of genetic material. Another way to achieve a multiple birth is if more than one ootid is available for fertilization, and the separate ootids are fertilized by separate spermatozoa. In this case the children would have no more resemblance to each other than would other children born at different times from the same parents. Such dizygotic twins are also known as *fraternal twins.*

More than two such twins would be known as *polyzygotic siblings*. Fraternal twins or multiple siblings, as with siblings born in different pregnancies, sometimes bear a striking resemblance to one another. However, unless they were monozygotic, they are not identical twins and do not have exact copies of all their chromosomes.

## SUMMARY

- Cells are made of protoplasm, which consists of proteins, carbohydrates, lipids, nucleic acids, water, and mineral salts (electrolytes).
  - Proteins are essential to growth, construction, and repair of tissue; they may function as hormones and antibodies.
  - Carbohydrates provide fuel for cell metabolism.
  - Lipids act as a reservoir for long-term storage of energy, guard the body against the environment, and protect organs.
  - Nucleic acids (DNA, RNA) carry genetic information necessary for cell replication.
  - Water constitutes the bulk of body weight, is essential to sustaining life, and serves as the transport medium for material the cell uses and eliminates.
  - Mineral salts maintain the correct portion of water in the cell, support cell function, aid in the conduction of nerve impulses, and prevent muscle cramping.
- Cells have several components.
  - The cell membrane surrounds the cell, functions as a barricade, and controls passage of water and other materials in and out of the cell.
  - Cytoplasm is the portion of a cell outside the nucleus in which all metabolic activity occurs.
  - The endoplasmic reticulum (ER) transports food and molecules from one part of the cell to another.
  - The Golgi apparatus unites large carbohydrate molecules with proteins to form glycoproteins.
  - Mitochondria contain enzymes that produce energy for cellular activity.
  - Lysosomes break down unwanted large molecules; they may rupture when they are exposed to radiation, with resulting cell death.
  - Ribosomes synthesize the various proteins that cells require.
  - The nucleus controls cell division, multiplication, and biochemical reactions.
- Somatic cells divide through the process of mitosis.
  - The cellular life cycle has four distinct phases of mitosis: pre-DNA synthesis, actual DNA synthesis, post-DNA manufacturing, and division.
  - Mitosis has four subphases: prophase, metaphase, anaphase, and telophase.
- Genetic cells divide through meiosis.
  - Meiosis is similar to mitosis, except no DNA replication occurs in telophase; the number of chromosomes in the daughter cell is reduced to half the number of chromosomes in the parent cell.
- The Human Genome Project has mapped the entire sequence of DNA base pairs on all 46 chromosomes.
  - There are 2.9 billion base pairs arranged into approximately 30,000 genes.

## REFERENCES

1. Ventner JC: The sequence of the human genome. *Science* 291:1304–1351, 2001.
2. Lee TF: *The Human Genome Project: cracking the genetic code of life*, New York, 1991, Plenum Press.
3. Stöppler MC: Electrolytes. Available at: www.medicinenet .com/electrolytes/article.htm. Accessed April 9, 2013.
4. Dowd SB, Tilson ER: *Practical radiation protection and applied radiobiology*, ed 2, Philadelphia, 1999, Saunders.

## GENERAL DISCUSSION QUESTIONS

1. What are the essential functions of water in the human body?
2. What role do antibodies fulfill for the human body?
3. Describe the structure of a DNA (deoxyribonucleic) macromolecule.

4. Name the four nitrogenous base pairs in a DNA (deoxyribose) macromolecule.
5. How do genes control the formation of proteins in every cell?
6. Describe the Human Genome Project.
7. Why is potassium of primary importance to the human body?
8. List the components of the normal cell, and explain their function.
9. Describe the processes of mitosis and meiosis.
10. How can multiple births occur from one pregnancy?

## REVIEW QUESTIONS

1. In a DNA macromolecule, the sequence of _____ determines the characteristics of every living thing.
   A. Sugars
   B. Phosphates
   C. Nitrogenous organic bases
   D. Hydrogen bonds
2. How many base pairs are there in the human genome?
   A. $2.58 \times 10^4$
   B. $2.58 \times 10^{-4}$
   C. $2.9 \times 10^9$
   D. $2.9 \times 10^{-9}$
3. Radiation-induced chromosome damage may be evaluated during which of the following processes?
   A. Prophase
   B. Metaphase
   C. Anaphase
   D. Telophase
4. If exposure to ionizing radiation damages the components involved in molecular synthesis beyond repair, cells do which of the following?
   A. Continue to function normally
   B. Function abnormally or die
   C. Repair themselves immediately because of the enzymatic proteins they contain
   D. Reproduce themselves in pairs

5. Which of the following produces antibodies?
   A. Erythrocytes
   B. Lymphocytes
   C. Thrombocytes
   D. Platelets
6. Water constitutes approximately _____ of the weight of the human body.
   A. 50% to 55%
   B. 60% to 70%
   C. 80% to 85%
   D. 90% to 95%
7. Which of the following must the human body provide to ensure efficient cell operation?
   1. Food as a source of raw material for the release of energy
   2. Oxygen to help break down food
   3. Water to transport inorganic substances into and out of the cell
   A. 1 and 2 only
   B. 1 and 3 only
   C. 2 and 3 only
   D. 1, 2, and 3
8. Which human cell component controls cell division and multiplication as well as biochemical reactions that occur within the cell?
   A. Endoplasmic reticulum
   B. Mitochondria
   C. Lysosomes
   D. Nucleus
9. What term is used to describe chemical secretions that are manufactured by various endocrine glands and carried by the bloodstream to influence the activities of other parts of the body?
   A. Amino acids
   B. Antibodies
   C. Hormones
   D. Disaccharides
10. Somatic cells divide through the process of:
   A. Meiosis.
   B. Mitosis.
   C. Mapping.
   D. Metabolism.

*Somatic - mitosis*
*genetic - meiosis*

# Molecular and Cellular Radiation Biology

## OBJECTIVES

*After completing this chapter, the reader will be able to perform the following:*

- List the three radiation energy transfer determinants, and explain their individual concepts.
- Explain why x-rays and gamma rays can also be referred to as a stream of particles called *photons.*
- Differentiate among the three levels of biologic damage that may occur in living systems as a result of exposure to ionizing radiation, and describe how the process of direct and indirect action of ionizing radiation on the molecular structure of living systems occurs.
- Draw a diagram to illustrate the various effects of ionizing radiation on a DNA macromolecule, and describe the effects of ionizing radiation on chromosomes, various types of cells, and ultimately the entire human body.
- Describe the target theory.
- Explain the purpose and function of survival curves for mammalian cells.
- List the factors that affect cell radiosensitivity.
- State and describe the law of Bergonié and Tribondeau.

Copyright © 2014, Elsevier Inc.

## KEY TERMS

apoptosis
cell survival curve
chromosome breakage
direct action
free radicals
indirect action

law of Bergonié and
    Tribondeau
linear energy transfer (LET)
mutation
oxygen enhancement ratio
    (OER)

point mutation
radiation weighting factor ($W_R$)
relative biologic effectiveness
    (RBE)
target theory
wave-particle duality

Radiation biology is the branch of biology concerned with the effects of ionizing radiation on living systems. Areas of study included in this science are the:

- Sequence of events occurring after the absorption of energy from ionizing radiation
- Action of the living system to make up for the consequences of this energy assimilation
- Injury to the living system that may be produced

The human body is a living system composed of large numbers of various types of cells, most of which may be damaged by radiation. Because the potentially harmful effects of ionizing radiation on living systems occur primarily at the cellular level, those who administer radiation to human patients for medical purposes should have a basic understanding of cell structure, composition, and function, as well as the adverse effects of ionizing radiation on these entities. This chapter provides the reader with a basic knowledge of aspects of molecular and cellular radiation biology that are relevant to the subject of radiation protection. It also provides a foundation for the radiation effects on organ systems that are covered in Chapters 8 and 9.

## IONIZING RADIATION

Ionizing radiation damages living systems by ionizing (removing electrons from) the atoms comprising the molecular structures of these systems. X-ray and gamma-ray photons can impart energy to orbital electrons in atoms if the photons happen to pass near the electrons. High-energy charged particles such as alpha and beta particles and protons also may ionize atoms by interacting electromagnetically with orbital electrons. The alpha particle (see Chapter 2), which is composed of two protons and two neutrons and therefore carries an electric charge of plus two, strongly attracts the negatively charged electron as it passes by.

Biologic damage, then, begins with the ionization produced by various types of radiation. An ionized atom does not bond properly in molecules. If the molecule in question is necessary for the normal functioning of an organism, then the entire organism may be affected.

## RADIATION ENERGY TRANSFER DETERMINANTS

Characteristics of ionizing radiation vary among different types of radiation. Characteristics include:

- Charge
- Mass
- Energy

These attributes determine the extent to which different radiation modalities transfer energy into biologic tissue. To understand the way ionizing radiation causes injury and how the effects can vary in biologic tissue, three important concepts must be studied:

1. Linear energy transfer
2. Relative biologic effectiveness
3. Oxygen enhancement ratio

## Linear Energy Transfer

When passing through a medium, ionizing radiation may interact with it during its passage and as a result lose energy along its path (called a *track*). The average energy deposited per unit length of track is called **linear energy transfer (LET)** (Fig. 7-1). The energy average is calculated by dividing the track into equal energy intervals and averaging the lengths of the tracks that contain that specific energy amount. LET is generally described in units of kiloelectron volts (keV) per micron (1 micron [$\mu$m] = $10^{-6}$ m). The rate of transfer of energy from ionizing radiation used for diagnostic purposes to soft biologic tissue is estimated to be 3 keV/$\mu$m. This is considered to be relatively low-LET radiation

compared with other types of radiation, which can have very much higher keV/$\mu$m values. Because the amount of ionization produced in an irradiated object corresponds to the amount of energy it absorbs and because both chemical and biologic effects in tissue coincide with the degree of ionization experienced by the tissue, LET is a very important factor in assessing potential tissue and organ damage from exposure to ionizing radiation. When LET increases, the chance of producing a significant biologic response in the radiosensitive DNA macromolecule grows.

**Radiation Categories According to Linear Energy Transfer.** Radiation may be divided into two general categories according to its LET (Box 7-1):

- Low
- High

***Low–Linear Energy Transfer Radiation.*** Low-LET radiation is electromagnetic radiation, such as:

- X-rays
- Gamma rays (short-wavelength, high-energy waves emitted by the nuclei of radioactive substances)

Because of a property known as **wave-particle duality** (described in Chapter 2, proof p. 2-28), x-rays and gamma rays can also be referred to as streams of particles called *photons*, each of which has no mass and no charge.

Although this electromagnetic radiation can be quite penetrating, it is sparsely ionizing and interacts randomly along the length of its track.

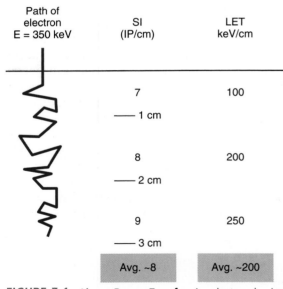

| Path of electron E = 350 keV | SI (IP/cm) | LET keV/cm |
|---|---|---|
| | 7 | 100 |
| — 1 cm | | |
| | 8 | 200 |
| — 2 cm | | |
| | 9 | 250 |
| — 3 cm | | |
| Avg. ~8 | | Avg. ~200 |

**FIGURE 7-1    Linear Energy Transfer.** An electron having energy (E) of 350 keV interacts in a tissuelike material. Its actual path is tortuous, changing direction a number of times, as the electron interacts with atoms of the material via excitations and ionizations. As interactions reduce the energy of the electron through excitation and ionization, the electron's energy is transferred to the material. The interactions that take place along the path of the particle may be summarized as specific ionization (SI; ion pairs/cm) or as linear energy transfer (LET; keV/cm) along the straight line continuation of the particle's trajectory beyond its point of entry.

| BOX 7-1 | General Categories of Linear Energy Transfer Radiation |
|---|---|

| **Low-LET Radiation** | **High-LET Radiation** |
|---|---|
| Gamma rays | Alpha particles |
| X-rays | Ions of heavy nuclei |
| | Charged particles released from interactions between neutrons and atoms |
| | Low-energy neutrons |

*LET,* Linear energy transfer.

It does not relinquish all its energy quickly. When low-LET radiation interacts with biologic tissue, it causes damage to a cell primarily through an *indirect* action that involves the production of molecules called **free radicals** (solitary atoms, e.g., an unpaired hydrogen atom [H], or most often a combination of atoms that are very chemically reactive single entities as a result of the presence of unpaired electrons). In addition, but much less likely, the radiation may *directly* induce single-strand breaks in the ladderlike DNA structure. (Both free radicals and their influences on DNA are discussed in detail later in this chapter.) Because low-LET radiation generally causes sublethal damage to DNA, repair enzymes can usually reverse the cellular damage.

**High–Linear Energy Transfer Radiation.** High-LET radiation includes particles that possess substantial:

• Mass
• Charge

This type of radiation, unlike low-LET radiation, can produce dense ionization along its path and therefore is much more likely to interact significantly with biologic tissue. Some typical examples of high-LET radiation are:

• Alpha particles
• Ions of heavy nuclei
• Charged particles released from interactions between neutrons and atoms

Low-energy neutrons, which carry no electrical charge, also are a form of high-LET radiation. All these types of high-LET radiation lose energy more rapidly than does low-LET radiation because they produce much more ionization per unit of distance traveled. As a result, they exhaust their energy in a shorter length of track and therefore, unless they are of extremely high energies, cannot travel or penetrate as far as x-ray and gamma ray photons. Even so, it is clear that high-LET radiation can be very destructive to biologic matter.

**Risk of Damage to DNA.** Figure 7-2 shows an electron and an alpha particle passing through the nucleus of a cell in the vicinity of a strand of DNA. The size of the entire area is only approximately 10 nanometers (10 billionths of a meter, or 10 millionths of a millimeter). The electron is either a Compton scattered electron or a photoelectron generated by the interaction of a photon from a diagnostic x-ray beam. The alpha particle represents one of the particles ejected from the nucleus of an atom after radioactive decay of an element such as radon.

*Probability of Interaction with DNA.* As mentioned previously, the parameter that describes the average energy deposited over small distances in the material is the LET. The presence of many more alpha particle interactions in the small region displayed is reflected in the finding that the LET for the alpha particle shown in Figure 7-2 is 1000 times the LET of the electron. Each time the particle interacts, it loses some energy and slows down in the cell. When enough interactions have occurred, the particle comes to a stop, and no further interactions take place. Because it does not interact as often, the electron, however, can travel significantly farther than the alpha particle. A Compton scattered electron or photoelectron set in motion in a patient exposed to diagnostic x-rays may travel through thousands of cells (interacting in only some of them), with a low probability that a significant number of interactions will occur by chance in the DNA. Conversely, an alpha particle, such as the one shown, may travel through only one or two cells but will have a high probability of interacting with the DNA of a cell it encounters.

*High–Linear Energy Transfer Radiation and Internal Contamination.* For radiation protection, high-LET radiation is of greatest concern when internal contamination is possible, that is, when a radionuclide has been:

• Implanted
• Ingested
• Injected
• Inhaled

Then the potential exists for irreparable damage because, with high-LET radiation, multiple-strand breaks in DNA are possible. For example, with a double-strand break in the same rung of

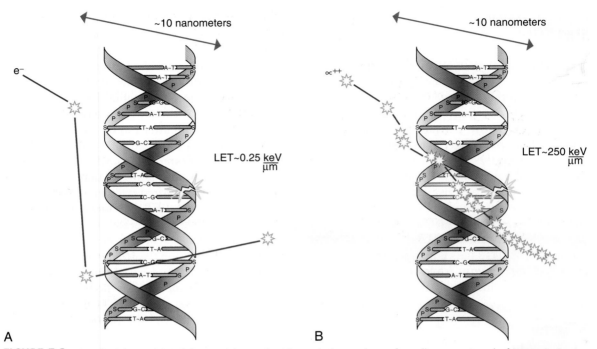

**FIGURE 7-2**   An electron and an alpha particle passing through the nucleus of a cell near a strand of DNA. **A,** For an electron, several interactions may occur in the vicinity of a DNA strand and create a risk of damage to the DNA. **B,** Because so many interactions may occur in the vicinity of a DNA strand, some damage is likely.

the DNA ladderlike structure, complete chromosome breakage occurs (see Fig. 7-8, *A* later in this chapter). Repair enzymes are not effective at undoing this damage, and hence cell death will probably occur.

## Relative Biologic Effectiveness

Biologic damage produced by radiation escalates as the LET of radiation increases. Identical doses of radiation of different LETs do not render identical biologic effects. The **relative biologic effectiveness (RBE)** describes the relative capabilities of radiation with differing LETs to produce a particular biologic reaction. RBE of the type of radiation being used is the ratio of the dose of a reference radiation (conventionally 250-kVp x-rays) to the dose of radiation of the type in question that is necessary to produce the same biologic reaction in a given experiment. The reaction is produced by a dose of the test radiation delivered under the same conditions.

Box 7-2 demonstrates how RBE can be expressed mathematically.

**Use of the Relative Biologic Effectiveness Concept for Specific Experiments.**   The concept of RBE is used to refer to specific experiments with specific cells or animal tissues (e.g., tumor cells in a Petri dish, skin of the left hind flank of a certain strain of laboratory rat). Because the various types of cells or tissues differ in their biologic response per unit quantity of absorbed dose, the concept of RBE is not practical for specifying radiation protection dose levels in humans. To overcome this limitation, a **radiation weighting factor** ($W_R$) is used to calculate the equivalent dose (EqD) to determine the ability of a dose of any kind of ionizing radiation to cause biologic damage. The $W_R$ values are similar to the values of RBE for any particular type of radiation. For example, the $W_R$ for x-radiation is 1, and the RBE for diagnostic x-rays is also 1. The $W_R$ values for different types of ionizing radiation are listed in Table 4-2 in Chapter 4.

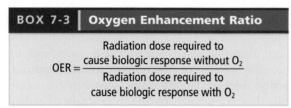

**BOX 7-2 | Mathematical Expression of Relative Biologic Effectiveness**

$$RBE = \frac{\text{Dose in Gy}_t \text{ from 250-kVp x-rays (reference radiation)}}{\text{Dose in Gy}_t \text{ of test radiation}}$$

**Example:** A biologic reaction is produced by 2 Gy$_t$ of a test radiation. It takes 10 Gy$_t$ of 250-kVp x-rays to produce the same biologic reaction. What is the RBE of the test radiation?

$$\frac{10}{2} = 5$$

The RBE is 5, which means that the test radiation is five times as effective in producing this biologic reaction as are 250-kVp x-rays.

*RBE*, Relative biologic effectiveness.

**BOX 7-3 | Oxygen Enhancement Ratio**

$$OER = \frac{\text{Radiation dose required to cause biologic response without O}_2}{\text{Radiation dose required to cause biologic response with O}_2}$$

*OER*, Oxygen enhancement ratio.

## Oxygen Enhancement Ratio

When irradiated in an oxygenated, or aerobic state, biologic tissue is more sensitive to radiation than when it is exposed to radiation under anoxic (without oxygen) or hypoxic (low-oxygen) conditions. This is known as the *oxygen effect*. The **oxygen enhancement ratio** (**OER**) describes this effect numerically.[1,2]

The OER is the ratio of the radiation dose required to cause a particular biologic response of cells or organisms in an oxygen-deprived environment to the radiation dose required to cause an identical response under normal oxygenated conditions. The OER formula is given in Box 7-3.

In general, x-rays and gamma rays, which are low-LET types of radiation, have an OER of approximately 3.0 when the radiation dose is high. The OER may be less (approximately 2.0) when radiation doses are lower than 2 Gy$_t$. This surprising result exists because a 2-Gy$_t$ dose is associated with the linear (i.e., straight-line) portion of the linear-quadratic dose-response relationship for cell killing (see Figure 9-3), whereas higher doses can fall on the curved (i.e., quadratic) portion of the dose-response curve.[3] The term *linear-quadratic* means that the equation that best fits the data has terms that depend on dose (linear) and also dose squared (quadratic). Because high-LET radiation such as alpha particles produces its biologic effects from direct action—namely, direct ionization and disruption of biomolecules—the presence or absence of oxygen is of no consequence. Therefore, the OER of high-LET radiation is approximately equal to 1. For low-LET radiation, a significant fraction of bioeffects is caused by indirect actions in which an entity of a chemical species called a *free radical* is formed. Free radicals dramatically increase the amount of biologic damage. (Both the direct and indirect actions of radiation and the resulting chemical agents are discussed later in this chapter.) However, the presence of oxygen in biologic tissues makes the damage produced by these free radicals permanent because oxygen reacts with them to produce organic peroxide compounds. The latter represent nonrestorable changes in the chemical composition of the target material. Without oxygen, damage produced by the indirect action of radiation on a biologic molecule may be repaired, but when damage occurs through an oxygen-mediated process, the end result is permanent, or fixed. This phenomenon has been called *the oxygen fixation hypothesis.*

## MOLECULAR EFFECTS OF IRRADIATION

In living systems, biologic damage resulting from exposure to ionizing radiation may be observed on three levels:

- Molecular
- Cellular
- Organic

Any visible radiation-induced injuries of living systems at the cellular or organic level always begin with damage at the molecular level. Molecular damage results in the formation of structurally changed molecules that may impair cellular functioning.

## Effects of Irradiation on Somatic and Genetic Cells

Cells of the human body are highly specialized. Each cell has a predetermined task to perform, and each cell's function is determined and defined by the structures of its constituent molecules. Because exposure to ionizing radiation can alter these structures, such exposure may disturb the cell's chemical balance and ultimately the way it operates. When this occurs, the cell no longer performs its normal tasks. If sufficient quantities of somatic cells (i.e., all cells in the body other than female and male germ cells) are affected, entire body processes can be disrupted. Conversely, if radiation damages the germ (reproductive) cells, the damage may be passed on to future generations in the form of genetic mutations (changes in the genes). (More information pertaining to somatic and genetic [hereditary] effects is presented later in this chapter and in Chapters 8 and 9.)

## Classification of Ionizing Radiation Interaction

When ionizing radiation interacts with a cell, ionizations and excitations (the addition of energy to a molecular system that transforms it from a ground state to a higher-energy, or excited, state) are produced either in vital biologic macromolecules (e.g., DNA), or in water ($H_2O$), the medium in which the cellular organelles are suspended. Based on the site of the interaction, the effect of radiation on the cell is classified as either (Fig. 7-3):

- Direct
- Indirect

In **direct action,** biologic damage occurs as a result of ionization of atoms on essential molecules

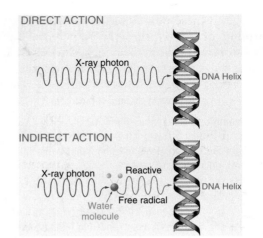

**FIGURE 7-3** The action of radiation on the cell can be direct or indirect. It is direct when ionizing particles interact with a vital biologic macromolecule such as DNA. The action is indirect when ionizing particles interact with a water molecule, thus resulting in the creation of ions and reactive free radicals that eventually produce toxic substances that can create biologic damage.

that may potentially cause these molecules to become inactive or functionally altered. **Indirect action** refers to the effects produced by free radicals that are created by the interaction of radiation with water ($H_2O$) molecules. These unstable agents are so highly reactive that they can substantially disrupt master molecules, with resulting cell death.

Direct action may possibly occur after exposure to any type of radiation. However, direct action is much more likely to happen after exposure to high-LET radiation such as alpha particles, which produce a very large number of ionizations in a very short distance of travel. This is in glaring contrast to exposure to low-LET radiation, such as x-rays, which are only sparsely ionizing.

## Direct Action

When ionizing particles interact directly with vital biologic macromolecules such as:

- DNA
- Ribonucleic acid (RNA)
- Proteins
- Enzymes

damage to these molecules occurs from the absorption of energy through photoelectric and Compton interactions. The ionization or excitation of the atoms of the biologic macromolecules results in breakage of the macromolecules' chemical bonds and causes them to become abnormal structures. This change could in turn lead to inappropriate chemical reactions. Therefore, when enzyme molecules are damaged by interaction with ionizing particles, essential biochemical processes may not occur in the cell at the appropriate time. For example, if an enzyme is inactivated, it will not be available to facilitate a particular biochemical reaction. Should this occur during the synthesis of a particular protein, the protein will not be manufactured, and if this protein was intended to perform a specific function, its failure to exist will hinder or prevent that function. In the event that other cell operations depend on the suppressed function, these operations will sustain some type of damage as well, and so a biologic chain reaction essentially occurs.

## Radiolysis of Water

**Ionization of Water Molecules.** X-ray photons can interact with and ionize water molecules contained within the human body, thereby separating them into other molecular components. For example, an interaction between an x-ray photon and a water molecule could create an ion pair consisting of a water molecule with a positive charge ($HOH^+$) and an electron ($e^-$). After the original ionization of the water molecule, several reactions are possible. One is that the positively charged water molecule ($HOH^+$) may recombine with the electron ($e^-$) to re-form a stable water molecule ($HOH^+ + e^- = H_2O$). If this happens, no damage will occur. Alternatively, the electron (the negative ion) may join with another water molecule to produce a negative water ion ($H_2O + e^- = HOH^-$).

**Production of Free Radicals.** The positive water molecule ($HOH^+$) and the negative water molecule ($HOH^-$) are basically unstable. Hence they will break apart into smaller molecules.

$HOH^+$ becomes a hydrogen ion ($H^+$) and a hydroxyl radical ($OH^*$), whereas $HOH^-$ becomes a hydroxyl ion ($OH^-$) and a hydrogen radical ($H^*$). The asterisk symbolizes a free radical. A free radical, which exists only for approximately 1 millisecond, is a configuration with one or more atoms having an unpaired electron but no net electrical charge. This short-lived object is highly interactive because the unpaired electron will pair up with another electron even if it has to break a chemical bond to do this. Hence the interaction of radiation with water results in the formation of an ion pair, $H^+$ and $OH^-$ (hydrogen ion and hydroxyl ion), and two free radicals, $H^*$ and $OH^*$ (a hydrogen radical and a hydroxyl radical) (Fig. 7-4).

**Production of Undesirable Chemical Reactions and Biologic Damage.** Because the hydrogen and hydroxyl ions usually recombine to form a normal water molecule, the existence of these ions as free agents within the human body is insignificant in terms of biologic damage. The presence of hydrogen and hydroxyl free radicals, however, is not insignificant. As molecules containing an unpaired electron in their outer shell, they are chemically unstable and very reactive. They can produce undesirable chemical reactions and cause biologic damage by transferring their excess energy to other molecules, thereby either breaking these molecules' chemical bonds or at the very least causing point lesions (i.e., altered areas caused by the breaking of a single chemical bond) in the molecule. Approximately two thirds of all radiation-induced damage is believed to be ultimately caused by the hydroxyl free radical ($OH^*$). In addition, because free radicals have excess energy and can travel through the cell, they are capable of destructively interacting with other molecules located at some distance from the radicals' place of origin.

**Production of Cell-Damaging Substances.** Hydrogen and hydroxyl radicals are not the only destructive substances produced during the radiolysis of water. A hydroxyl radical ($OH^*$) can bond with another hydroxyl radical ($OH^*$) and form hydrogen peroxide ($OH^* + OH^* = H_2O_2$), a substance that is very poisonous to the cell.

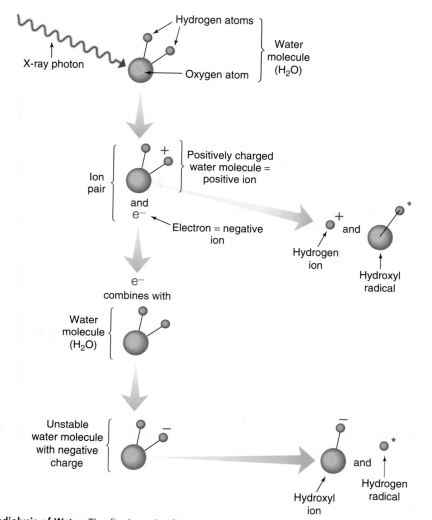

**FIGURE 7-4**    **Radiolysis of Water.** The final result of the interaction of radiation with water is the formation of an ion pair ($H^+$ and $OH^-$) and two free radicals ($H^*$ and $OH^*$).

In addition, a hydroperoxyl radical ($HO_2^*$) is formed when a hydrogen free radical ($H^*$) combines with molecular oxygen ($O_2$). This radical and hydrogen peroxide are believed to be among the primary substances that produce biologic damage directly after the interaction of radiation with water.

**Organic Free Radical Formation.** Absorption of radiation can cause a normal organic molecule (for simplicity, let us call it *RH*, in which *H* stands for hydrogen and *R* can be any organic molecule) to form the free radicals R*

(an organic neutral free radical) and $H^*$. Without oxygen or a force to attract an electron, these radicals usually react with each other to reform the original organic molecule (RH). When oxygen is present, however, R* and $H^*$ may react with oxygen molecules ($O_2$) to form the radicals $RO_2^*$ and $HO_2^*$. Hence the original organic molecule (RH) is destroyed and replaced by the radicals $RO_2^*$ and $HO_2^*$. These radicals can react with other organic molecules to cause biologic damage. Thus a small-scale chain reaction of destructive events results when radiation deposits energy within tissue in the presence of oxygen.

## Indirect Action

When free radicals previously produced by the interaction of radiation with water molecules act on a molecule such as DNA, the damaging action of ionizing radiation is indirect in the sense that the radiation is not the immediate cause of injury to the macromolecule. The by-products of the radiation, the free radicals, are the immediate cause of this damage. Because the human body is 80% water and less than 1% DNA, essentially all effects of irradiation in living cells result from indirect action.[1]

In summary, the process of indirect action involves the breakdown of a water molecule into smaller molecules, a process that produces both ions and free radicals (Fig. 7-5). As described previously, the free radicals produced can recombine to form hydrogen peroxide, a cellular poison, and a hydroperoxyl radical, another toxic substance. Both these agents are highly reactive and therefore very capable of producing biologic damage. By themselves, free radicals such as OH* also may transfer excess energy to other molecules, thereby breaking their chemical bonds.

## Effects of Ionizing Radiation on DNA

**Single-Strand Break.** If ionizing radiation interacts with a DNA macromolecule, the energy transferred could rupture one of its chemical bonds and possibly sever one of the sugar-phosphate chain side rails, or strands, of the ladderlike molecular structure (single-strand break) (Fig. 7-6). This type of injury to DNA is called a **point mutation.** Such a single alteration along the sequence of nitrogenous bases can result in a gene abnormality. Point mutations commonly occur with low-LET radiation. Repair enzymes, however, are often capable of reversing this damage.

**Double-Strand Break.** Further exposure of the affected DNA macromolecule to ionizing

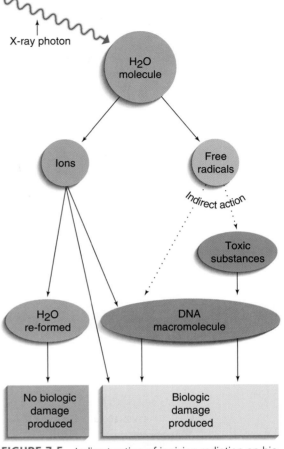

**FIGURE 7-5**   Indirect action of ionizing radiation on biologic molecules. X-ray photons interact directly with a water ($H_2O$) molecule. The $H_2O$ molecule breaks down into ions and free radicals. The ions can recombine to form a water molecule, thereby creating no biologic damage. The free radicals can migrate to another molecule, such as a DNA molecule located at some distance from the site of the initial ionization, and destructively interact with it by ionizing it or rupturing some chemical bonds. This creates molecular or point lesions in the DNA macromolecule. Free radicals can spread biologic damage by combining with other molecules to form toxic substances that also can migrate to distant DNA molecules and destructively interact.

radiation can lead to additional breaks in the sugar-phosphate molecular chain(s). These breaks may also be repaired, but double-strand breaks (one or more breaks in each of the two sugar-phosphate chains) (Fig. 7-7) are not fixed as

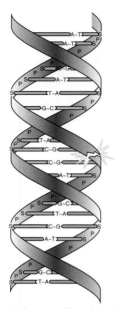

**FIGURE 7-6**   A single-strand break in the ladderlike DNA molecular structure.

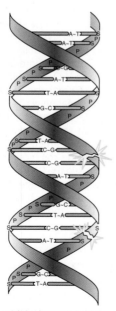

**FIGURE 7-7**   A widely spaced double-strand break in the ladderlike DNA molecular structure.

easily as single-strand breaks. If repair does not take place, further separation may occur in the DNA chains, threatening the life of the cell. Double-strand breaks occur more commonly with densely ionizing (high-LET) radiation and often are associated with the loss or gain of one or more nitrogenous bases. When high-LET radiation interacts with DNA molecules, the ionization interactions may be so closely spaced that, by chance, both strands of the DNA chain are broken. If both strands are broken at the same nitrogenous base "rung," the result is the same as if both side rails of the ladder were cut at the same step, or rung—the ladder would be cut into two pieces. If the DNA is cut into two pieces, the chromosome, which is composed of a long chain of twisted strands of DNA ladders, is itself broken. Thus some types of chromosomal damage that are specifically associated with high-LET radiation are related to double-strand breaks of DNA. Because the chance of reversing this type of damage is very low, the possibility of a lethal alteration of nitrogenous bases within the genetic sequence is far greater.

**Double-Strand Break in the Same Rung of DNA.** When two interactions (hits), one on each of the two sugar-phosphate chains, occur within the same rung of the DNA ladderlike configuration (Fig. 7-8, *A*), the result is a cleaved or broken chromosome (Fig. 7-8, *B*), with each new portion containing an unequal amount of genetic material. If this damaged chromosome divides, each new daughter cell will receive an incorrect amount of genetic material. This will culminate in either death or impaired functioning of the new daughter cell.

**Mutation.** In general, the interaction of high-energy radiation with a DNA molecule causes a loss of or change in a nitrogenous base on the DNA chain. The direct consequence of this damage is an alteration of the base sequence (Fig. 7-9). Because the genetic information to be passed on to future generations is contained in the strict sequence of these bases, the loss or change of a base in the DNA chain represents a **mutation.** It may not be reversible and may generate acute consequences for the cell, but, more

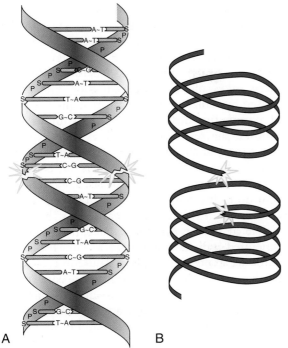

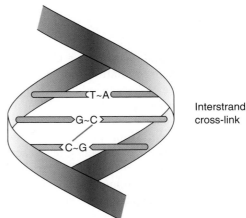

FIGURE 7-10 Interstrand covalent cross-link produced by high-energy radiation acting directly on a DNA molecule.

FIGURE 7-8 A double-strand break in same rung of the DNA ladderlike molecular structure (**A**) causes complete chromosome breakage, resulting in a cleaved or broken chromosome (**B**).

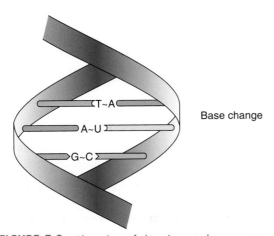

FIGURE 7-9 Alteration of the nitrogen base sequence on the DNA chain caused by the action of high-energy radiation directly on a DNA molecule.

important, if the cell remains viable, incorrect genetic information will be transferred to one of the two daughter cells when the cell divides.

**Covalent Cross-Links.** Covalent cross-links are chemical unions created between atoms by the single sharing of one or more pairs of electrons. Covalent cross-links involving DNA comprise another effect directly initiated by high-energy radiation. At low energies, however, covalent cross-links are probably caused by the process of indirect action. Following irradiation, some molecules can fragment or change into small, spurlike molecules that become very interactive ("sticky") when they themselves are exposed to radiation. Such sticky molecules attach to other macromolecules or to other segments of the same macromolecule chain. Cross-linking can occur in many different patterns. For example, a cross-link can form between two places on the same DNA strand. This joining is termed an *intrastrand cross-link*. Cross-linking may also happen between complementary DNA strands (Fig. 7-10) or between entirely different DNA molecules. These joinings are termed *interstrand cross-links*. Finally, DNA molecules also may become covalently linked to a protein molecule.[4] All these linkages are potentially fatal to the cell if they are not properly repaired.

# Effects of Ionizing Radiation on Chromosomes

Large-scale structural changes in a chromosome produced by ionizing radiation may be as grave for the cell as are radiation-induced changes in DNA. When changes occur in the DNA molecule, the chromosome exhibits the variation. Because DNA modifications are discrete, they do not inevitably result in observable structural chromosome revisions. However, if these discrete effects are numerous enough, such as may be brought about by exposure to very high-LET radiation, then an observable structural chromosome alteration is possible.

**Radiation-Induced Chromosome Breaks.** After irradiation and during cell division, some radiation-induced chromosome breaks may be viewed microscopically. These changes manifest during the metaphase and anaphase of the cell division cycle, when the length of the chromosomes is visible. Because the events that precede these phases of cell division are not visible, they can only be assumed to have occurred. What can be seen, however, is the effect of these events—the gross or visible differences in the structure of the chromosome. Both somatic cells and reproductive cells are subject to chromosome breaks induced by radiation.

**Chromosomal Fragments.** After chromosome breakage, two or more chromosomal fragments are produced. Each of these fragments has a fractured extremity. These broken ends are chemically very active and therefore have a strong tendency to adhere to another similar sticky end. The broken fragments can:

• Rejoin in their original configuration
• Fail to rejoin and create an aberration (lesion or anomaly) or
• Join to other broken ends and thereby create new chromosomes that may not look structurally altered compared with the chromosome before irradiation.

**Chromosome Anomalies.** Two types of chromosome anomalies have been observed at metaphase. They are called:

• Chromosome aberrations
• Chromatid aberrations

Chromosome aberrations result when irradiation occurs early in interphase, before DNA synthesis takes place. In this situation, the break caused by ionizing radiation is in a single strand of chromatin; during the DNA synthesis that follows, the resultant break is replicated when this strand of chromatin lays down an identical strand adjacent to itself if repair is not complete before the start of DNA synthesis. This situation leads to a chromosome aberration in which both chromatids exhibit the break. This break is visible at the next mitosis. Each daughter cell generated will have inherited a damaged chromatid as a consequence of a failure in the repair mechanism. Chromatid aberrations, conversely, result when irradiation of individual chromatids occurs later in interphase, after DNA synthesis has taken place. In this situation, only one chromatid of a pair may undergo a radiation-induced break. Therefore, only one daughter cell is affected.

**Structural Changes in Biologic Tissue Caused by Ionizing Radiation.** Ionizing radiation interacts randomly with matter transferring energy in the process. Because of this phenomenon, exposure to radiation can lead to the occurrence of a variety of deleterious effects in biologic tissue, including the following:

• A single-strand break in one chromosome
• A single-strand break in one chromatid
• A single-strand break in separate chromosomes
• A strand break in separate chromatids
• More than one break in the same chromosome
• More than one break in the same chromatid
• Chromosome stickiness, or clumping together

## Consequences to the Cell from Structural Changes in Biologic Tissue

1. *Restitution,* whereby the breaks rejoin in their original configuration with no visible damage (Fig. 7-11). In this case, no damage to the cell occurs because the chromatid has been

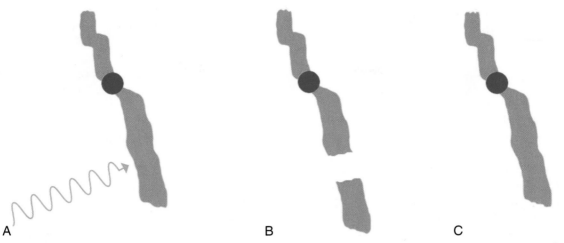

A                                          B                                          C

**FIGURE 7-11**   The process of restitution, whereby the breaks rejoin in the original configuration with no visible damage. **A,** The chromatid break occurs because of a photon interaction. **B,** The fragment is fully separated from the rest of the chromatid. This same type of damage could occur to a chromosome if S phase had already occurred. **C,** The broken fragment has reattached in its original location through the action of repair enzymes.

restored to the condition it was in before irradiation. The process of healing by restitution is believed to be the way in which 95% of single-chromosome breaks mend.[4]

2. *Deletion,* whereby a part of the chromosome or chromatid is lost at the next cell division, thus creating an aberration known as an *acentric fragment* (Fig. 7-12). This results in a cell mutation.

3. *Broken-end rearrangement,* whereby a grossly misshapen chromosome may be produced. Ring chromatids, dicentric chromosomes, and anaphase bridges are examples of such distorted chromosomes and chromatids (Fig. 7-13). This results in a cell mutation.

4. *Broken-end rearrangement without visible damage to the chromatids,* whereby the chromatid's genetic material has been rearranged even though the chromatid appears normal. Translocations are examples of such rearrangements (Fig. 7-14). This results in a cell mutation.

Changes such as those outlined in items 2, 3, and 4 in the previous list inevitably result in mutation because the positions of the genes on the chromatids have been rearranged, thus altering the heritable characteristics of the cell.

## Target Theory

As described earlier, the biologic effects of exposure to radiation stem primarily from the ionizations occurring at sensitive cellular points secondary to energy transfers from that radiation. These affected locations in a cell or, more specifically, on a vital molecule within the cell are known as "targets." Whether or not such locations are struck by radiation is a random process. From all existing evidence, it appears that producing a serious effect usually requires more than one radiation "hit" on a specific target. The damage from a single hit normally is not conclusive because of repair mechanisms. This concept of radiation damage resulting from discrete and random events is known as **target theory.**

Amid the many different types of molecules that lie within the cell, a master, or key, molecule that maintains normal cell function is believed to be present (Fig. 7-15). This master molecule is

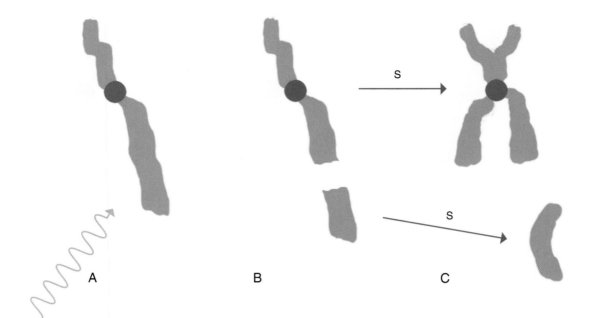

**FIGURE 7-12**    The process of deletion, in which part of a chromosome is lost at the next cell division, thus creating an acentric fragment. **A,** The chromatid break results from a photon interaction. **B,** The fragment is fully separated from the rest of the chromatid. **C,** After the next DNA synthesis phase of the cell cycle (labeled S), the remainder of the chromosome has been replicated normally but with fragments missing from the two arms of the chromosome. The replicated fragment is acentric, a section of genetic material without a centromere.

necessary for the survival of the cell. Because this molecule is unique in any given cell, no similar molecules in the cell are available to replace it; if a critical location on the master molecule is a target receiving multiple hits from ionizing radiation, the master molecule may well be inactivated. Normal cell function will then cease, and the cell will die (Fig. 7-16). If, conversely, it receives only a single hit, then the master molecule most likely will still be operational. Experimental data strongly support this concept and also indicate that DNA is the irreplaceable master, or key, molecule that serves as the preeminent vital target. Destruction of some of the molecules that are plentiful in the cell does not result in cell death. The reason for this is simply that cells have an abundance of similar molecules to take over and perform necessary functions for them in the event of their destruction. Consequently, if only a few non-DNA cell molecules are made dysfunctional by radiation exposure,

the cell will probably not show any evidence of injury after irradiation.

In its passage through the molecular structure of living systems, radiation does not preferentially seek out master molecules in cells to destroy them; it interacts with these key molecules only by chance. The target theory concept then is useful for explaining cell death and nonfatal cell abnormalities caused by exposure to radiation.

Interactions between ionizing radiation and molecular targets such as DNA occur through both direct and indirect action. However, discerning which of the two types of effects or actions has been at work in any given case of cell death is virtually impossible.

## CELLULAR EFFECTS OF IRRADIATION

Ionizing radiation adversely affects the cell primarily by transferring energy to the cell's nucleus.

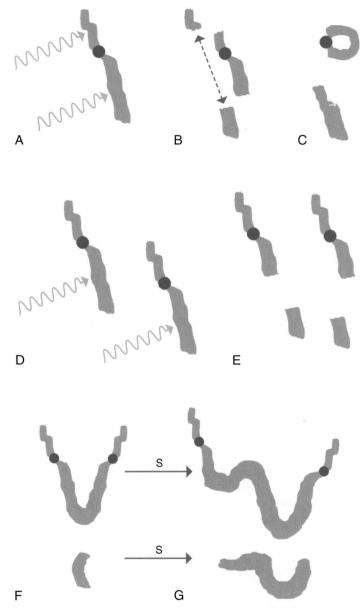

**FIGURE 7-13** The process of broken-end rearrangement may result in grossly misshapen chromatids. **A,** Two chromatid breaks occur in a single chromatid as a result of the interactions of two photons. **B,** The fragments from opposite ends unite before the DNA synthesis phase. **C,** The ends of the chromatid that are still attached to the centromere also unite and form a "ring" chromatid. **D,** Chromatid breaks occur in two different chromatids. **E,** The fragments are fully separated from the rest of their respective chromatids. **F,** The ends of the chromatids and the ends of the fragments have joined before DNA synthesis, thus forming a dicentric (two centromeres) and an acentric (no centromere) fragment. **G,** After DNA synthesis (labeled S), the chromatid is elongated but cannot split in two. The two centromeres are "bridged." This type of chromatid damage leads to reproductive death of the cell (i.e., it cannot replicate or divide into two cells).

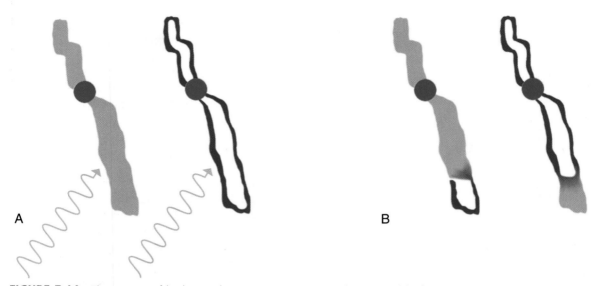

**FIGURE 7-14**    The process of broken-end rearrangement may result in no visible damage to the chromatid, although the chromatid's genetic material has been rearranged—a result that will drastically alter its function within the cell and probably lead to cell death or failure to replicate. This same type of damage could occur to a chromosome if S phase had already occurred. In this case, the cell may divide, but the genetic material in the daughter cells is compromised, and those cells may not function properly.

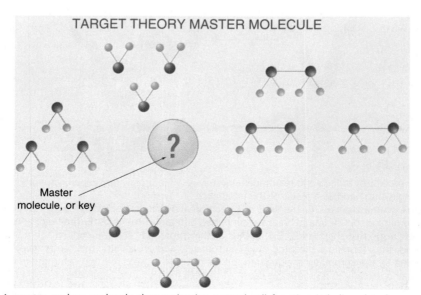

**FIGURE 7-15**    A master, or key, molecule that maintains normal cell function is believed to be present in every cell. This molecule is vital to the survival of the cell and is presumed to be DNA.

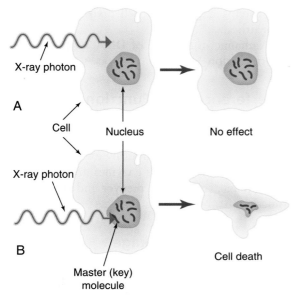

**FIGURE 7-16** The target theory holds that the cell will die after exposure to ionizing radiation only if the master, or key, molecule (DNA) is inactivated in the process. **A,** An x-ray photon passes through the cell without interacting with the master molecule, which is located in the cell nucleus; no measurable effect results. **B,** An x-ray photon enters the nucleus and interacts with and inactivates the master molecule; the cell dies as a result.

Damage to the cell's nucleus reveals itself in one of the following ways:

1. Instant death
2. Reproductive death
3. Apoptosis, or programmed cell death (interphase death)
4. Mitotic, or genetic, death
5. Mitotic delay
6. Interference with function
7. Chromosome breakage

## Instant Death

Instant death of large numbers of cells occurs when a volume is irradiated with an x-ray or gamma-ray dose of approximately 1000 $Gy_t$ in a period of seconds or a few minutes. This large influx of energy causes gross disruption of cellular form and structure and severe changes in chemical machinery. As a result of receiving such a massive dose of ionizing radiation, a cell's DNA macromolecule breaks up, and cellular proteins coagulate. Radiation doses high enough to cause this type of damage are vastly greater than those used for diagnostic examinations or even therapeutic treatments.

## Reproductive Death

Reproductive death generally results from exposure of cells to doses of ionizing radiation in the range of 1 to 10 $Gy_t$. Although the cell does not die when reproductive death occurs, it permanently loses its ability to procreate but continues to metabolize and also to synthesize nucleic acids and proteins. The termination of the cell's reproductive abilities does, however, prevent the transmission of damage to future generations of cells.

## Apoptosis

A nonmitotic, or nondivision, form of cell death that occurs when cells die without attempting division during the interphase portion of the cell life cycle is termed **apoptosis,** or programmed cell death. This was formerly called *interphase death*. Apoptosis occurs spontaneously in both normal tissue and in tumors. It can occur in human beings and other vertebrate animals and amphibians, both in the embryo and in the adult. An example of this process is the sequence of events during embryonic development whereby tadpoles lose their tails.

**Programmed Cell Death for Development and Maintenance of Organisms.** Certain types of *programmed cell death* are integral to the development and maintenance of organisms. Many types of cells are destined to die for the good of the organism. For example, human beings lose webbing between their digits during embryonic development, and all through life human skin cells die and form the protective outer coating we usually refer to as *skin*. In apoptosis the cell shrinks and produces tiny membrane-enclosed structures called *blebs*. The cell nucleus breaks up and then the cell itself breaks up, and its fragments are usually ingested by neighboring cells.

**Apoptosis Research.** Researchers believe that apoptosis may be instigated by radiation under some circumstances. The mechanisms of apoptosis and its relationship with radiosensitivity are areas of active research in radiobiology. A new type of radiation therapy may involve activation of the genes that regulate apoptosis so that the occurrence of apoptosis becomes much more likely after irradiation in a tumor.

**Radiosensitivity.** Radiosensitivity of the individual cell governs the dose required to induce apoptosis; the more radiosensitive the cell is, the smaller the dose required to cause apoptotic death during interphase. A few hundred centigray ($cGy_t$) can kill very sensitive cells such as lymphocytes or spermatogonia. For less radiosensitive cells, such as those in bone, apoptosis may require radiation doses of several thousand $cGy_t$.

## Mitotic Death

Ionizing radiation can adversely affect cell division. It may retard the mitotic process or permanently inhibit it; cell death follows permanent inhibition. *Mitotic,* or *genetic, death* occurs when a cell dies after one or more divisions. Even relatively small doses of radiation can cause this type of cell death. The radiation dose required to produce mitotic death is less than the dose needed to produce apoptosis in slowly dividing cells or nondividing cells.

## Mitotic Delay

Exposing a cell to as little as 0.01 $Gy_t$ of ionizing radiation just before it begins dividing can cause *mitotic delay,* the failure of the cell to start dividing on time. After this delay the cell may resume its normal mitotic function. The underlying cause of this phenomenon is not known. Possible reasons for the delay are as follows:

1. Irradiation causing alteration of a chemical involved in mitosis

2. Proteins required for cell division not being synthesized
3. A change in the rate of DNA synthesis after irradiation

## Interference with Function

Permanent or temporary interference with cellular function independent of the cell's ability to divide can be brought about by exposure to ionizing radiation. If repair enzymes are able to fix the damage, the cell can recover and continue to function.

## Chromosome Breakage

**Chromosome breakage** is a potential outcome when ionizing radiation interacts with a DNA macromolecule. These breaks may occur in one or both strands (sugar-phosphate chains) of the DNA ladderlike structure and are discussed previously in the discussion of direct action.

If cells are irradiated during mitosis and chromosome breakage occurs, permanent chromosome abnormalities will be evident in future mitotic cycles. Because chromosome breakage results in a loss of genetic material, this may lead to genetic mutations in succeeding generations.

# SURVIVAL CURVES FOR MAMMALIAN CELLS

Cells vary in their radiosensitivity. This fact is particularly important in determining the types of cancer cells that will respond to radiation therapy. A classic method of displaying the sensitivity of a particular type of cell to radiation is the **cell survival curve.**[5] A cell survival curve is constructed from data obtained by a series of experiments. First, the cells are made to grow "in culture," meaning in a laboratory environment such as a Petri dish. Then the cells are exposed to a specified dose of radiation. After radiation exposure, the ability of the cells to divide, or form new "colonies" of cells, is measured. The fraction of cells that are able to form new colonies through cell division is then reported as the

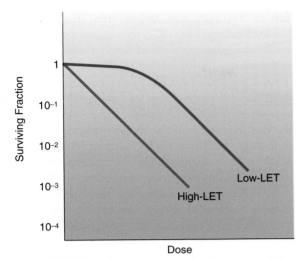

**FIGURE 7-17**   Cell survival curves for the same cell line irradiated with both low- and high-linear energy transfer (LET) radiation. With low-LET radiation, a "shoulder" to the curve at lower doses indicates the cell's ability to repair some damage at low doses. High-LET radiation typically has no shoulder, thus indicating that little or no repair takes place.

---

fraction of cells that have survived irradiation. The process is repeated for a range of radiation doses, and the results are graphed with the logarithm* of the surviving fraction on the vertical axis and the dose on the horizontal axis.

Figure 7-17 shows two cell survival curves, one for high-LET radiation and one for low-LET radiation. The curve for low-LET radiation shows very little change in survival at low doses, followed by a linear portion in which survival decreases in regular proportions at higher doses. This indicates that at low doses the cell is able to find and repair some of the damage. At higher doses the repair mechanism is overwhelmed. For the high-LET curve, no survival shoulder exists. If damage occurs, it is usually so extensive that it is irreparable.

---

*In our ordinary decimal counting system, the logarithm (log) of a number $N$ is by definition the power to which 10 must be raised to give $N$ (e.g., log 1000 = 3 because $10^3 = 1000$).

| BOX 7-4 | Examples of Radiosensitive and Radioinsensitive Cells |
|---|---|

| Radiosensitive Cells | Radioinsensitive Cells |
|---|---|
| Basal cells of the skin | Brain cells |
| Blood cells such as lymphocytes and erythrocytes | Muscle cells |
| | Nerve cells |
| Intestinal crypt cells | |
| Reproductive (germ) cells | |

## CELL RADIOSENSITIVITY

### Cell Maturity and Specialization

The human body is composed of different types of cells and tissues, which vary in their degree of radiosensitivity. Immature cells are nonspecialized (undifferentiated) and undergo rapid cell division, whereas more mature cells are specialized in their function (highly differentiated) and divide at a slower rate or do not divide. These factors affect the cells' degree of radiosensitivity. Examples of radiosensitive and radioinsensitive cells are listed in Box 7-4. Because combinations of both immature and mature cells in various ratios form the different body tissues and organs, radiosensitivity varies from one tissue and organ to another.

### Amount of Radiation Energy Transferred to Biologic Tissue

When ionizing radiation interacts with cell atoms and molecules, the amount of radiation energy transferred to the tissue (i.e., the radiation absorbed dose) plays a major role in determining the amount of biologic response. As its LET increases (i.e., as the radiation transfers more energy per unit length of track), the ability of the radiation to cause biologic effects also generally increases until it reaches a maximal value. Hence LET can influence cell radiosensitivity.

## Oxygen Enhancement Effects

As addressed earlier in this chapter, oxygen enhances the effects of ionizing radiation on biologic tissue by increasing tissue radiosensitivity. If oxygen is present when a tissue is irradiated, more free radicals will be formed in the tissue; this increases the indirect damage potential of the radiation.

During imaging procedures, fully oxygenated human tissues are exposed to x-radiation or gamma radiation. However, both radiographic and nuclear medicine procedures employ low doses of radiation that is also low LET. Consequently, very few cells are killed by the types of radiation used in these procedures.

In radiotherapy, the presence of oxygen plays a significant role in radiosensitivity. When radiation is used to treat certain types of cancerous tumors, high-pressure (hyperbaric) oxygen has sometimes been used in conjunction with it to increase tumor radiosensitivity. Cancerous tumors often contain both hypoxic cells, which lack an adequate amount of oxygen, and normally aerated cells. The poorly oxygenated cells severely inhibit the indirect mechanism of radiation interaction with cells and therefore are radioresistant (particularly to low-LET radiation); hence, hypoxic cells are more difficult to destroy than normally oxygenated cells. However, when oxygen tensions in capillaries are increased by hyperbaric oxygenation, hypoxic cells may reoxygenate and become sensitive to radiation; consequently, the chances of their being destroyed by therapeutic radiation increase. Radiosensitization also may be accomplished with chemical-enhancing agents such as misonidazole.[3]

## Law of Bergonié and Tribondeau

In 1906, two French scientists, J. Bergonié and L. Tribondeau, observed the effects of ionizing radiation on testicular germ cells of rabbits they had exposed to x-rays. These researchers established that radiosensitivity was a function of the metabolic state of the cell receiving the exposure. Their findings eventually became known as the law of Bergonié and Tribondeau. It states that the radiosensitivity of cells is directly proportional to their reproductive activity and inversely proportional to their degree of differentiation. Thus the most pronounced radiation effects occur in cells having the least maturity and specialization or differentiation, the greatest reproductive activity, and the longest mitotic phases.[6] Although the law was originally applied only to germ cells, it is actually true for all types of cells in the human body. Consequently, within the realm of diagnostic imaging, the embryo-fetus, which contains a large number of immature, nonspecialized cells, is much more susceptible to radiation damage than is an adult or even a child. All imaging professionals should be ever mindful of this.

## Effects of Ionizing Radiation on Human Cells

As already discussed, equal doses of ionizing radiation produce different degrees of damage in different kinds of human cells because of differences in cell radiosensitivity. The more mature and specialized in performing functions a cell is, the less sensitive it is to radiation. In the following sections, the radiation response of some of the most important cell groups is examined in detail.

### Blood Cells

***Hematologic Depression.*** Ionizing radiation adversely affects blood cells by depressing the number of cells in the peripheral circulation. A whole-body dose of 0.25 $Gy_t$ delivered within a few days produces a measurable hematologic depression. This dose by far exceeds normal doses sustained by the working population of the radiation industry. Therefore, the use of blood tests for purposes of dosimetry is not valid.

***Depletion of Immature Blood Cells.*** Most blood cells are manufactured in bone marrow. Radiation causes a decrease in the number of immature blood cells (stem, or precursor) produced in bone marrow and hence a reduction, ultimately, in the number of mature blood cells in the bloodstream. The higher is the radiation dose received by the bone marrow, the greater is the severity of the resulting cell depletion.

### Repopulation after a Period of Recovery.
If the bone marrow cells have not been destroyed by exposure to ionizing radiation, they can repopulate after a period of recovery. The time necessary for recovery depends on the magnitude of the radiation dose received. If a relatively low dose (less than 1 $Gy_t$) of radiation is received, bone marrow repopulation occurs within weeks after irradiation. Moderate (1 to 10 $Gy_t$) to high (10 or more $Gy_t$) doses, which severely deplete the number of bone marrow cells, require a longer recovery period. Very high doses of radiation can cause a permanent decrease in the number of stem cells.

### Effects on Stem Cells of the Hematopoietic System.
Radiation affects primarily the stem cells of the hematopoietic (blood-forming) system. Erythrocytes (precursors of red blood cells) are among the most sensitive of human tissues. As with all cells that transform from an immature, undifferentiated state to a mature, functional state, the mature red blood cells are much less radiosensitive. Because the population of circulating red blood cells is high and their life span is long, depletion of red cells is not usually the cause of death in high-dose irradiation (i.e., several $Gy_t$ delivered to the whole body). Death, if it occurs, is more typically caused by infection that cannot be overcome by the immune system because of the destruction of myeloblasts (precursors of granulocytes, a type of white blood cell) and internal hemorrhage resulting from destruction of megakaryoblasts (precursors of platelets).

### Whole-Body Doses in Excess of 5 $Gy_t$.
Human beings who receive whole-body doses in excess of 5 $Gy_t$ may die within 30 to 60 days because of effects related to initial depletion of the stem cells of the hematopoietic system. The use of antibiotics or isolation from pathogens in the environment (e.g., placing the patient in a sterile environment, feeding only sterilized food) has been shown to mitigate these effects in animals and humans. Human, however, recover more slowly than do laboratory animals. Thus the lethal dose in animals is usually specified as LD 50/30 (dose that produces death in 50% of the subjects within 30 days). The lethal dose in human beings is usually given as LD 50/60 because a human's recovery is slower than that of the laboratory animals, and death may still occur at a later time following a substantial whole-body exposure. Whether survival lasts for 30 days or 60 days, the lethal whole-body dose for humans is generally estimated to be 3.0 to 4.0 $Gy_t$ without treatment and higher if medical intervention is available. Table 7-1 presents an overview of LD 50/30 for various species. Additional information pertaining to the measurement of acute radiation lethality is presented in Chapter 8.

### Effects of Ionizing Radiation on Lymphocytes.
White blood cells are collectively called *leukocytes*. Lymphocytes are a very important subgroup of white blood cells. These cells defend the body against foreign objects (antigens) by producing protective proteins (antibodies) to combat disease. Lymphocytes, which live for only approximately 24 hours, have the shortest life span of all the blood cells. Lymphocytes manufactured in bone marrow are the most radiosensitive blood cells in the human body. A radiation

| TABLE 7-1 | LD 50/30 Values for Various Species | |
|---|---|---|
| | | LD 50/30 |
| Species | | $Gy_t$ |
| Human being | | 3.0-4.0* |
| Monkey | | 4.0-4.75 |
| Dog | | 3.0 |
| Hamster | | 7.0 |
| Rabbit | | 7.25 |
| Rat | | 9.0 |
| Turtle | | 15.0 |
| Newt | | 30.0 |

*Depending on the source of the radiation exposure, LD 50/30 (dose that produces death in 50% of the subjects within 30 days) varies. LD 50 may be higher if medical intervention is available. For humans, LD 50/60 may be more realistic because humans are more likely to survive longer than 30 days after an acute whole-body exposure, especially if medical treatment is provided.

dose as low as 0.25 $Gy_t$ is sufficient to noticeably depress the number of such cells present in the circulating blood. When significant numbers of lymphocytes are damaged by radiation exposure, the body loses its natural ability to combat infection and becomes very susceptible to bacteria and viral antigens.

The normal white blood cell count for an adult ranges from 5000 to 10,000/mm³ of blood. At this dose level of 0.25 $Gy_t$ or less, complete blood cell recovery occurs shortly after irradiation. However, when a higher dose range of whole-body radiation (0.5 to 1 $Gy_t$) is received, the lymphocyte count decreases to zero within a few days. Full recovery generally requires a period of several months after this level of exposure.

**Effects of Ionizing Radiation on Neutrophils.** Neutrophils, another kind of white blood cell, also play an important role in fighting infection. A decrease in the number of these cells brought on by radiation exposure also increases a person's susceptibility to infection. A dose of 0.5 $Gy_t$ of ionizing radiation reduces the number of neutrophils present in the circulating blood. When they receive larger doses of radiation (2 to 5 $Gy_t$), however, these cells decrease in number to 10% or less within a few weeks of irradiation. A few months after the exposure, the number of neutrophils present in the blood returns to its original value.

**Effects of Ionizing Radiation on Granulocytes.** Granulocytes are a scavenger type of white blood cells that fight bacteria. They remain in the circulating blood for only a few days. These cells respond to irradiation by suddenly increasing in number. After this sudden increase, the granulocytes decrease in number, rapidly at first and then more slowly. Depending on the dose of radiation received, these cells may fully repopulate within approximately 2 months after their irradiation.

**Effects of Ionizing Radiation on Thrombocytes (Platelets).** Thrombocytes, or platelets, initiate blood clotting and prevent hemorrhage. They have a life span of approximately 30 days. The normal platelet count in the human adult ranges from 150,000 to 350,000/mm³ of blood. A dose of radiation greater than 0.5 $Gy_t$ lessens the number of platelets in the circulating blood, but when exposed to radiation in the range of 1 to 10 $Gy_t$, these cells may become significantly depleted and begin to regain their original numbers only approximately 2 months after being irradiated.

**Radiation Exposure during Diagnostic Imaging Procedures.** Neither the blood nor the blood-forming organs of patients should undergo appreciable damage from radiation exposure received during diagnostic imaging procedures. However, numerous studies indicate chromosome aberrations in circulating lymphocytes that received radiation doses within the diagnostic radiology range. Prime candidates for such aberrations are patients either for whom high-level fluoroscopy was employed or for whom very long fluoroscopic exposure times occurred (e.g., cardiac catheterization and other specialized invasive procedures).

**Monitoring of Patients Undergoing Radiation Therapy Treatment.** A therapeutic dose of ionizing radiation decreases the blood count. Patients who are undergoing radiation therapy treatment are monitored frequently (in the form of weekly or biweekly blood counts) to determine whether their platelet counts are adequate.

**Occupational Radiation Exposure Monitoring.** As previously discussed, a periodic blood count is not recommended as a method for monitoring occupational radiation exposure because biologic damage has already been sustained when an irregularity is seen in the blood count. In addition, a blood count is a relatively insensitive test that is unable to indicate exposures of less than 10 $cGy_t$. Traditional film badge dosimetry and state-of-the-art optically stimulated luminescence (OSL) dosimetry (see Chapter 5) detect effective doses in the millirem range and therefore may be used to discover potentially hazardous working conditions before actual hazards appear.

**Epithelial Tissue.** Epithelial tissue lines and covers body tissue. The cells of these tissues lie close together, with few or no substances between them. Epithelial tissue contains no blood vessels, and it regenerates through the process of mitosis. These cells are found in the lining of the intestines, the mucous lining of the respiratory tract, the pulmonary alveoli, and the lining of blood and lymphatic vessels. Because the body constantly regenerates epithelial tissue, the cells that comprise this tissue are highly radiosensitive.

**Muscle Tissue.** Muscle tissue contains fibers that affect movement of an organ or part of the body. Because muscle tissue cells are highly specialized and do not divide, they are relatively insensitive to radiation.

**Nervous Tissue.** Nervous tissue (conductive tissue) is found in the brain and spinal cord. A nerve cell (neuron) (Fig. 7-18) consists of a cell body and two kinds of very fine stringlike tissue segments, called *processes,* that extend outward— namely, dendrites (tentacle-like extensions from the cell body that carry impulses toward the cell) and the axon (a long, single tentacle from the cell body that carries impulses away from it). Nerve cells relay messages to and from the brain. A message enters the nerve cell through the

dendrites. It passes through the cell body and exits the cell through the axon, which transmits the message across a synapse, the communicating area leading to the next nerve cell in the chain.

***Nerve Tissue in the Human Adult.*** In the adult, nerve cells are highly specialized. They perform specific functions for the body and, similar to muscle cells, do not divide. Nerve cells contain a nucleus. If the nucleus of one of these cells is destroyed, the cell dies and is never restored. If the cell nucleus has been damaged but not destroyed by exposure to radiation, the damaged nerve cell may still be able to function but in a partially impaired fashion. Radiation also can cause temporary or permanent damage to a nerve's processes (dendrites and axon). When this occurs, communication with and control of some areas of the body may be disrupted. Whole-body exposure to very high doses of radiation causes severe damage to the central nervous system. A single exposure in excess of 50 $Gy_t$ of ionizing radiation may lead to death within a few hours or days.

***Nerve Tissue in the Embryo-Fetus.*** Developing nerve cells in the embryo-fetus are more radiosensitive than are the mature nerve cells of the adult. Irradiation of the embryo may lead to central nervous system anomalies, microcephaly (small head circumference), and mental retardation. Study of the Japanese atomic bomb survivors provides strong evidence of a "window of maximal sensitivity" extending from 8 to 15 weeks after gestation. This time span covers the end of *neuron organogenesis* (a period of development and change of the nerve cells) into the beginning of the fetal period. After this a lower level of risk remains until week 25, at which time the risk is not found to be significantly different from that of young adults. During the window of maximal sensitivity, a 0.1-Sv fetal EqD is associated with as much as a 4% chance of mental retardation. This level is considered significant compared with risks during a normal pregnancy. Therefore, special consideration is given to the irradiation of the abdomen or pelvis of a pregnant patient, particularly during the period of greatest sensitivity. The fetal EqD associated with

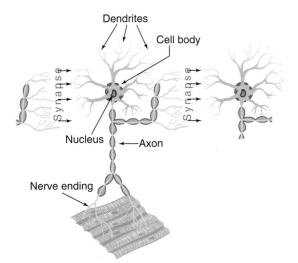

**FIGURE 7-18  A Nerve Cell (Neuron).** Nerve cells relay messages to and from the brain. A message enters a nerve cell through its dendrites, passes through the cell body, and exits the cell through the axon, which transmits the message across a synapse, the communication area leading to the next nerve cell in the chain.

abdominal fluoroscopy, however, is generally in the range of 0.05 Sv. Thus, if the referring physician and radiologist believe that the diagnostic imaging procedure is vital to the medical management of the mother or embryo-fetus, the risk associated with the needed radiation exposure may be justified.

### Reproductive Cells

*Spermatogonia.* Human reproductive cells (germ cells) are relatively radiosensitive, although the exact responses of male and female germ cells to ionizing radiation differ because their processes of development from immature to mature status differ. The male testes contain both mature and immature spermatogonia. Because the mature spermatogonia are specialized and do not divide, they are relatively insensitive to ionizing radiation. The immature spermatogonia, however, are unspecialized and divide rapidly, and therefore these germ cells are extremely radiosensitive. A radiation dose of 2 $Gy_t$ may cause temporary sterility for as long as 12 months, and a dose of 5 or 6 $Gy_t$ can cause permanent sterility. Even small doses of ionizing radiation (doses as low as 0.1 $Gy_t$) could depress the male sperm population. Male reproductive cells that have been exposed to a radiation dose of 0.1 $Gy_t$ or more may cause genetic mutations in future generations. To prevent mutations from being passed on to children, male patients receiving this level of testicular radiation dose should refrain from unprotected sex for a few months after such an exposure. By that time, cells that were irradiated during their most sensitive stages will have matured and disappeared. It is highly unlikely that germ cells of patients undergoing diagnostic imaging procedures would ever receive doses of 0.1 $Gy_t$, and radiographers working under normal occupational conditions would never receive a gonadal dose of this level.

*Ova.* The ova, the mature female germ cells, do not divide constantly. After puberty, one of the two ovaries expels a mature ovum approximately every 28 to 36 days (the exact number of days varies among women). During the reproductive life of a woman (from approximately 12 to

50 years old), 400 to 500 mature ova are produced. Radiosensitivity of ova varies considerably throughout the lifetime of the germ cell. Immature ova are very radiosensitive, whereas more mature ova have little radiosensitivity. After irradiation, a mature ovum can still unite with a male germ cell during conception. However, these irradiated cells may contain damaged chromosomes. If fertilization of an ovum with damaged chromosomes occurs, hereditary damage can be passed on to the child. A child who receives damaged chromosomes may be born with congenital abnormalities. In general, whenever chromosomes in male or female germ cells are damaged by exposure to ionizing radiation, it is possible for mutations to be passed on to succeeding generations. Even low doses received from diagnostic imaging procedures could cause chromosomal damage. For this reason, the reproductive organs should be shielded whenever possible.

Exposure to ionizing radiation also may cause female sterility. The dose necessary to produce this consequence depends partly on the age of the patient. Sterility occurs when radiation exposure destroys new and/or mature ova. The ovaries of the female fetus and those of a young child are very radiosensitive because they contain a large number of stem cells (oogonia) and immature cells (oocytes). As the female child matures from birth to puberty, the number of immature cells (oocytes) decreases. Hence the ovaries become less radiosensitive. This decrease continues up to the age of 30 years; women between the ages of 20 and 30 years exhibit the lowest level of sensitivity. After a woman reaches age 30 years, the overall sensitivity of the ovaries increases constantly until menopause because the new ova being destroyed are not replenished.[7-9] Because the ovaries of a younger woman are less sensitive overall than the ovaries of an older woman, a higher dose of radiation is required to cause sterility in the younger woman.

Temporary sterility usually results from a single radiation dose of 2 $Gy_t$ to the ovaries. If the radiation dose is fractionated (i.e., given as a combination of smaller doses with time between doses) over a period of several weeks, thus permitting the cells to repair some of the damage, doses as high as 20 $Gy_t$ may be tolerated.[10,11] A single dose of 5 $Gy_t$ generally causes permanent sterility in mature women. Even small doses of ionizing radiation (doses as low as 0.1 $Gy_t$) could cause menstrual irregularities such as delay or suppression of menstruation. Although some evidence suggests that immature ova are capable of repairing radiation damage, women who have received 0.1 $Gy_t$ or more are sometimes advised to postpone attempting conception for 30 days or more to allow the damaged immature ova to be expelled. Because all the ova a woman will ever possess are present from birth until the time they are fertilized or expelled, the best solution is to avoid substantial exposures in the first place.

## SUMMARY

- Linear energy transfer (LET)
  - LET is the average energy deposited per unit length of track by ionizing radiation as it passes through and interacts with a medium along its path.
    - It is described in units of keV per micron (1 micron [$\mu$m] $=10^{-6}$ m).
  - Because of a property known as wave-particle duality, x-rays and gamma rays can also be referred to as a stream of particles called photons.
  - Low-LET radiation (x-rays and gamma rays) mainly causes indirect damage to biologic tissues that usually can be reversed by repair enzymes.
  - High-LET radiation (alpha particles, ions of heavy nuclei, and low-energy neutrons) can cause irreparable damage to deoxyribonucleic acid (DNA) because multiple-strand breaks in DNA that cannot be undone by repair enzymes may result.
- Relative biologic effectiveness (RBE)
  - RBE for the type of radiation being used is the ratio of the dose of a reference

radiation (conventionally 250-kVp x-rays) to the dose of radiation of the type in question that is necessary to produce the same biologic reaction in a given experiment; the reaction is produced by a dose of test radiation delivered under the same conditions.
  - As the LET of radiation increases, so do biologic effects; RBE quantitatively describes this relative effect.
  - RBE describes the relative capabilities of radiation with differing LETs to produce a particular biologic reaction.
- Oxygen enhancement ratio (OER)
  - OER is a comparative measure used to obtain the amount of cellular injury for a species of ionizing radiation.
- Radiation-induced damage is observed on molecular, cellular, and organic levels.
- Radiation action on the cell is either direct or indirect, depending on site of interaction.
  - Action is direct when biologic damage occurs as a result of the ionization of atoms on DNA, thus causing them to become inactive or functionally altered.
  - Action is indirect when effects are produced by reactive free radicals created by the interaction of radiation with water molecules; these unstable, highly reactive molecules can cause substantial disruption to DNA molecules that results in cell death.
  - High-LET radiation is more likely to cause biologic damage through direct action than is low-LET radiation.
    - Most x-ray damage to macromolecules is the result of indirect action.
  - Point mutations commonly occur with low-LET radiation and are reversible through the action of repair enzymes.
  - Double-strand breaks of DNA are associated with high-LET radiation, and repair of this type of damage is not likely to occur.
  - Target theory states that when cell DNA is directly or indirectly inactivated by exposure to radiation, the cell will die.

- When a cell nucleus is significantly damaged by exposure to ionizing radiation, the cell can die or experience reproductive death, apoptosis, mitotic death, mitotic delay, interference with function, or chromosome breakage.
- The cell survival curve is used to display the radiosensitivity of a particular type of cell, which helps determine the types of cancer cells that will respond to radiation therapy.
- The law of Bergonié and Tribondeau states that the most pronounced radiation effects occur in cells having the least maturity and specialization, the greatest reproductive activity, and the longest mitotic phases.
  - The embryo-fetus is very susceptible to radiation damage, which can cause central nervous system (CNS) anomalies, microcephaly, and mental retardation.
  - Lymphocytes are the most radiosensitive blood cells, and when they are damaged the body loses its natural ability to combat infection and becomes more susceptible to bacterial and viral antigens.
  - Human germ cells are relatively radiosensitive; temporary sterilization occurs at 2 $Gy_t$; permanent sterilization occurs at 5 to 6 $Gy_t$.

# REFERENCES

1. Bushong SC: *Radiologic science for technologists: physics, biology and protection*, ed 10, St. Louis, 2013, Elsevier.
2. Forshier S: *Essentials of radiation biology and protection.* Albany, NY, 2002, Delmar.
3. Hall EJ: *Radiobiology for the radiologist*, ed 5, Philadelphia, 2000, Lippincott Williams & Wilkins.
4. Travis EL: *Primer of medical radiobiology*, ed 2, Chicago, 1989, Year Book.
5. Puck TT, Marcus PI: Action of x-rays on mammalian cells. *J Exp Med* 103:653, 1956.
6. Bergonié J, Tribondeau L: De quelques résultats de la radiothérapie et assai de fixation d'une technique rationelle. *CR Acad Sci (Paris)* 143:983, 1906.
7. United Nations Scientific Committee on the Effects of Atomic Radiation (UNSCEAR): *Ionizing radiation sources and biologic effects*, Report E.82.IX.8. New York, 1992, United Nations.
8. International Commission on Radiological Protection (ICRP): *Non-stochastic effects of ionizing radiation*, ICRP Publication No. 41. Oxford, 1984, Pergamon.
9. Upton AR: Cancer induction and non-stochastic effects. *Br J Radiol* 60:1, 1987.
10. Lushbaugh CC, Ricks RC: Some cytokinetic and histopathologic consideration of irradiated male and female gonadal tissue. In Vath JM, editor: *Frontiers of radiation therapy and oncology*, vol 6, Basel, 1972, Karger.
11. Lushbaugh CC, Casarett GW: The effects of gonadal irradiation in clinical radiation therapy: a review. *Cancer* 37:1111, 1976.

# GENERAL DISCUSSION QUESTIONS

1. Why is it necessary for persons who administer radiation to humans for medical purposes to have a basic understanding of cell structure, composition, and function, as well as the adverse effects of ionizing radiation on these entities?
2. What will an ionized atom of biologic tissue not be able to do?
3. Why is LET an important factor in assessing potential tissue and organ damage from exposure to ionizing radiation?
4. Why is high-LET radiation more destructive to biologic matter than low-LET radiation?
5. Why is the concept of relative biologic effectiveness (RBE) not practical for specifying radiation protection dose levels in humans?
6. Why does the presence of oxygen in biologic tissue make the damage produced in that tissue by free radicals permanent?
7. What consequences can occur if ionizing radiation damages germ (reproductive) cells?
8. How can ionizing radiation interact with a DNA macromolecule and create a point mutation?
9. Why is the embryo-fetus more susceptible to radiation damage than either the child or the adult?

10. Why is LD 50/60 a more accurate way to assess lethal dose for humans than LD 50/30?

## REVIEW QUESTIONS

1. For radiation protection, high-LET radiation is of *greatest* concern when a radionuclide has been implanted, ingested, injected, or inhaled because:
   A. Only single-strand breaks in DNA are possible.
   B. The potential exists for reparable damage of single-strand breaks in DNA.
   C. The potential exists for irreparable damage because multiple-strand breaks in DNA are possible.
   D. The potential exists for reparable damage in DNA resulting from multiple-strand breaks.
2. Free radicals behave as an extremely reactive single entity as a result of the presence of:
   A. Paired electrons.
   B. Unpaired electrons.
   C. Paired neutrons and protons.
   D. Unpaired neutrons and protons.
3. Which of the following are classified as high-LET radiation?
   1. Alpha particles
   2. Gamma rays
   3. X-rays
   A. 1 only
   B. 2 only
   C. 3 only
   D. 1, 2, and 3
4. A biologic reaction is produced by 3 $Gy_t$ of a test radiation. It takes 12 $Gy_t$ of 250-kVp x-radiation to produce the same biologic reaction. What is the relative biologic effectiveness (RBE) of the test radiation?
   A. 2.5
   B. 3
   C. 4
   D. 8

5. Which action of ionizing radiation is *most* harmful to the human body?
   A. Direct action
   B. Indirect action
   C. Epidemiologic action
   D. Mitotic action
6. Which molecules in the human body are most commonly directly acted on by ionizing radiation to produce molecular damage through an indirect action?
   A. Protein
   B. Carbohydrate
   C. Fat
   D. Water
7. When does ionizing radiation cause complete chromosome breakage?
   A. When a single strand of the sugar-phosphate chain sustains a direct hit
   B. When two direct hits occur in the same rung of the DNA macromolecule
   C. When two direct hits occur in different rungs of the DNA macromolecule
   D. When two direct hits are sustained at opposite ends of the DNA macromolecule
8. When significant numbers of lymphocytes are damaged by exposure from ionizing radiation, the body:
   1. Loses its natural ability to combat infection.
   2. Becomes more susceptible to bacteria.
   3. Becomes more susceptible to viral antigens.
   A. 1 and 2 only
   B. 1 and 3 only
   C. 2 and 3 only
   D. 1, 2, and 3

9. With respect to the law of Bergonié and Tribondeau, which of the following would *best* complete this statement? "The most pronounced radiation effects occur in cells having the _____."
   A. Least reproductive activity, shortest mitotic phases, and most maturity.
   B. Greatest reproductive activity, shortest mitotic phases, and most maturity.
   C. Greatest reproductive activity, longest mitotic phases, and least maturity.
   D. Least reproductive activity, shortest mitotic phases, and least maturity.

10. What do basal cells of the skin, intestinal crypt cells, and reproductive cells have in common?
    A. All cells are hypoxic.
    B. All cells are premalignant.
    C. All cells are radioinsensitive.
    D. All cells are radiosensitive.

# Early Deterministic Radiation Effects on Organ Systems

## OBJECTIVES

*After completing this chapter, the reader will be able to perform the following:*

- List four factors on which the amount of somatic and genetic (hereditary) biologic damage resulting from radiation exposure depends.
- List and describe the various early deterministic somatic effects of ionizing radiation on living systems.
- Describe acute radiation syndrome, and list three separate dose-related syndromes that occur as part of this total-body syndrome.
- Identify and describe the four major response stages of acute radiation syndrome.
- Recall the LD 50/30 for human adults, explain its significance, and explain why LD 50/60 is more accurate for humans as a measure of lethality.
- Explain why cells that are exposed to sublethal doses of ionizing radiation recover after irradiation, and discuss the cumulative effect that exists after repeated radiation injuries.
- Describe local tissue damage that occurs when any part of the human body receives high radiation exposure.
- List three factors on which organ and tissue responses to radiation exposure depend.
- Describe radiation-induced skin damage from a historical perspective, and identify the

person who became known as the first advocate of radiation protection.
- Differentiate among the three layers of human skin, and identify other related accessory structures.
- State the single absorbed dose of ionizing radiation that can cause radiation-induced skin erythema within 24 to 48 hours after irradiation, and describe how this dose first manifests.
- Explain the difference between moderate and large radiation doses with regard to epilation.
- State the energy range of grenz rays, and give a historical example of their use in treating disease.
- Discuss the concept of orthovoltage radiation therapy treatment, and identify how this radiation energy range affects human skin.
- Discuss the impact on human skin when high-level fluoroscopy is used for extended periods of time during cardiovascular or therapeutic interventional procedures.
- State the radiation dose that is capable of depressing the male sperm population and also has the potential to cause genetic mutations in future generations, and identify the radiation dose in girls or women that may delay or suppress menstruation.
- Explain the progression of both male and female germ cells from elementary stem cells

Copyright © 2014, Elsevier Inc.

to mature cells, and describe how this development affects cell radiosensitivity.
- State the dose of ionizing radiation necessary to cause both temporary and permanent sterility in male and female humans.
- Identify consequences other than impaired fertility for male and female humans, and discuss the benefit of gonadal shielding.
- State the whole-body radiation dose that would produce measurable hematologic depression, and identify the blood cells that are most sensitive to radiation exposure.
- List the components of the hematopoietic system, and identify the cells of this system that develop from a single pluripotential cell.

- Discuss the impact on the human body if radiation exposure causes a decrease in the cells that protect it against disease.
- Define *cytogenetics*, and explain how cytogenetic analysis of chromosomes may be accomplished.
- Explain the process of karyotyping, and identify the phase of cell division in which chromosome damage caused by radiation exposure can be evaluated.
- List two types of aberrations that can be caused by exposure to ionizing radiation, and explain what determines the rate of production of chromosome aberrations.

## CHAPTER OUTLINE

**Somatic and Genetic (Hereditary) Damage Factors**
**Somatic Effects**
    Early Deterministic Somatic Effects

Lethal Dose
Repair and Recovery
Local Tissue Damage

Hematologic Effects
Cytogenetic Effects
**Summary**

## KEY TERMS

acute radiation syndrome (ARS)
biologic dosimetry
chromosomal abnormalities
cytogenetics
desquamation
early deterministic somatic effects

epilation
genetic mutations
grenz rays
karyotype
latent period
manifest illness

metaphase
pluripotential stem cell
prodromal, or initial, stage
radiodermatitis
recovery
somatic effects

When biologic effects of radiation occur relatively soon after humans receive high doses of ionizing radiation, the biologic responses demonstrated are called *early effects*. Numerous laboratory animal studies and data from observation of some irradiated human populations provide substantial evidence of the consequences of such responses. Although early effects are not common in diagnostic imaging, they are discussed in this

chapter to provide the learner with a broader and more complete understanding of the impact of high radiation exposure on the human body.

## SOMATIC AND GENETIC (HEREDITARY) DAMAGE FACTORS

The amount of somatic and genetic (hereditary) biologic damage a human undergoes as a result of radiation exposure depends on several factors (Box 8-1). Ionizing radiation produces the greatest amount of biologic damage in the human body when a large dose of densely ionizing (high–linear energy transfer [LET]) radiation is delivered to a large or radiosensitive area of the body.

## SOMATIC EFFECTS

When living organisms, such as humans, experience biologic damage from exposure to radiation, the results of this exposure are classified as **somatic effects.** Depending on the length of time from the moment of irradiation to the first appearance of symptoms of radiation damage, the effects are classified as either:

1. Early somatic effects
2. Late somatic effects

This chapter discusses *early* radiation effects on organ systems. If the consequences include

*[handwritten: nonstochastic = deterministic]*

cell killing and are directly related to the dose received, they are termed **deterministic somatic effects** (formerly called *nonstochastic somatic effects*). (See Chapters 9 and 10 for additional information.) As the radiation dose increases, the severity of early deterministic somatic effects also increases. These results have a threshold, a point at which they begin to appear and below which they are absent (Fig. 8-1). The amount of biologic damage depends on the actual absorbed dose of ionizing radiation.

Late radiation effects on organ systems are discussed in Chapters 9 and 10. The two categories of late effects which are covered are:

- Late deterministic somatic effects
- Late stochastic (probabilistic) effects

Both of these types of late radiation-induced changes are consequences of high-level radiation exposure or of low doses of radiation delivered over a long interval of time.

### Early Deterministic Somatic Effects

**Early deterministic somatic effects** depend on the time of exposure to ionizing radiation. They appear within:

- Minutes
- Hours
- Days
- Weeks

---

| BOX 8-1 | Somatic and Genetic (Hereditary) Damage Factors |
|---|---|

1. The quantity of ionizing radiation to which the subject is exposed
2. The ability of the ionizing radiation to cause ionization of human tissue
3. The amount of body area exposed
4. The specific body parts exposed

---

*[handwritten: cell death directly related to dose = deterministic somatic effects]*

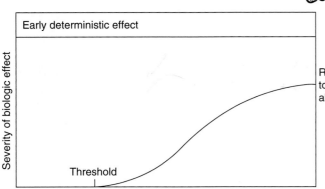

**FIGURE 8-1** This graph demonstrates the existence of a threshold whereby early deterministic effects of an absorbed dose of ionizing radiation begin and increase in severity as the dose of radiation received increases.

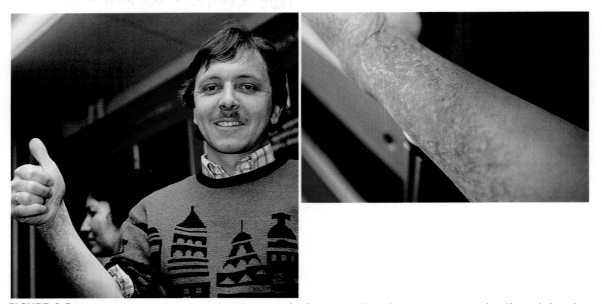

**FIGURE 8-2**  Radiation burn or erythema on the arm of a former worker who was present at the Chernobyl nuclear power plant during the 1986 radiation accident.

A substantial dose of ionizing radiation is required to produce biologic changes soon after irradiation. The severity of these is dose related. Early effects are precipitated by cell death.

With the exception of certain lengthy high–dose-rate fluoroscopic procedures, diagnostic imaging examinations do not usually impose radiation doses sufficient to cause early deterministic effects. Therefore, they are of little concern in this modality. Possible high-dose consequences include:

- Nausea
- Fatigue
- Erythema (diffuse redness over an area of skin after irradiation) (Fig. 8-2)
- Epilation (loss of hair)
- Blood disorders
- Intestinal disorders
- Fever
- Dry and moist desquamation (shedding of the outer layer of skin) (Fig. 8-3)
- Depressed sperm count in the male
- Temporary or permanent sterility in the male and female

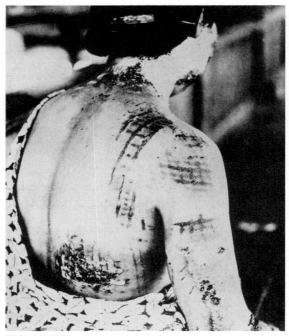

**FIGURE 8-3**  **Dry and Moist Desquamation.** The back of this female Japanese atomic bomb survivor demonstrates the pattern of the kimono she was wearing at the time of the bombing. Radiation burns resulting in the shedding of the outer layer of skin are visible.

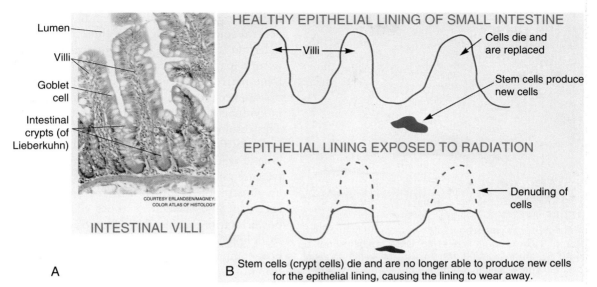

Lumen

Villi

Goblet cell

Intestinal crypts (of Lieberkuhn)

COURTESY ERLANDSEN/MAGNEY: COLOR ATLAS OF HISTOLOGY

INTESTINAL VILLI

HEALTHY EPITHELIAL LINING OF SMALL INTESTINE

Villi

Cells die and are replaced

Stem cells produce new cells

EPITHELIAL LINING EXPOSED TO RADIATION

Denuding of cells

A

B   Stem cells (crypt cells) die and are no longer able to produce new cells for the epithelial lining, causing the lining to wear away.

**FIGURE 8-4**   **A,** Intestinal villi. **B,** The *top drawing* depicts the healthy lining of the small intestine. The *bottom drawing* shows the epithelial lining of the small intestine after it has been exposed to radiation. Stem cells (crypt cells) die and are no longer able to produce new cells for the epithelial lining, thus causing the lining to wear away.

- Injury to the central nervous system (at extremely high radiation doses)

The various types of organic damage may be related to the cellular effects discussed in Chapter 7. For example, intestinal disorders are caused by damage to the sensitive epithelial tissue lining the intestines (Fig. 8-4). When the whole body is exposed to a dose of 6 $Gy_t$ of ionizing radiation, many of these manifestations of organic damage occur soon thereafter and in succession. These early deterministic somatic effects are called **acute radiation syndrome (ARS).**

**Acute Radiation Syndrome.** ARS, or radiation sickness, occurs in humans after whole-body reception of large doses of ionizing radiation delivered over a short period of time. Data from epidemiologic studies of human populations exposed to doses of ionizing radiation sufficient to cause this syndrome have been obtained from:

- Atomic bomb survivors of Hiroshima and Nagasaki
- Marshall Islanders who were inadvertently subjected to high levels of fallout during an atomic bomb test in 1954

- Nuclear radiation accident victims, such as those injured in the 1986 Chernobyl disaster
- Patients who have undergone radiation therapy

*Symptoms of Acute Radiation Syndrome.* *Syndrome* is the medical term that defines a collection of symptoms. ARS is a collection of symptoms associated with high-level radiation exposure. Three separate dose-related syndromes occur as part of the total-body syndrome:

- Hematopoietic syndrome
- Gastrointestinal syndrome
- Cerebrovascular syndrome

*Hematopoietic Syndrome.* The hematopoietic form of ARS, or "bone marrow syndrome," occurs when people receive whole-body doses of ionizing radiation ranging from 1 to 10 $Gy_t$ (Fig. 8-5). The hematopoietic system manufactures the corpuscular elements of the blood and is the most radiosensitive vital organ system in humans. Radiation exposure causes the number of red blood cells, white blood cells, and platelets in the circulating blood to decrease. Dose levels that cause this syndrome also may damage cells in

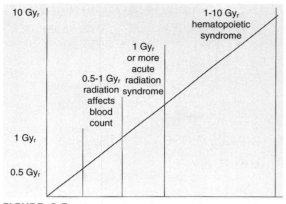

**FIGURE 8-5** The prodromal stage of acute radiation syndrome occurs within hours after a whole-body absorbed dose of 1 $Gy_t$ or more is received. Doses ranging from 1 to 10 $Gy_t$ are responsible for causing the hematopoietic form of acute radiation syndrome.

other organ systems and cause the affected organ or organ system to fail. For example, radiation doses ranging from 1 to 10 $Gy_t$ decrease the number of bone marrow stem cells. When the cells of the lymphatic system are damaged, the body loses some of its ability to combat infection. Because the number of platelets also decreases with loss of bone marrow function, the body loses a corresponding amount of its blood-clotting ability. This makes the body more susceptible to hemorrhage.

For persons with hematopoietic syndrome, survival time shortens as the radiation dose increases. Because additional bone marrow cells are destroyed, as the radiation dose escalates, the body becomes more susceptible to infection (mostly from its own intestinal bacteria) and more prone to hemorrhage. When death occurs, it is a consequence of bone marrow destruction.

Death may occur 6 to 8 weeks after irradiation in some sensitive human subjects who receive a whole-body dose exceeding 2 $Gy_t$. As the whole-body dose increases from 2 to 10 $Gy_t$, irradiated individuals die sooner. If the radiation exposure is not lethal, perhaps in the range of 1 to 2 $Gy_t$, bone marrow cells will eventually repopulate to a level adequate to support life in most individuals. Many of these people recover 3 weeks to 6 months after irradiation. The actual dose of

radiation received and the irradiated person's general state of health at the time of irradiation determine the possibility of recovery. When death occurs in exposed individuals, it results from bone marrow destruction. The severe reduction of blood cells causes anemia and permits exposed individuals to become susceptible to infection. This results in death of those individuals.

Survival probability of patients with hematopoietic syndrome is enhanced by intense supportive care and special hematologic procedures. As an illustration, victims who received doses in excess of 5 $Gy_t$, such as those of the nuclear power station accident in Chernobyl, benefited from bone marrow transplants from appropriate histocompatible donors. During the operation, hematopoietic stem cells are transplanted to facilitate bone marrow recovery. This operation, however, is not an absolute cure for patients with hematopoietic syndrome because many individuals undergoing bone marrow transplant die of burns or other radiation-induced damage they sustained before the transplanted stem cells have had a chance to support recovery.

***Gastrointestinal Syndrome.*** In humans, the gastrointestinal form of ARS appears at a threshold dose of approximately 6 $Gy_t$ and peaks after a dose of 10 $Gy_t$. Without medical support to sustain life, exposed persons receiving doses of 6 to 10 $Gy_t$ may die 3 to 10 days after being exposed. Even if medical support is provided, the exposed person will live only a few days longer. Survival time does not change with dose in this syndrome.

A few hours after the dose required to cause the gastrointestinal syndrome has been received, the prodromal stage occurs. Severe nausea, vomiting, and diarrhea persist for as long as 24 hours. This is followed by a latent period, which lasts as long as 5 days. During this time, the symptoms disappear. The manifest illness stage follows this period of false calm. Again, the human subject experiences:

- Severe nausea
- Vomiting
- Diarrhea

Other signs and symptoms that may occur include:

- Fever (as in hematopoietic syndrome)
- Fatigue
- Loss of appetite
- Lethargy
- Anemia
- Leukopenia (decrease in the number of white blood cells)
- Hemorrhage (gastrointestinal tract bleeding occurs because the body loses its blood-clotting ability)
- Infection
- Electrolyte imbalance
- Emaciation

Death occurs primarily because of catastrophic damage to the epithelial cells that line the gastrointestinal tract. Such severe damage to these cells causes the death of the exposed person within 3 to 5 days of irradiation as a result of infection, fluid loss, or electrolytic imbalance. Death from gastrointestinal syndrome is not exclusively from damage to the bowel, but it also can be induced by damage to the bone marrow. Bone marrow damage is usually sufficient to cause death in hematopoietic syndrome.

The small intestine is the most severely affected part of the gastrointestinal tract. Because epithelial cells function as an essential biologic barrier, their breakdown leaves the body vulnerable to:

- Infection (mostly from its own intestinal bacteria)
- Dehydration
- Severe diarrhea

Some epithelial cells regenerate before death occurs. However, because of the large number of epithelial cells damaged by the radiation, death may occur before cell regeneration is accomplished. The workers and firefighters at Chernobyl are examples of humans who died as a result of gastrointestinal syndrome.

***Cerebrovascular Syndrome.*** The cerebrovascular form of ARS results when the central nervous system and cardiovascular system receive doses of 50 $Gy_t$ or more of ionizing radiation. A

dose of this magnitude can cause death within a few hours to 2 or 3 days after exposure. After irradiation, the prodromal stage begins. Signs and symptoms include:

- Excessive nervousness
- Confusion
- Severe nausea
- Vomiting
- Diarrhea
- Loss of vision
- Burning sensation of the skin
- Loss of consciousness

A latent period lasting up to 12 hours follows. During this time, symptoms lessen or disappear. After the latent period, the manifest illness stage occurs. During this period, the prodromal syndrome recurs with increased severity, and other symptoms appear, including:

- Disorientation and shock
- Periods of agitation alternating with stupor
- Ataxia (confusion and lack of muscular coordination)
- Edema in the cranial vault
- Loss of equilibrium
- Fatigue
- Lethargy
- Convulsive seizures
- Electrolytic imbalance
- Meningitis
- Prostration
- Respiratory distress
- Vasculitis
- Coma

Damaged blood vessels and permeable capillaries permit fluid to leak into the brain and cause an increase in fluid content. This creates an increase in intracranial pressure, which causes additional tissue damage. The final result of this damage is failure of the central nervous and cardiovascular systems, which causes death in a matter of minutes. Because the gastrointestinal and hematopoietic systems are more radiosensitive than the central nervous system, they also are severely damaged and fail to function after a dose of this magnitude. However, because death

| Stage | Dose ($Gy_t$) | Average Survival Time | Symptoms |
|---|---|---|---|
| Prodromal | 1 | — | Nausea, vomiting, diarrhea, fatigue, leukopenia |
| Latent | 1-100 | — | None |
| Hematopoietic | 1-10 | 6-8 wk (doses over 2 $Gy_t$) | Nausea; vomiting; diarrhea; decrease in number of red blood cells, white blood cells, and platelets in the circulating blood; hemorrhage; infection |
| Gastrointestinal | 6-10 | 3-10 days | Severe nausea, vomiting, diarrhea, fever, fatigue, loss of appetite, lethargy, anemia, leukopenia, hemorrhage, infection, electrolytic imbalance, and emaciation |
| Cerebrovascular | 50 and above | Several hours to 2-3 days | Same as hematopoietic and gastrointestinal, plus excessive nervousness, confusion, lack of coordination, loss of vision, burning sensation of the skin, loss of consciousness, disorientation, shock, periods of agitation alternating with stupor, edema, loss of equilibrium, meningitis, prostration, respiratory distress, vasculitis, coma |

**TABLE 8-1** | **Overview of Acute Radiation Lethality**

occurs quickly, the consequences of the failure of these two systems are not demonstrated.

An overview of acute radiation lethality is presented in Table 8-1. The radiation dose required to cause a particular syndrome and the average survival time are the most important measures used to quantify human radiation lethality. The progression of each syndrome, the length of time required for the consequential chain of events to occur, and the final outcome depend on the effective dose received.

***Major Response Stages of Acute Radiation Syndrome.*** ARS presents in four major response stages:

- Prodromal (initial)
- Latent period
- Manifest illness
- Recovery or death (Fig. 8-6)

The **prodromal, or initial, stage,** also called *prodromal syndrome*, occurs within hours after a whole-body absorbed dose of 1 $Gy_t$ or more (see Fig. 8-6). This initial stage is characterized by:

- Nausea
- Vomiting

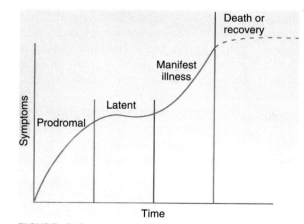

**FIGURE 8-6** The graph depicts the stages of acute radiation syndrome following whole-body reception of large doses of ionizing radiation delivered over a short period of time. The length of time involved for the syndrome to run its course and the final outcome of the syndrome depend on the dose received.

- Diarrhea
- Fatigue
- Leukopenia (an abnormal decrease in white blood corpuscles, usually to less than 5000/mm³)

The severity of these symptoms is dose related; the higher the dose, the more severe the symptoms. The length of time involved for this stage to run its course may be hours or a few days. After the prodromal stage, a **latent period** of approximately 1 week follows during which no visible symptoms occur. Actually, it is during this period that either recovery or lethal effects begin. Toward the end of the first week, the next stage commences. This stage is called **manifest illness** because it is the period when signs and symptoms that affect the hematopoietic, gastrointestinal, and cerebrovascular systems become visible. Some of these signs and symptoms are:

- Apathy
- Confusion
- Decreased numbers of red and white blood cells and platelets in the circulating blood
- Fluid loss
- Dehydration
- Epilation
- Exhaustion
- Vomiting
- Severe diarrhea
- Fever
- Headaches
- Infection
- Hemorrhage
- Cardiovascular collapse

In severe high-dose cases, emaciated human beings eventually die.

If, after a whole-body sublethal dose such as 2 to 3 $Gy_t$, exposed persons pass through the first three stages but show less severe symptoms than those seen after superlethal doses of 6 to 10 $Gy_t$, recovery may occur in approximately 3 months. However, persons who recover may show some signs of radiation damage and experience late effects.

***Acute Radiation Syndrome as a Consequence of the Chernobyl Nuclear Power Plant Accident.*** The massive explosion that blew apart a reactor (unit 4) at the nuclear power station in Chernobyl in the Soviet Union (see Fig. 2-7) on April 26, 1986, provides an example of humans developing ARS. During the explosion,

several tons of burning graphite, uranium dioxide fuel, and other contaminants such as cesium-137, iodine-131, and plutonium-239 were ejected vertically into the atmosphere in a 3-mile–high radioactive plume of intense heat. Of 444 people working at the power plant at the time of the explosion, 2 died instantly, and 29 died within 3 months of the accident as a consequence of thermal trauma (burns) and severe injuries from doses of whole-body ionizing radiation of approximately 6 $Gy_t$ or more.[1-3]

Without effective physical monitoring devices, biologic criteria such as the occurrence of nausea and vomiting played an important role in the identification of radiation casualties during the first 2 days after the nuclear disaster. ARS caused the hospitalization of at least 203 people.[3,4] A determination of the lapse of time from the incidental exposure of the victims to the onset of nausea and/or regurgitation completed the biologic criteria. Dose assessment was determined from **biologic dosimetry.** This included serial measurements of levels of lymphocytes and granulocytes in the blood and a quantitative analysis of dicentric chromosomes (chromosomes having two centromeres) in blood and hematopoietic cells, coming from bone marrow. The data were compared with doses and effects from earlier radiation mishaps.[2,3]

***Acute Radiation Syndrome as a Consequence of the Atomic Bombing of Hiroshima and Nagasaki.*** The Japanese atomic bomb survivors of Hiroshima and Nagasaki are examples of a human population affected by ARS as a consequence of war. Follow-up studies of the survivors who did not die of ARS demonstrated late deterministic (e.g., cataracts) and stochastic effects of ionizing radiation. The atomic bombing of Japan and the nuclear accident at Chernobyl made the medical community recognize the need for a thorough understanding of ARS and appropriate medical support of persons affected.

## Lethal Dose (LD)

**LD 50/30.** The term *LD 50/30* signifies the whole-body dose of radiation that can be lethal to 50% of the exposed population within 30 days. This is a quantitative measurement that is fairly precise when applied to experimental animals. Humans exposed to substantial whole-body doses of ionizing radiation, however, take longer to recover than do laboratory animals. Hence the LD 50 for humans may require more than 30 days for its full expression. As stated in Chapter 7, the LD 50/30 for adult humans is estimated to be 3.0 to 4.0 Gy$_t$ without medical support (Fig. 8-7). For x-rays and gamma rays, this is equal to an equivalent dose of 3.0 to 4.0 Sv. Whole-body doses greater than 6 Gy$_t$ may cause the death of the entire population in 30 days without medical support. With medical support, human beings have tolerated doses as high as 8.5 Gy$_t$.[5]

**LD 10/30, LD 50/60, and LD 100/60.** Other measures of lethality also are quoted, such as *LD 10/30, LD 50/60,* and *LD 100/60.* All these measures refer to the percentage of subjects who die after a certain number of days. The values reported in the literature vary widely because most lethal dose data represent an estimate of the role played by radiation in fatalities in which other factors (e.g., fire at Chernobyl, physical effects of a large explosion at Hiroshima and Nagasaki, chemical contamination in a few nuclear accidents) were present. Specifications of lethal effects are further complicated by the medical treatment that the patient may receive during the prodromal and latent stages, before many of the symptoms of ARS appear. When medical treatment is given promptly, the patient is supported through initial symptoms, but the question of long-term survival may simply be delayed. Thus survival over a 60-day period may be a more relevant indicator of outcome for humans than is survival over a 30-day period. For this reason, LD 50/60 for humans may be more accurate. Table 8-2 gives estimates of lethal doses, including the treatment given in populations studied. Regardless of treatment,

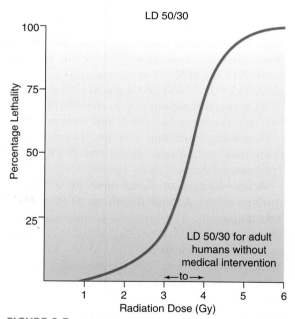

LD 50/30

**FIGURE 8-7** *LD 50/30* refers to the whole-body dose of radiation that can be lethal to 50% of the exposed population within 30 days. As can be seen in the graph, no deaths are expected below 1 Gy$_t$. In this particular graph, which represents the human response to radiation exposure, LD 50/30 is reached at 3.5 Gy$_t$, a dose that falls between 3.0 and 4.0 Gy$_t$. This is the point at which half of those exposed to 3.5 Gy$_t$ of ionizing radiation would die. The graph also demonstrates that at a dose of 6 Gy$_t$ no one is expected to survive. In reality, survival is possible with extensive medical intervention.

| TABLE 8-2 | Lethal Dose Values for Healthy Adults Who Receive the Specified Medical Treatment after Exposure to Low–Linear Energy Transfer Radiation at Dose Rates of More Than 100 mGy$_a$/min |
|---|---|

| Effect | Treatment | Dose (Gy$_a$) |
|---|---|---|
| LD 50/60 | Minimal | 3.2-4.5 |
| LD 50/60 | Optimal supportive | 4.8-5.4 |
| LD 50/60 | Autologous bone marrow transplantation | 11 |

From Fry RJM: Acute radiation effects. In Wagner LK Fabrikant JI, Fry RJM, editors: *Radiation bioeffects and management: test and syllabus,* Reston, Va, 1991, American College of Radiology.

whole-body equivalent doses of greater than 12 Gy$_t$ are considered fatal.[6]

## Repair and Recovery

Because cells contain a repair mechanism inherent in their biochemistry (repair enzymes), repair and recovery can occur when cells are exposed to sublethal doses of ionizing radiation. After irradiation, surviving cells begin to repopulate. This process permits an organ that has sustained functional damage as a result of radiation exposure to regain some or most of its functional ability. However, the amount of functional damage sustained determines the organ's potential for recovery. In the repair of sublethal damage, oxygenated cells, which receive more nutrients, have a better prospect for recovery than do hypoxic (poorly oxygenated) cells that consequently receive fewer nutrients. When both oxygenated and hypoxic cells are exposed to a comparable dose of low-LET radiation, the oxygenated cells are more severely damaged, but those that survive repair themselves and recover from the injury. Even though they are less severely damaged, the hypoxic cells do not repair and recover as efficiently.

Research has shown that repeated radiation injuries have a cumulative effect. Hence a percentage (approximately 10%) of the radiation-induced damage is irreparable, whereas the remaining 90% may be repaired over time. When the processes of repair and repopulation work together, they aid in healing the body from radiation injury and promote recovery.

## Local Tissue Damage

A destructive response in biologic tissue can occur when any part of the human body receives a high radiation dose. Significant cell death usually results after such a substantial partial-body exposure. This leads to the shrinkage of organs and tissues, a process referred to as *atrophy.* Organs and tissues sustaining such damage can lose their ability to function, or they may possibly recover. If recovery of the irradiated biologic structures does occur, it may be partial or complete, depending on the types of cells involved and the dose of radiation received. If organ or tissue recovery fails to occur, necrosis, or death, of the irradiated biologic structure results.

Organ and tissue response to radiation exposure depends on factors such as:

- Radiosensitivity
- Reproductive characteristics
- Growth rate

Some local tissues suffer immediate consequences from high radiation doses. Examples of such tissues include the following:

- Skin
- Male and female reproductive organs
- Bone marrow

**Effects on the Skin.** From the unfortunate experiences of early pioneers (see Chapter 4), radiation accident victims, atomic bomb survivors (discussed earlier in this chapter; see Figs. 8-2 and 8-3), and patients who have received radiation therapy in certain areas, a considerable amount of information is available on radiation-induced skin damage. As stated in Chapter 4, many early radiologists and dentists developed **radiodermatitis**, a significant reddening of the skin caused by excessive exposure to ionizing radiation that eventually led to cancerous lesions on the hands and fingers (see Fig. 4-5). In 1898, after suffering severe burns attributed to radiation exposure, William Herbert Rollins, a Boston dentist, began investigating the hazards of radiation exposure and became the first known advocate of radiation protection. Rollins performed experiments on guinea pigs that led to "three important safety practices: wear radiopaque glasses; enclose the x-ray tube in protective housing; and irradiate only areas of interest on the patient, covering adjacent areas with radiopaque materials."[7] Unfortunately, at the time Rollins made the recommendations, they were not given much attention. The misfortune of ignoring his suggestions led to continuing radiation-induced injuries. Eventually, however, our pioneers did learn from their misfortunes.

THICK SKIN

THIN SKIN

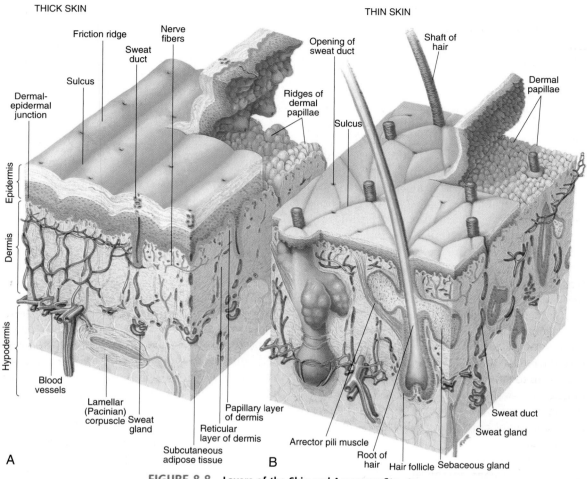

**FIGURE 8-8    Layers of the Skin and Accessory Structures.**

The skin consists of three layers (Fig. 8-8):

- Epidermis, or outer layer
- Dermis, or middle layer composed of connective tissue
- Hypodermis, a subcutaneous layer of fat and connective tissue

Accessory structures include hair follicles, sensory receptors, sebaceous glands, and sweat glands. All the layers of the skin, as well as its accessory structures, are actively involved in the response of the tissue to radiation exposure.

Because the skin functions as an ongoing regeneration system, it is relatively radiosensitive. Approximately 2% of the body's surface

skin cells are replaced daily by stem cells from an underlying basal layer. The characteristics of these stem cells are actually responsible for the radiosensitivity of the skin. A single absorbed dose of 2 $Gy_t$ can cause radiation-induced skin erythema within 24 to 48 hours after irradiation (see Table 2-2). As time progresses, over the next week or two, the erythema becomes much greater until it reaches its maximal intensity. **Desquamation,** or shedding of the outer layer of skin, occurs at higher radiation doses. It generally manifests first as moist desquamation, and then dry desquamation may develop (see Fig. 8-3).

**Epilation,** or hair loss (also called alopecia), can be caused when individuals are exposed to radiation because hair follicles are growing tissue. Moderate doses of radiation may result in temporary hair loss, whereas large radiation doses can result in permanent hair loss.

Historically, skin diseases, such as ringworm, were treated and successfully cured by irradiating the affected area with **grenz rays** (x-rays in the energy range of 10 to 20 kVp).[5] These soft, low-energy rays were adequate to cure the disease. However, if the ringworm was located on the scalp, the local irradiation of that area also caused the hair to fall out for a period of time. This would normally be followed by regrowth, provided the radiation dose delivered to the patient was not sufficient to cause permanent hair loss.

Significant evidence of skin damage, as a consequence of exposure to orthovoltage radiation therapy (x-rays in the range of 200 to 300 kVp), comes from oncology patients who underwent such treatments in earlier years for deep-seated tumors. With orthovoltage irradiation used for this purpose, the ability of an individual person's skin to tolerate this exposure actually determined the total amount of treatment radiation the individual could receive, especially when only one radiation entrance surface portal was employed.

The overall goal of the treatment was to deposit the radiant energy at a predetermined, specific location within a specified treatment volume enclosing the tumor while sparing as much healthy surrounding tissue as possible. Orthovoltage radiation treatments caused the patient's skin to receive a higher radiation dose than the dose received by the tumor volume because radiation in this energy range was substantially absorbed while traversing the skin and other intervening tissue layers before it reached the tumor. Thus, to deliver a specific dose to the tumor, the superficial, or skin dose, would unavoidably be increased significantly. This often resulted in an area of diffuse redness, or *erythema*, of the skin at the treatment entrance site. If that radiation dose was high enough, moist desquamation of the irradiated skin would occur, followed by dry desquamation of the skin.

During cardiovascular or therapeutic interventional procedures that use high-level fluoroscopy for extended periods of time, the effects of ionizing radiation on the skin are significant. Patient exposure rates have been estimated to range from 100 to 200 $mGy_a$/min and sometimes even greater. A list of radiation-induced skin injuries may be found in Table 11-2. Additional information on high-level fluoroscopy may also be found in Chapter 11. As a result of numerous reported injuries to patients that were associated with the use of high-level fluoroscopy, imposing strict controls on its use is essential.

**Effects on the Reproductive System.** Some of the early deterministic effects of ionizing radiation are discussed in Chapter 7.

Human germ cells are relatively radiosensitive. Doses as low as 0.1 $Gy_t$ can depress the male sperm population, and this same dose has the potential to cause **genetic mutations** in future generations. In girls and women, a gonadal dose of 0.1 $Gy_t$ may delay or suppress menstruation.

Because the reproductive organs of both the male and female produce the germ cells that control fertility and heredity, many studies have been performed to document this important information. Animal experiments and data from irradiated human populations have provided significant information on gonadal response to radiation exposure. Irradiated human populations include:

- Patients who have undergone radiation therapy
- Radiation accident victims
- Volunteer convicts[8,9]

The testes of the male and ovaries of the female do not respond in the same way to irradiation because of the difference in the way in which these cells are produced and progress from elementary stem cells to mature cells. The spermatogonia, the stem cells of the testes, constantly reproduce. They mature and become spermatocytes. These cells then multiply and develop into spermatids that eventually differentiate and become spermatozoa, or sperm, which are the functionally mature germ cells (Fig. 8-9).

**Male:**

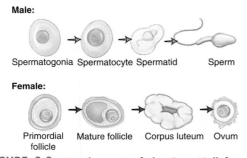

Spermatogonia   Spermatocyte   Spermatid        Sperm

**Female:**

Primordial    Mature follicle   Corpus luteum   Ovum
follicle

**FIGURE 8-9   Development of the Germ Cell from the Stem Cell Phase to the Mature Cell.**

The development of the male stem cell into a functionally mature germ cell takes 3 to 5 weeks.[5]

In the female, the oogonia, the ovarian stem cells, multiply to millions of cells only during fetal development, before birth, and then they steadily decline in number throughout life. During the later part of fetal development, the oogonia become encapsulated by numerous primordial (primary) follicles that actually grow around them. The oogonia eventually become oocytes, which contain follicles that are nests of cells, some of which eventually mature during the reproductive life of a woman. Before these primary oocyte-containing follicles grow into mature follicles, they actually remain dormant until puberty. However, just before puberty, the oocytes are reduced in number to only several hundred thousand. Some of the cells of the primary follicles proliferate in response to stimulation by hormones from the pituitary gland, and these cells begin to mature. At the same time, the ovum contained within each of the follicles undergoes meiosis. As puberty begins, the developed ova, or mature female germ cells, within the follicles are ejected when the follicles themselves rupture. Usually only one follicle will fully mature and move toward the surface of the ovary to be expelled, and the others disintegrate. This process occurs at regular time intervals of approximately 28 days. Of the mature ova that are actually enclosed within the follicles, only 400 to 500 are produced, matured, and made available for fertilization during a woman's reproductive life cycle.

Follicles range in size from small to large. Of these, the intermediate-size follicles are the most radiosensitive, and the small follicles are least radiosensitive. Large mature follicles possess a moderate degree of radiosensitivity.[10] During the female menstrual cycle, the mature follicle releases an ovum during the period of ovulation, when a ripe ovum is expelled into the pelvic cavity. If the ovum is not fertilized by a male sperm, it will be lost during menstruation and not replaced.

*Testes.* The male testes contain both mature and immature spermatogonia. Mature spermatogonia are specialized, nondividing cells that are relatively radioresistant. Immature spermatogonia, however, are unspecialized cells that divide rapidly and are extremely radiosensitive. Irradiation of these immature cells can lead to damage and reduction in the number of spermatogonia produced. This reduction in the number of spermatogonia eventually causes depletion of mature sperm. This is referred to as *maturation depletion.* Temporary sterility may occur and last for as long as 12 months when the testes receive a radiation dose of 2 Gy$_t$. The infertility actually begins approximately 2 months after the initial irradiation because the maturing cells that are present, the spermatocytes and spermatids, are relatively insensitive to radiation and continue to mature. Because of this, fertility continues during this period of time.

Permanent sterility is most likely to be induced by a radiation dose of 5 or 6 Gy$_t$ to the testes. High radiation doses to the testes can also result in atrophy. When sterility is temporary, fertility will return; however, it is possible that there could be **chromosomal abnormalities** in the functional spermatogonia that may be passed on to future generations. Imaging procedures generally produce relatively low doses of gonadal radiation for the patient and for imaging personnel. Therefore, the chance of causing sterility is negligible. However, because any dose of radiation to the gonads could cause chromosomal abnormalities, the testes should be protected with lead shielding whenever possible.

***Ovaries.*** As discussed in Chapter 7, radiosensitivity of the ova varies considerably throughout the lifetime of the germ cell. During the fetal stage of life and during early childhood, the ovaries are very radiosensitive because they contain a large number of stem cells (oogonia) and immature cells (oocytes). If the ovaries are irradiated during this period of time, germ cell death will occur as a consequence of ovarian atrophy. After puberty and the onset of menstruation, one of the two ovaries expels a mature ovum approximately every 28 to 36 days (the exact number of days varies among women). From approximately 12 to 50 years of age, as previously mentioned, only a total of 400 to 500 mature ova are produced. A dose of 0.1 $Gy_t$ to the gonads may delay or suppress menstruation. Radiosensitivity of the ovaries declines between ages 20 and 30 years, and then, after approximately age 30 years, radiosensitivity increases constantly with age until menopause commences because new ova are not replenished after they have been lost. A single radiation exposure of 2 $Gy_t$ to the ovaries usually results in temporary sterility of the woman, whereas a dose of 5 to 6 $Gy_t$ results in permanent sterility.

For the female, impaired fertility may not be the only consequence of gonadal irradiation. Genetic mutations are possible. They have been produced in experimental animals when their ovaries were irradiated with doses as low as 0.25 $Gy_t$. Fertility usually recurs, following irradiation of the ovaries with low to moderate radiation doses. The functional ova, however, may have chromosomal damage that can be passed on to future generations. For this reason, the ovaries should be shielded during all imaging procedures whenever possible.

## Hematologic Effects

Radiation protection programs have long since abandoned relying on hematologic depression as a means for monitoring imaging personnel, to assess whether they have sustained any degree of radiation damage from occupational exposure. During the 1920s and 1930s, periodic blood counts were the only means of radiation exposure monitoring for radiation workers engaged in radiologic practices. The use of personnel dosimeters for monitoring of occupational exposure made the practice of requiring periodic blood counts for monitoring radiation damage obsolete.

As determined during the years when such monitoring was employed, a whole-body dose as low as 0.25 $Gy_t$ would produce measurable hematologic depression. This dose could cause a decrease in the number of lymphocytes in the blood and, as a consequence, leave the body vulnerable to infection by foreign invaders because the body simply did not produce sufficient antibodies to combat disease.

**Hematopoietic System.** The hematopoietic system consists of:

- Bone marrow
- Circulating blood
- Lymphoid organs (lymph nodes, spleen, and thymus gland)

Cells of this system all develop from a single precursor cell, the **pluripotential stem cell.** The following are other types of cells that originate from this one type of elementary cell: lymphocytes; granulocytes (white blood cells that act as scavengers to fight bacteria); thrombocytes, or platelets (blood cells that initiate blood clotting and prevent hemorrhage); and erythrocytes (red blood cells that through their hemoglobin carry oxygen from the lungs to all body tissue and cells as blood circulates). Figure 8-10 demonstrates the progressive development of these cells from a single pluripotential stem cell. Most of these blood cells are manufactured in bone marrow at different intervals, and when they mature, they enter the blood capillaries and peripheral circulation. Even though blood cells are constantly being produced, the life span of each individual type of blood cell differs, varying on average from only a few hours (e.g., lymphocytes) to almost 120 days (e.g., erythrocytes).

Because the hematopoietic system is a cell regeneration system, the effects of ionizing radiation on this system are governed by normal

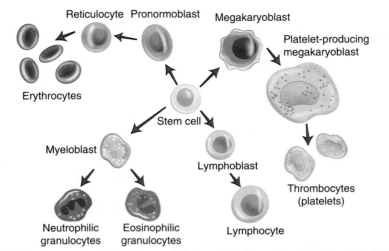

**FIGURE 8-10** **Progressive Development of Various Cells from a Single Pluripotential Stem Cell.**

cell growth and development. The most pronounced effect of radiation on this system is a reduction in the number of blood cells in the peripheral circulation. Highly specialized, nondividing cells in the circulating blood, with the exception of lymphocytes, are relatively insensitive to radiation.

If the number of radiosensitive stem cells in bone marrow is reduced as a consequence of irradiation, this decrease will manifest as a reduction in the number of mature circulating blood cells, thus indicating the presence of radiation damage in the bone marrow. The individual sensitivity of each type of precursor cell and the life span of cells of each of these different types in the circulating blood are factors in determining the degree of bone marrow damage. When precursor cells are irradiated with a radiation dose as low as 0.1 $Gy_t$, the number of lymphocytes in the blood will lessen before other blood cells are affected. Although lymphocytes are first in radiation sensitivity and response, neutrophils (leukocytes that fight infection) are second to respond and demonstrate a decrease in number if they are exposed to a dose of 0.5 $Gy_t$. Thrombocytes, or platelets, and red blood cells may be considered third to respond when the radiation dose received is greater than 0.5 $Gy_t$.[11]

Lymphocytes receiving low radiation doses, however, demonstrate only a slight depression in number. This depression is followed by recovery and then a return to preexposure normal values. If lymphocytes receive a moderate dose of radiation (e.g., 0.25 $Gy_t$, which is considered moderate), the lymphocyte count will come close to zero within just a few days, but this minuscule count will return to normal values within a few months after exposure, thus indicating full recovery.

For thrombocytes and erythrocytes, radiation doses in the moderate range have very slight effects. However, higher doses cause a significant cell depression; recovery commences only approximately 4 weeks after exposure and then takes a few months to complete.

The human body may experience health-related consequences throughout life if there is a decrease in the numbers of these various cells. If cells that protect the body against disease are noticeably reduced in number, the body's ability to combat infection will worsen substantially, and vulnerability to aggressive infectious organisms will increase dramatically. If cells that are needed to clot blood are depleted, the risk for hemorrhage will increase. A decrease in the number of red blood cells in the circulating blood

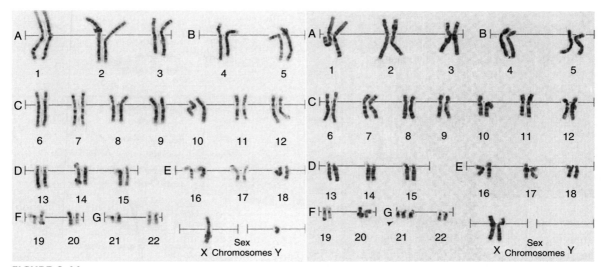

**FIGURE 8-11**   A photomicrograph of the human cell nucleus at metaphase that shows each chromosome individually demonstrated. The karyotype is constructed by cutting out the individual chromosomes and pairing them with their sister chromosomes. These chromosome pairs are usually aligned by size, beginning with the largest pair and ending with the smallest pair. The left karyotype is male, and the right is female.

can result in a lack of vitality and a condition known as *anemia.*

Radiation doses resulting from diagnostic imaging procedures during which appropriate radiation protection methods have been employed for patients and all personnel result in negligible damage to the blood and the blood-forming organs. However, in this dose range, some chromosomal changes in circulating lymphocytes have been observed.

## Cytogenetic Effects

In simple terms, **cytogenetics** may be defined as the study of cell genetics with an emphasis on cell chromosomes. The techniques used to study and observe the chromosomes of each human cell have greatly contributed to genetic analysis and radiation genetics and have led to numerous observations on radiation-induced chromosome damage.

A cytogenetic analysis of chromosomes may be accomplished through the use of a chromosome map called a **karyotype.** This map consists of a photograph, or *photomicrograph,* that is

taken of the human cell nucleus during metaphase, when each chromosome can be individually demonstrated. The karyotype is constructed by cutting out the individual chromosomes and pairing them on the map with their sister chromosomes. These chromosome pairs are usually aligned by size, beginning with the largest pair and ending with the smallest pair (Fig. 8-11).

**Metaphase** is the phase of cell division in which chromosome damage caused by radiation exposure can be evaluated. *Chromosome aberrations* (deviation from normal development or growth) and *chromatid aberrations* have been observed at metaphase.

Both low and high radiation doses can cause chromosomal damage that may not be apparent immediately. Most chromosomal damage results from the process of indirect action of ionizing radiation on vital biologic macromolecules. Chromosome breakage occurs as a consequence of this damage. Only a very small percentage of chromosome breakage occurs from the direct action of ionizing radiation on a macromolecule such as deoxyribonucleic acid (DNA). The mechanisms of direct and indirect action of ionizing radiation on biologic macromolecules and the early effects of ionizing radiation on chromosomes are discussed in Chapter 7.

Almost every type of chromosome aberration can be brought about by exposure to ionizing radiation. However, some aberrations can also be produced "only" by radiation exposure.[5] The total radiation dose received to a somatic or genetic (hereditary) cell and the period of time in which that dose was delivered determine the rate of production of chromosome aberrations.

Attempts have been made to measure chromosome aberrations after diagnostic x-ray imaging procedures, but successful results have not been achieved in these studies. For imaging procedures that involve somewhat higher radiation dose rates, studies demonstrated that radiation-induced chromosome imperfections were observed shortly after the imaging procedure was completed.

Increased frequency of chromosome translocations is an established radiation biomarker and may also suggest increased cancer risk.[12] An occupational epidemiologic study of 146,000 U.S. radiologic technologists began in 1982 and is still in progress. This study is a collaborative effort of the University of Minnesota School of Public Health, the National Cancer Institute, and the American Registry of Radiologic Technologists.[13,14] The purpose of the research is "to determine whether their personal cumulative exposure to diagnostic x-rays was associated with increased frequencies of chromosome translocations"[12] and possible associated cancer risk. Included in the study were mail surveys, telephone interviews, and a collection of 150 blood samples for testing purposes. Results of the blood tests indicated increased chromosome damage as a consequence of cumulative work-related exposure from routine x-ray procedures[12] (see Chapter 9 for additional discussion of the U.S. radiologic technologists study). For patients, increased computed tomography (CT) and nuclear medicine procedures can contribute substantially to higher radiation exposure. "Some studies have found increased chromosome abnormalities

immediately after radiation exposure from CT scanning"[12,15] or in patients with unusually high numbers of diagnostic procedures.[12,16]

## SUMMARY

- The amount of somatic and genetic biologic damage a human undergoes as a result of radiation exposure depends on the quantity of ionizing radiation to which the subject is exposed, the ability of that radiation to cause ionization of the biologic tissue, the amount of body area exposed, and the specific body parts exposed.
- Early deterministic somatic effects occur within a short period of time after exposure to ionizing radiation.
  - These effects include nausea, fatigue, erythema, epilation, and blood and intestinal disorders.
- Acute radiation syndrome (ARS) occurs when the whole body is exposed to 1 $Gy_t$ of ionizing radiation or more.
  - ARS can manifest as hematopoietic syndrome, gastrointestinal syndrome, and cerebrovascular syndrome.
  - ARS presents in four major response stages: prodromal, latent period, manifest illness, and recovery or death.
- LD (lethal dose) 50/30 signifies the whole-body dose of ionizing radiation that can be lethal to 50% of an exposed population within 30 days.
  - LD in humans is usually given as LD 50/60 and is estimated to be 3 to 4 $Gy_t$.
  - When cells are exposed to sublethal doses of ionizing radiation, repair and recovery are possible.
  - Surviving cells begin to repopulate.
  - Approximately 90% of radiation-induced damage may be repaired over time; 10% is irreparable.
- High radiation doses to any part of the human body can result in local tissue damage.
  - Cell death results after a substantial partial-body exposure, leading to atrophy of organs and tissues.

- Depending on the types of cells involved and the dose of radiation received, recovery may be partial or complete, or it may fail to occur, resulting in death of the irradiated biologic structure.
- Factors such as radiosensitivity, reproductive characteristics, and growth rate govern organ and tissue response to radiation exposure.
- Many early radiologists and dentists developed radiodermatitis as a consequence of radiation exposure to the skin that eventually led to the development of cancerous lesions.
  - Human skin consists of three layers and several accessory structures, all of which are actively involved in the response of tissue to radiation exposure.
  - A single absorbed dose of 2 $Gy_t$ can cause radiation-induced skin erythema within 24 to 48 hours after irradiation.
  - High radiation doses can cause moist and then dry desquamation.
  - Moderate radiation doses can cause temporary hair loss, and large radiation doses can result in permanent hair loss.
  - Study of patients who underwent radiation therapy and who received orthovoltage radiation therapy treatments provides significant evidence of skin damage caused by radiation exposure.
  - The use of high-level fluoroscopy for extended periods of time can result in radiation-induced skin injuries for patients.
- Human germ cells are relatively radiosensitive.
  - In males, a radiation dose of 0.1 $Gy_t$ can depress the sperm population and possibly cause genetic mutations in future generations.
  - A radiation dose of 2 $Gy_t$ may result in temporary sterility for up to a period of 1 year, and a dose of 5 or 6 $Gy_t$ may result in permanent sterility.
  - In females, a gonadal dose of 0.1 $Gy_t$ may delay or suppress menstruation. A single dose of 2 $Gy_t$ to the ovaries can result in

temporary sterility, and a dose of 5 to 6 $Gy_t$ to the ovaries can result in permanent sterility.
  - Gonadal irradiation of the ovaries can result in genetic mutations that can be passed on to future generations. For this reason the ovaries should be shielded whenever possible during all imaging procedures.
- Periodic blood counts have been replaced by personnel dosimeters as a means to monitor occupational radiation exposure.
  - Measurable hematologic depression can be caused by a whole-body dose of radiation as low as 0.25 $Gy_t$.
  - Lymphocytes are very radiosensitive. A radiation dose as low as 0.1 $Gy_t$ can cause a decrease of these cells in the blood.
  - A radiation dose of 0.5 $Gy_t$ causes a decrease in neutrophils, and a dose greater than 0.5 $Gy_t$ can cause a decrease in the number of thrombocytes (platelets).
  - A depletion of cells that protect the body against disease causes the body to lose its ability to fight infection.
- Mapping of chromosomes is called *karyotyping*.
  - Karyotyping is done during metaphase, when each chromosome can be individually demonstrated and radiation-induced chromosome and chromatid aberrations can be observed.
  - Chromosomal damage can be caused by both low and high radiation doses.
  - Chromosome aberrations have been observed in individuals after completion of imaging procedures in which high radiation dose rates were administered.

## REFERENCES

1. Finch SC: Acute radiation syndrome. *JAMA* 258:666, 1987.
2. Gale RP: Immediate medical consequences of nuclear accidents: lessons from Chernobyl. *JAMA* 258:625, 1987.
3. Perry AR, Iglar AF: The accident at Chernobyl: radiation doses and effects. *Radiol Technol* 61:290, 1990.

4. Linnemann RE: Soviet medical response to Chernobyl nuclear accident. *JAMA* 258:639, 1987.
5. Bushong SC: *Radiologic science for technologists: physics, biology and protection*, ed 10, St. Louis, 2013, Mosby.
6. Fry RJM: Acute radiation effects. In Wagner LK, Fabrikant JI, Fry RJM, editors: *Radiation bioeffects and management: test and syllabus*, Reston, Va, 1991, American College of Radiology.
7. Hidden giants. *ASRT Scanner* 41:1, 2008.
8. George Washington University: *Staff memo: experiments on prisoners*. Available at: http://www.gwu.edu/~nsarchiv/radiation/dir/mstreet/commeet/meet1/brief1/br1n.txt. Accessed April 10, 2013.
9. Advisory Committee on Human Radiation Experiments (ACHRE) report: *Chapter 9: The Oregon and Washington experiments*. Available at: http://www.hss.energy.gov/healthsafety/ohre/roadmap/achre/chap9_2.html. Accessed April 10, 2013.
10. Forshier S: *Essentials of radiation biology and protection*. Albany, NY, 2002, Delmar.
11. Travis EL: *Primer of medical radiobiology*, ed 2, Chicago, 1989, Year Book.
12. Sigurdson AJ, Bhatti P, Preston DL, et al: *Routine diagnostic x-ray examinations and increased frequency of chromosome translocations among U.S. radiologic technologists*. Available at: http://www.ncbi.nlm.nih.gov/pubmed/18974125. Accessed April 15, 2013.
13. University of Minnesota, Health Science Section: *U.S. Radiologic Technologists Study*, vol 2, Minneapolis, 2004, University of Minnesota.
14. University of Minnesota, Health Studies Section: *U.S. Radiologic Technologists Study*. Available at: www.radtechstudy.org. Accessed April 10, 2013.
15. M'kacher R, Violot D, Aubert B, et al: Premature chromosome condensation associated with fluorescence in situ hybridization detects cytogenic abnormalities after a CT scan: evaluation of the low-dose effect. *Radiat Prot Dosimetry* 103:35, 2003.
16. Weber J, Scheid W, Traut H: Biological dosimetry after extensive diagnostic exposure. *Health Phys* 68:266, 1995.

## GENERAL DISCUSSION QUESTIONS

1. What type of diagnostic imaging procedure could possibly cause a radiation dose sufficient to cause early deterministic effects?
2. Why is LD 50/60 a more accurate indicator of outcome for humans receiving large radiation exposures than LD 50/30?
3. How can a cytogenetic analysis of chromosomes be accomplished?
4. What factors govern the response of organs and tissues to radiation exposure?
5. How have scientists become aware of radiation-induced skin damage in early pioneers?
6. What are the three separate dose-related syndromes that occur as part of acute radiation syndrome, and what are the four major response stages?
7. What is radiodermatitis?
8. After the reception of a single absorbed dose of 2 $Gy_t$ of radiation, approximately how long will it take to cause radiation-induced skin erythema?
9. How has information on the gonadal response to radiation exposure been acquired?
10. How significant is the chance of causing sterility in imaging personnel who perform routine procedures?

## REVIEW QUESTIONS

1. The lethal dose of ionizing radiation for humans is usually given as follows:
   A. LD 50/30
   B. LD 50/60    *See p.174*
   C. LD 50/90
   D. LD 50/120
2. Acute radiation syndrome presents in four major response stages. In what order do these stages occur?
   A. Latent period, prodromal, manifest illness, recovery or death
   B. Manifest illness, prodromal, latent period, recovery or death
   C. Prodromal, latent period, manifest illness, recovery or death
   D. Manifest illness, latent period, prodromal, recovery or death
3. Which of the following systems is the *most* radiosensitive vital organ system in human beings?
   A. Cerebrovascular
   B. Gastrointestinal
   C. Hematopoietic
   D. Skeletal

4. When cells are exposed to sublethal doses of ionizing radiation, approximately _____ of radiation-induced damage may be repaired over time, and about _____ is irreparable.
   A. 25%, 75%
   B. 50%, 50%
   C. 75%, 25%
   D. 90%, 10%
5. As radiation dose increases, the severity of early deterministic effects:
   A. Also increases.
   B. Gradually decreases.
   C. Increases sharply and then gradually decreases.
   D. Remains constant.
6. The total radiation dose received by a somatic or genetic cell and the dose rate determine the:
   A. Cell growth reduction rate.
   B. Cause of chromosome aberrations.
   C. Mechanism of action of ionizing radiation on biologic macromolecules.
   D. Production of chromosome aberrations.
7. In 1898, after developing burns attributed to radiation exposure, this Boston dentist began investigating the hazards of radiation exposure and became the first advocate of radiation protection. Who is this person?
   A. William Herbert Rollins
   B. Wilhelm Conrad Roentgen
   C. Thomas Alva Edison
   D. Clarence Madison Dally

8. In the female, the ovarian stem cells:
   A. Begin as a single cell during fetal development, before birth, and then gradually increase in number throughout life.
   B. Multiply to a few hundred cells during fetal life, before birth, and then gradually increase in number throughout life.
   C. Multiply to millions of cells only during fetal development, before birth, and then steadily decline in number throughout life.
   D. Multiply to millions of cells only during fetal development, before birth, and then steadily continue to increase in number throughout life.
9. Which of the following types of cells develop from a single precursor cell, the pluripotential stem cell?
   1. Lymphocytes and granulocytes
   2. Thrombocytes and erythrocytes
   3. Platelets
   A. 1 only
   B. 2 only
   C. 3 only
   D. 1, 2, and 3
10. With regard to radiation exposure, which part of the gastrointestinal tract is *most* severely affected?
   A. Esophagus
   B. Stomach
   C. Small intestine — bc cells are rapidly dividing
   D. Large intestine

# Late Deterministic and Stochastic Radiation Effects on Organ Systems

## OBJECTIVES

*After completing this chapter, the reader will be able to perform the following:*

- Explain how scientists use epidemiologic studies to predict the risk of cancer in human populations exposed to low doses of ionizing radiation.
- Explain the purpose of a radiation dose-response curve.
- Draw diagrams demonstrating various dose-response relationships.
- Explain why regulatory agencies continue to use the linear dose-response model for establishing radiation protection standards.
- Differentiate between threshold and nonthreshold relationships.
- List and describe the various late deterministic somatic effects and late stochastic effects of ionizing radiation on living systems.

- Describe the concept of risk for radiation-induced malignancies, and explain the models that are used to give risk estimates.
- Identify ionizing radiation-exposed human populations or groups that prove radiation induces cancer.
- Explain how spontaneous mutations occur, discuss the concept of radiation-induced genetic (hereditary) effects, and also explain how ionizing radiation causes these effects and how they can be passed on to future generations.
- Differentiate between dominant and recessive gene mutations.
- Explain the doubling dose concept, and give an example of how the number of mutations increases as dose increases.

## CHAPTER OUTLINE

Copyright © 2014, Elsevier Inc.

Natural Spontaneous
  Mutations
Mutagens Responsible for
  Genetic Mutations
Radiation Interaction with
  DNA Macromolecules

Cellular Damage Repair by
  Enzymes
Incapacities of Mutant
  Genes
Dominant or Recessive
  Point Mutations

Ionizing Radiation as a
  Cause of Genetic
  (Hereditary) Effects
Doubling Dose Concept
**Summary**

## KEY TERMS

absolute risk
carcinogenesis
cataractogenesis
doubling dose
embryologic effects (birth
  defects)
epidemiology
genetic (hereditary) effects

late deterministic somatic
  effects
late somatic effects
late stochastic effects
linear nonthreshold curve
linear-quadratic nonthreshold
  curve
nonthreshold

organogenesis
radiation dose-response
  relationship
relative risk
sigmoid, or S-shaped
  (nonlinear), threshold curve
threshold

Radiation-induced damage at the cellular level may lead to measurable somatic and hereditary damage in the living organism as a whole later in life. As mentioned previously, these outcomes are called *late effects* and are the long-term results of radiation exposure. Some examples of measurable late biologic damage are:

• Cataracts
• Leukemia
• Genetic mutations

Cataracts are considered to be a deterministic effect, whereas leukemia and genetic mutations are viewed as stochastic consequences. Hence this chapter focuses on organic damage from ionizing radiation that occurs months or years following radiation exposure.

## EPIDEMIOLOGY

**Epidemiology** is defined as a "science that deals with the incidence, distribution, and control of disease in a population."[1] Epidemiologic studies consist of observations and statistical analysis of data, such as the incidence of disease within groups of people. The latter studies include the risk of radiation-induced cancer. The incident

rates at which these irradiation-related malignancies occur are determined by comparing the natural incidence of cancer occurring in a human population with the incidence of cancer occurring in an irradiated population. Risk factors are then determined for the general human population.

In the early years after Roentgen's discovery of x-rays, pioneers working and experimenting with this virtually unknown form of radiant energy soon learned that radiation was a cancer-causing agent. Many cases of radiation-induced skin cancer among radiation workers in the early 1900s were documented. In addition, available data demonstrate that ionizing radiation is also responsible for causing other types of cancers.

Study of exposed populations, such as the Japanese atomic bomb survivors, provided proof that high radiation doses can certainly induce cancer in humans. Low radiation doses, such as those currently received by occupationally exposed individuals, are not actually measurable. Additional information about risk estimates for cancer are addressed later in this chapter.

Epidemiologic studies are of significant value to scientists, who use the information from these studies to formulate dose-response estimates to predict the risk of cancer in human populations exposed to low doses of ionizing radiation.

## RADIATION DOSE-RESPONSE RELATIONSHIP

### Dose-Response Curves

Radiobiologists engaged in research have a common goal to establish relationships between radiation and dose response. The information obtained can be used to attempt to predict the risk of occurrence of malignancies in human populations that have been exposed to low levels of ionizing radiation. The **radiation dose-response relationship** is demonstrated graphically through a curve that maps the observed effects of radiation exposure in relation to the dose of radiation received. As the dose escalates, so do most effects. In such a dose-response curve the variables, or numbers, are plotted along the axes of the graph to demonstrate the relationship between the dose received (horizontal axis) and the biologic effects observed (vertical axis). The curve is either linear (straight line) or nonlinear (curved to some degree), and it depicts either a threshold dose or a nonthreshold dose (Fig. 9-1).

### Threshold and Nonthreshold Relationships

The term **threshold** may be defined as a point at which a response or reaction to an increasing stimulation first occurs. With reference to ionizing radiation, this means that below a certain radiation level or dose, no biologic effects are observed. Biologic effects begin to occur only when the threshold level or dose is reached. A **nonthreshold** relationship indicates that any radiation dose has the capability of producing a biologic effect. Therefore, if ionizing radiation functions as the stimulus and the biologic effect it produces is the response, and if a nonthreshold relationship exists between radiation dose and a biologic response (Fig. 9-2), some biologic effects will be caused in living organisms by even the

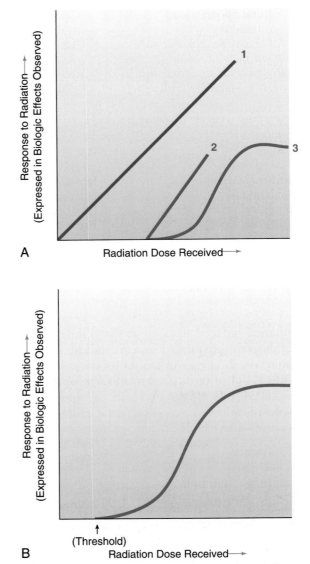

FIGURE 9-1 **A**, *1* represents a hypothetical linear (straight-line) nonthreshold curve of radiation dose-response relationship; *2* represents a hypothetical linear (straight-line) threshold curve of radiation dose-response relationship; *3* represents a hypothetical nonlinear threshold curve of radiation dose-response relationship. **B**, Hypothetical sigmoid (S-shaped, hence nonlinear) threshold curve of radiation dose-response relationship generally employed in radiation therapy to demonstrate high-dose cellular response.

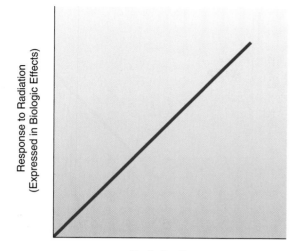

**FIGURE 9-2**  Hyopthetical linear (straight-line) non-threshold curve of radiation dose-response relationship. The straight-line curve passing through the origin in this graph indicates both that the response to radiation (in terms of biologic effects) is directly proportional to the dose of radiation and that no known level of radiation dose exists below which the chance of sustaining biologic damage is zero. In contrast to a cell-survival curve (see Chapter 7), both the vertical and horizontal axes of a dose-response curve are ordinary linear scales.

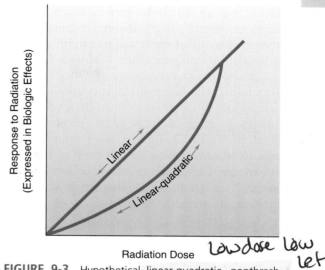

**FIGURE 9-3**  Hypothetical linear-quadratic, nonthreshold dose-response relationship. The curve estimates the risk associated with low-dose levels from low-linear energy transfer (LET) radiation.

smallest dose of ionizing radiation. Thus no radiation dose can be considered absolutely "safe."

## Risk Models Used to Predict Cancer Risk and Genetic (Hereditary) Damage in Human Populations

In a 1980 report, the Committee on the Biological Effects of Ionizing Radiation (BEIR), under the auspices of the National Academy of Sciences, revealed that most stochastic effects (e.g., cancer) and genetic (hereditary) effects at low-dose levels from low–linear energy transfer (LET) radiation, such as the type of radiation used in diagnostic radiology, appear to follow a linear-quadratic nonthreshold curve (Fig. 9-3). The term *linear-quadratic* states that the equation that best fits the data has components that depend on dose to the first power (linear or straightline behavior) and also dose squared (quadratic or

curved behavior). Newer risk models and updated dosimetry techniques provided a better follow-up study of Hiroshima and Nagasaki atomic bomb survivors. In 1990, the BEIR Committee's revised risk estimates indicated that the risk from radiation exposure was about three to four times greater than previously projected. Currently, the committee recommends the use of the **linear nonthreshold curve** of radiation dose-response for most types of cancers. The term *linear nonthreshold (LNT) curve* implies that the chance of a biologic response to ionizing radiation is directly proportional to the dose received. For example, if the absorbed dose is doubled, the biologic response probability, and therefore its actual occurrence in a large population sample, is also doubled (see Fig. 9-2).

## Risk Models Used to Predict Leukemia, Breast Cancer, and Heritable Damage

According to the LNT curve, no radiation exposure level is assumed to be "absolutely" safe. Currently, advocates of this point of view theorize that because all radiation exposure levels possess the potential to cause biologic damage, then radiographers must never fail to employ aggressive radiation safety measures whenever humans are exposed to radiation during diagnostic imaging procedures. The **linear-quadratic nonthreshold curve (LQNT)** (see Fig. 9-3) estimates the risk associated with low-level radiation. As previously stated, the BEIR Committee believes the LQNT curve to be a more accurate reflection of stochastic and genetic effects at low-dose levels from low-LET radiation. The following health concerns are presumed to follow this curve:

- Leukemia
- Breast cancer
- Heritable damage

For leukemia, the LQNT curve is supported by an analysis of the leukemia occurrences in Nagasaki and Hiroshima that used a more recent reevaluation of the radiation dose distribution in these two cities.[2,3]

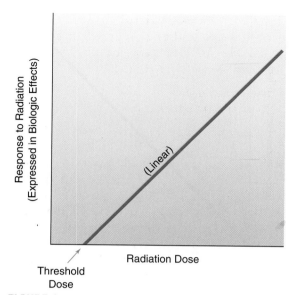

**FIGURE 9-4**  Hypothetical linear threshold curve of radiation dose-response. This depicts those cases for which a biologic response does not occur below a specific radiation dose.

## Rationale for Risk Model Selection

The continued use of the linear dose-response model for radiation protection standards has the potential to exaggerate the seriousness of radiation effects at lower dose levels from low-LET radiation. However, it accurately reflects the effects of high-LET radiation (neutrons and alpha particles) at higher doses. In establishing radiation protection standards, the regulatory agencies have chosen to be conservative—that is, to use a model that may overestimate risk but is not expected to underestimate risk.

## Risk Model Used to Predict High-Dose Cellular Response

Deterministic effects of significant radiation exposure such as skin erythema and hematologic depression may be demonstrated graphically through the use of a radiation *linear threshold dose-response curve* (Fig. 9-4). In this model, a biologic response does not occur below a specific dose level. Laboratory experiments on animals

and data from human populations observed after acute high doses of radiation provided the foundation for this curve. The **sigmoid, or S-shaped (nonlinear), threshold curve** of the radiation dose-response relationship (see Fig. 9-1, *B*) is generally employed in radiation therapy to demonstrate high-dose cellular response to the radiation within specific tissues such as skin, lens of the eye, and various types of blood cells. Different effects require different minimal doses. The tail of the curve indicates that limited recovery occurs at lower radiation doses. At the highest radiation doses, the curve gradually levels off and then veers downward because the affected living specimen or tissue dies before the observable effect appears.

## SOMATIC EFFECTS

When living organisms that have been exposed to radiation sustain biologic damage, the effects of this exposure are classified as *somatic (i.e., body) effects*. An example of a *non-somatic* effect is irradiation of an individual's genetic material (sperm or eggs) leading to a genetic malformation in offspring. The classification of somatic effects may be subdivided into:

- Stochastic effects
- Deterministic effects

In stochastic effects, the probability that the effect happens depends upon the received dose, but the severity of the effect does not. The occurrence of a cancer is an instance of a stochastic somatic effect. In deterministic effects, however, both the probability and the severity of the effect depend upon the dose. An example of a deterministic somatic effect is a cataract. The more radiation absorbed dose to the lens of the eye, the worse the cataract will become.

## Late Somatic Effects

**Late somatic effects** are consequences of radiation exposure that appear months or years after such exposure. These effects may result from the following:

- Previous whole- or partial-body acute exposure
- Previous high radiation doses
- Long-term low-level doses sustained over several years.

These late effects can be directly related to the dose received. Such slowly developing changes to the body from radiation exposure received are therefore classified as:

- **Late deterministic somatic effects**

Late responses in the body to radiation exposure that do not have a threshold, occur in an arbitrary or probabilistic manner, and have a severity that does not depend on dose, and are classified as:

- **Late stochastic effects**

Examples of both classes of late effects are listed in Box 9-1.

**Risk Estimate for Contracting Cancer from Low-Level Radiation Exposure.** Low-level doses are a consideration for patients and personnel

| BOX 9-1 | Late Effects of Radiation |
| --- | --- |

**Late Deterministic Somatic Effects**
Cataract formation
Fibrosis
Organ atrophy
Loss of parenchymal cells
Reduced fertility
Sterility

**Teratogenic Effects**
(i.e., effects of radiation on the embryo-fetus in utero that depend on the fetal stage of development and the radiation dose received)
Embryonic, fetal, or neonatal death
Congenital malformations
Decreased birth weight
Disturbances in growth and/or development
Increased stillbirths
Infant mortality
Childhood malignancy
Childhood mortality

**Late Stochastic Effects**
Cancer
Genetic (hereditary) effects

exposed to ionizing radiation as a result of diagnostic imaging procedures. The risk estimate for humans contracting cancer from low-level radiation exposure is still controversial. No conclusive proof exists that low-level ionizing radiation doses below 0.1 Sv cause a significant increase in the risk of malignancy. The risk, in fact, may be negligible or even nonexistent. Low-level radiation must be defined in broad terms to encompass the various sources of ionizing radiation, such as:

- X-rays and radioactive materials used for diagnostic purposes in the healing arts
- Employment-related exposures in medicine and industry
- Natural background exposure

Such low-level radiation has been defined as "an absorbed dose of 0.1 Sv or less delivered over a short period of time" and as "a larger dose delivered over a long period of time—for instance, 0.5 Sv in 10 years."[4] The effective dose of a typical routine two-view chest radiograph is approximately 0.06 mSv (can be greater or lesser, depending on the patient's body habitus), so this is considered far lower than what is considered a low-level exposure.[5] Numerous laboratory experiments on animals and studies on human populations exposed to high doses of ionizing radiation were conducted to determine adverse health effects. Using all data available on high radiation exposure, members of the scientific and medical communities determined that three categories of adverse health consequences require study at low levels of exposures:

- Cancer induction
- Damage to the unborn from irradiation in utero
- Genetic (hereditary) effects

**Late Effects Summary.** Cells that survive the initial irradiation and then retain a "memory" (i.e., some form of damage that persists and is passed on to future generations of the cell) of that event are responsible for producing late effects. Theoretically, radiation damage to one or more cells could actually produce a cancer or hereditary disorder. It is important to the reader to understand that late deterministic effects are not likely to occur from diagnostic imaging procedures. Late stochastic effects, on the other hand, could be initiated by even the smallest amount of radiation exposure if many low-probability occurrences were to be simultaneously realized. Stochastic and deterministic effects are also discussed in Chapter 10.

**Major Types of Late Effects.** To summarize, the three major types of late effects are:

- Carcinogenesis
- Cataractogenesis
- Embryologic effects (birth defects)

Of these, carcinogenesis and embryologic effects are considered stochastic events, and cataractogenesis is regarded as deterministic.

**Risk Estimates for Cancer.** Exposure to ionizing radiation may cause cancer as a late stochastic effect. At high doses, for groups such as the atomic bomb survivors, the risk is measurable

in human populations. At low doses, below 0.1 Sv, which includes groups such as occupationally exposed individuals and virtually all patients in diagnostic radiology, this risk is not directly measurable in population studies. Either the risk is overshadowed by other causes (e.g., environmental exposures, genetic predisposition, lifestyle factors such as smoking) of cancer in humans or the risk is zero. Current radiation protection philosophy assumes that risk still exists and may be determined by extrapolating (scaling down the risk-versus-dose curve) from high-dose data, in which risk has been directly observed, down to low doses, in which it has not been observed. This remains a very controversial concept.

**Absolute Risk and Relative Risk Models.** Risk estimates to predict cancer incidence may be given in terms of absolute risk or relative risk caused by a specific exposure to ionizing radiation (over and above background exposure). Both models predict the number of excess cancers, or cancers that would not have occurred in the population in question without the exposure to ionizing radiation. The **absolute risk** model predicts that a specific number of excess cancers will occur as a result of exposure (Fig. 9-5). The **relative risk** model predicts that the number of

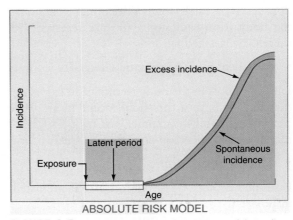

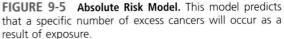

**FIGURE 9-5   Absolute Risk Model.** This model predicts that a specific number of excess cancers will occur as a result of exposure.

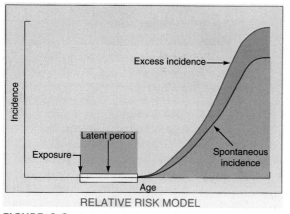

RELATIVE RISK MODEL

**FIGURE 9-6 Relative Risk Model.** This model predicts that the number of excess cancers will increase as the natural incidence of cancer increases with advancing age in a population.

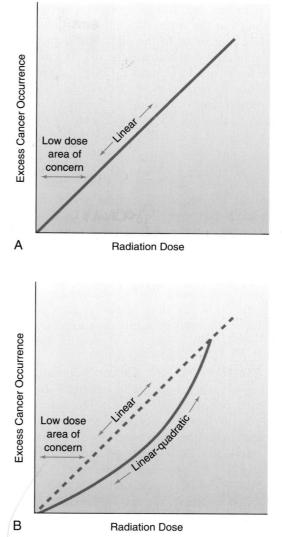

**FIGURE 9-7 A,** Hypothetical linear model used to extrapolate the occurrence of cancer from high-dose information to low doses. This model suits current high-dose information satisfactorily but exaggerates the actual risk at low doses and dose rates. **B,** Hypothetical linear-quadratic model used to extrapolate the occurrence of cancer from high-dose information to low doses. This model suits current high-dose information satisfactorily, but risk at low doses may be underestimated.

excess cancers will increase as the natural incidence of cancer increases with advancing age in a population (Fig. 9-6). It is relative in the sense that it predicts a percentage increase in incidence rather than a specific number of cases. More recent studies of atomic bomb survivors tend to support the relative risk model over the absolute risk model.

***Epidemiologic Studies for Determining the Risk of Cancer.*** Epidemiologic studies suggest that although the radiation doses encountered in diagnostic radiology should be considered, the benefit to the patient of the information gained from an imaging procedure greatly exceeds the minimal theoretical risk to the patient for developing cancer as a late stochastic response to radiation exposure. Even at the relatively high doses encountered by the Japanese atomic bomb survivors, the probability of causation of an excess fatal cancer is surprisingly low—approximately 5% per sievert.[6]

***Models for Extrapolation of Cancer Risk from High-Dose to Low-Dose Data.*** Researchers commonly use two models for extrapolation of risk from high-dose to low-dose data. These are linear and linear-quadratic models. In the linear model (Fig. 9-7, *A*), the risk per centigray is constant; the occurrence of cancer follows a

*[handwritten notes: Stochastic - probablistic (possibly) / nonstochastic - deterministic (guaranteed)]*

straight-line or dose-proportional progression throughout the entire dose range. Although this model appears to fit the high-dose data, it may substantially overestimate the risk at low doses. The linear-quadratic model (Fig. 9-7, *B*) includes additional mathematical terms that produce a deviation from straight-line behavior at low doses so that the risk per additional centigray at low doses is predicted to be less than at high doses. The 1989 BEIR V report supported the linear-quadratic model for leukemia only. For all other cancers, the BEIR V Committee recommended adoption of the linear model to fit the available data.[7]

**Carcinogenesis.** Cancer is the most important late stochastic effect caused by exposure to ionizing radiation. As previously discussed, this effect is a random occurrence that does not seem to have a threshold and for which the severity of the disease is not dose related (e.g., a patient's leukemia induced by a low-dose exposure is no different from a person's leukemia that was caused by a high-dose exposure).

***Radiation-Induced Cancer.*** Laboratory experiments with animals and statistical studies of human populations (e.g., the Japanese atomic bomb survivors) prove that radiation induces cancer. In humans, this may take 5 or more years to develop. Distinguishing radiation-induced cancer by its physical appearance is difficult because it does not appear different from cancers initiated by other agents. Cancer from natural causes frequently occurs, and the number of cancers induced by radiation is small compared with the natural incidence of malignancies even at doses many times those encountered in diagnostic radiology. Therefore, cancer caused by low-level radiation is difficult to identify. Human evidence of radiation-induced carcinogenesis comes from the observation of irradiated humans and from epidemiologic studies conducted many years after subjects were exposed to high doses of ionizing radiation. Examples of these data are listed in Box 9-2. An explanation of each example follows.

***Radium Watch-Dial Painters.*** During the early years of the last century (1920s and 1930s),

| BOX 9-2 | **Human Evidence for Radiation Carcinogenesis** |
|---|---|

1. Radium watch-dial painters (1920s and 1930s)
2. Uranium miners (early years, and Navajo people of Arizona and New Mexico during the 1950s and 1960s)
3. Early medical radiation workers (radiologists, dentists, technologists) (1896 to 1910)
4. Patients injected with the contrast agent Thorotrast (1925 to 1945)
5. Infants treated with x-radiation to reduce an enlarged thymus gland (1940s and 1950s)
6. Children of the Marshall Islanders inadvertently subjected to high levels of fallout during an atomic bomb test in 1954
7. Japanese atomic bomb survivors, 1945
8. Patients with benign postpartum mastitis who were given radiation therapy treatments
9. Evacuees from the Chernobyl nuclear power station disaster in 1986

a radium* watch-dial painting industry flourished in some factories in New Jersey. Young, unprotected, and ill-informed young women employed in these factories hand-painted the luminous numerals on watches and clocks with a radium-containing paint. The girls used sable brushes to apply the paint. To do the fine work required, some would place the paint-saturated brush tip on their lips to draw the bristles to a fine point. The girls who followed this procedure unfortunately ingested large quantities of radium. Because it is chemically similar to calcium, the radium was incorporated into bone tissue. Eventually the accumulation of this toxic substance caused:

- Development of osteoporosis (decalcification of bone)
- Osteogenic sarcoma (bone cancer)
- Other malignancies such as:
  - Carcinoma of the epithelial cells lining the nasopharynx and paranasal sinuses

---

*Radium (atomic number [Z] = 88) has an unstable nucleus and decays with a half-life of 1622 years by alpha particle emission to the radioactive element radon (Z = 86).

The bones most frequently affected by cancer included the pelvis, femur, and mandible. Doses of 5 Gy$_t$ or more are assumed to have induced the aforementioned malignancies. The number of head carcinomas attributed to the radium watch-dial painting industry, although small, is statistically significant. Of 1474 women in the industry, 61 were diagnosed with cancer of the paranasal sinuses and 21 with cancer of the mastoid air cells. Studies attributed the death of at least 18 of the radium watch-dial painters to radium poisoning.

***Uranium Miners.*** During the early years of the last century, people worked in European mines to extract pitchblende, a uranium ore. Uranium is a radioactive element with a very long half-life (the half-life of uranium-238 [$^{238}$U] is 4.5 billion years); it decays through a series of radioactive nuclides by emitting alpha, beta, and gamma radiation. One of the most important members of its decay family is radium, which decays to the radioactive element radon (Z = 86). As discussed in Chapter 2, radon is a gas that decays with a half-life of 3.8 days by way of alpha particle emission. This gas emanates through tiny gaps in rocks and created an insidious airborne hazard to miners. Throughout many years of employment, some miners inevitably inhaled significant amounts of radon. Possessing high LET, alpha particles passing through a person's lungs have a high probability of producing a great deal of cellular damage. About 50% of the miners eventually succumbed to lung cancer.

During the 1950s and 1960s, at the height of the Cold War between the United States and the Soviet Union, the U.S. government needed fuel for nuclear weapons and power plants. The Navajo people of Arizona and New Mexico mined uranium to meet this need. Because the government did not regulate working conditions in the mines to ensure safety from exposure—despite an awareness of risk—some 15,000 Navajo and white workers in the uranium mines sustained lethal doses of ionizing radiation by breathing radioactive dust and drinking radioactive water. Experts estimate that each miner unknowingly received an approximate equivalent dose of 10 Sv or more.[8] As a result, an alarmingly high number of miners died of cancer and other respiratory diseases. Compounding this tragedy, the families of the miners also were affected. Given that the miners had no knowledge of the adverse effects of ionizing radiation, they did not promptly change their work clothing on returning home. Because the clothing was contaminated by radioactive material, the miners' immediate families were extremely vulnerable to radiation-induced cancers.

***Early Medical Radiation Workers.*** Many of the first generation of radiation workers (radiologists, dentists, and technologists) were exposed to large amounts of ionizing radiation without realizing the dangers of the exposure. This resulted in more than a few severe radiation injuries to these individuals. An example was the development of cancerous skin lesions on the hands of radiologists and dentists (Fig. 9-8). When compared with their nonradiologist counterparts, substantial numbers also had a higher incidence of blood disorders such as:

- Aplastic anemia
- Leukemia

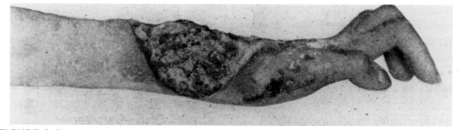

**FIGURE 9-8** Carcinoma of the distal arm and hand developing after an x-ray burn (in 1904).

Because all worked without the benefit of protective devices and some received doses estimated at more than 1 Gy/year, the occurrence of these radiation-induced injuries is understandable. Today, as a result of programs stressing radiation safety education, appropriate use of protective devices, and improvements in x-ray imaging equipment, radiation workers employed in medical imaging need not experience any adverse health effects as a consequence of their work. Studies of radiographers and physicians who began their careers in radiology after the 1940s demonstrated that these radiation workers had no increase in adverse health effects as a result of their occupational exposure. This finding is attributed to increased knowledge and use of proper protective measures and devices.

### Patients Injected with the Contrast Agent Thorotrast.

Between 1925 and 1945, Thorotrast was used as a contrast agent for diagnostic angiography. This medium contained a radioactive colloidal suspension that was approximately 25% thorium dioxide ($ThO_2$) by weight.[9] When administered by intravascular injection, the radioactive material emitted alpha particles that were deposited in the patient's reticuloendothelial system. The liver and spleen became the primary recipients of this adverse substance. After a latent period of 15 to 20 years, the cumulative destruction wrought by the alpha particle–emitting contrast agent resulted in many cases of:

- Liver cancer
- Spleen cancer
- Angiosarcomas
- Biliary duct carcinomas

When the contrast agent was administered by extravascular injection, the tissue surrounding the injection site eventually became cancerous.

### Infants Treated for an Enlarged Thymus Gland.

During the 1940s and early 1950s, physicians diagnosed thymus gland enlargement in many infants with respiratory distress. The thymus is located adjacent to the thyroid in the mediastinal cavity, which extends into the neck as far as the lower edge of the thyroid gland. Functioning as a vital part of the immune mechanism, this gland plays a crucial role in the body's defense against infection. Shortly after birth, the thymus gland in these infants responded to infection by enlarging. To reduce the size of the gland, physicians treated the infants with therapeutic doses (1.2 to 60 $Gy_t$) of x-radiation. Because the thyroid is adjacent to the thymus, the thyroid gland also received a substantial radiation dose. This resulted in the development, some 20 years later, of thyroid nodules and carcinomas in many of these treated infants.

### Incidence of Breast Cancer in Radiation Treatment of Benign Postpartum Mastitis.

Studies showed that postpartum patients treated with ionizing radiation for relief of mastitis are another group of individuals in whom the results of radiation exposure to healthy breast tissue indicate that radiation can cause breast cancer. In a particular study of 531 women who received a mean dose of 247 $cGy_t$, "breast cancer incidence doubled from 3.2% expected to 6.3% actual."[10] Because there is ongoing concern that mammography performed for either screening or diagnostic purposes could possibly cause the development of breast cancer, epidemiologic studies that provide such statistical information continue to be a high priority.

### Children of the Marshall Islanders.

Thyroid cancer also occurred in the children of the Marshall Islanders who were inadvertently subjected to high levels of fallout during an atomic bomb test (code name BRAVO) on March 1, 1954. During the detonation of a 15-megaton thermonuclear device on Bikini Atoll, the wind shifted and carried the fallout over the neighboring islands. As a consequence of this exposure, the children received substantial absorbed doses to the thyroid from both external exposure and internal ingestion of radioiodine. Estimates indicate that inhabitants of Rongelap Atoll received a mean dose of radiation to the thyroid gland of 21 $Gy_t$, and the inhabitants of Utrik Atoll received 2.80 $Gy_t$.[11,12] Hence a dose of 12 $Gy_t$ is considered to be representative of a population average dose for these two areas combined.

## Japanese Atomic Bomb Survivors

### Atomic Bomb Detonation on Hiroshima and Nagasaki.

On August 6, 1945, the United States dropped the first atomic bomb on the Japanese city of Hiroshima, thus marking the pivotal moment in the latter stages of World War II. Three days later, on August 9, 1945, a second bomb was dropped on the city of Nagasaki. Of the 300,000 people living in these 2 cities at the time of these bombings, approximately 88,000 people were killed and at least 70,000 more were injured. Many of those who died were killed by the heat and the blast (Fig. 9-9). Many of those who survived became victims of radiation injuries. These individuals have been observed since that time for signs of late stochastic effects of radiation.

### Data Obtained from Epidemiologic Studies.

Epidemiologic studies of approximately 100,000 Japanese survivors of the atomic bombings at Hiroshima and Nagasaki indicate that ionizing radiation causes leukemia (proliferation of the white blood cells). According to estimates, atomic bomb survivors (hibakusha) exposed to radiation doses of about 1 $Gy_t$ or more showed a significant increase in the incidence of leukemia. When compared with the spontaneous incidence of leukemia in the Japanese population at the time of the bomb, the incidence of leukemia in the irradiated population increased about 100-fold. "Studies of the atomic bomb survivors in both Hiroshima and Nagasaki show a statistically significant increase in leukemia incidence in the exposed population compared with the non-exposed population. In the period 1950 to 1956, 117 new cases of leukemia were reported in the Japanese survivors; approximately 64 of these can be attributed to radiation exposure."[1]

### Incidence of Leukemia and Occurrence Rate of Other Radiation-Induced Malignancies.

The incidence of leukemia has slowly declined since the late 1940s and early 1950s. However, the occurrence rates of other radiation-induced malignancies have continued to escalate since the late 1950s and early 1960s. Among these are a variety of solid tumors such as:

- Thyroid cancer
- Breast cancer

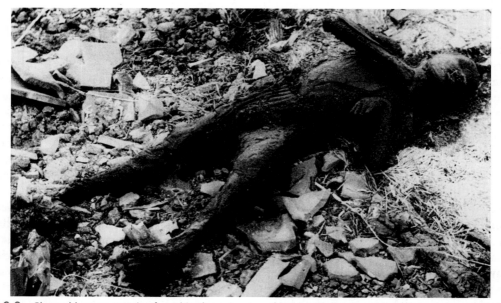

**FIGURE 9-9**  Charred human remains found in the epicenter of Nagasaki after the detonation of the atomic bomb on August 9, 1945.

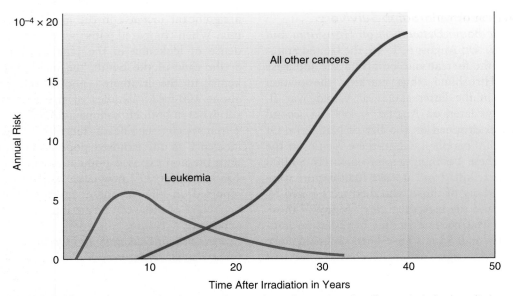

**FIGURE 9-10**    Nominal risk of malignancy from a dose of 0.01 $Gy_t$ of uniform whole-body radiation.

- Lung cancer
- Bone cancers

Figure 9-10 demonstrates the nominal risk of malignancy, as identified by Warren K. Sinclair, from a dose of 0.01 $Gy_t$ of uniform whole-body radiation.[13] The graph indicates that leukemia occurs approximately 2 years after the initial exposure, rises to its highest level of incidence between 7 and 10 years, and then declines to almost zero at about 30 years. Unlike leukemia, solid tumors take approximately 10 years to develop and generally increase in occurrence at the same rate that cancer increases as people age. Whether the risk for solid tumors continues to rise beyond 40 years or declines, as with leukemia, is still unknown. Follow-up studies of the atomic bomb survivors may eventually provide the answer.

***Incidence of Breast Cancer in Japanese Women.*** In general, Japanese women have a lower natural incidence of breast cancer than U.S. and Canadian women.[14] Studies of the female Japanese atomic bomb survivors provide strong evidence that ionizing radiation can induce breast cancer. The incidence of breast cancer in these women rises with radiation dose. It follows a linear nonthreshold curve. Numerous studies of female survivors indicate a relative risk for breast cancer ranging from 4:1 to as high as 10:1.

***Effectiveness of Ionizing Radiation as a Cancer-Causing Agent.*** Although studies from Hiroshima and Nagasaki confirm that high doses of ionizing radiation cause cancer, radiation is not a highly effective cancer-causing agent. For example, follow-up studies of approximately 82,000 atomic bomb survivors from 1950 to 1978 reveal an excess of only 250 cancer deaths attributed to radiation exposure. Instead of the expected 4500 cancer deaths, 4750 actually occurred. This indicates that of about every 300 atomic bomb survivors, 1 died of a malignancy attributed to an average whole-body radiation dose of approximately 0.14 Sv.

***Radiation Dose and Radiation-Induced Leukemia.*** Epidemiologic data about the Hiroshima atomic bomb survivors also indicate that a linear relationship exists between radiation dose and radiation-induced leukemia. In other words, the chance of contracting leukemia as a result of exposure to radiation is directly proportional to the magnitude of the radiation exposure.

Available information of the kind necessary to establish the existence of a threshold dose-response relationship (i.e., whether a harmless dose exists) is inconclusive. Hence radiation-induced leukemia is assumed to follow a linear nonthreshold dose-response relationship compared with leukemia in a population that has not been exposed to ionizing radiation.[9] More recent reevaluation of the quantity and type of radiation that was released in the cities of Hiroshima and Nagasaki provides a better foundation for radiation dose and damage assessment. Originally, neutrons were credited with the damage in Hiroshima. However, when more recent studies revealed that the uranium-fueled bomb dropped on Hiroshima provided more gamma radiation exposure and less neutron exposure than previously believed, data on the survivors were updated to reflect this more accurate information. Researchers, as a result, have established that gamma radiation and neutrons each provided about 50% of the radiation dose inflicted on the population of Hiroshima. Conversely, the inhabitants of Nagasaki, who were exposed to a plutonium bomb, received only 10% of their exposure from neutrons and 90% from gamma radiation. Based on the revised atomic bomb data, radiation-induced leukemias and solid tumors in the survivors may be attributed predominantly to gamma radiation exposure. The impact of the atomic bomb dosimetry revision is a significant increase in cancer risk estimates for both gamma and x-ray irradiation. The BEIR V report provides a summary of the newer estimates.

### Evacuees from the Chernobyl Nuclear Disaster

*Need for Follow-up Studies.* The 1986 nuclear power station accident at Chernobyl requires long-term follow-up studies to assess the magnitude and severity of late effects on the exposed population. Detailed observations investigating potential increases in the incidence of leukemia, thyroid problems, breast cancer, and other possible radiation-induced malignancies will continue.

*Evacuation of People within 36 Hours after the Accident.* Within 36 hours of the nuclear

catastrophe, 49,360 people residing at Pripyat, a city 2 miles from the plant, were evacuated. An additional 85,640 people, most of whom were living in a 10-mile (30-km) radial zone of Chernobyl, also were evacuated over a period of 14 days after the disaster. In general the 135,000 evacuees received an average equivalent dose of 0.12 Sv per person. Of the 135,000, approximately 24,000 people received an equivalent dose of about 0.45 Sv. The remaining 111,000 people received from 0.03 to 0.06 Sv.[15,16] If the evacuees are monitored for at least 30 years, important estimates of radiation-induced leukemias, thyroid cancers, and other malignancies may be obtained.

*Worldwide Effects of the Accident.* The possibility of late effects occurring from the Chernobyl power station disaster is still a source of concern worldwide. Because winds carried the radioactive plume in several different directions during the 10 days after the accident, more than 20 countries received fallout as a consequence of the catastrophe. Approximately 400,000 people received some exposure to fallout. In February 1989, Dr. Richard Wilson, professor of physics at Harvard University in Cambridge, Massachusetts, estimated "that about 20,000 people throughout the world" will develop a radiation-induced malignancy from the Chernobyl accident.[17]

*Attempts by Physicians to Prevent Thyroid Cancer in Children.* Iodine-131 ($^{131}$I) is one of the radioactive materials that became airborne in the radioactive plume. $^{131}$I concentrates in the thyroid gland and may cause cancer many years after the initial exposure. In an attempt to prevent thyroid cancer resulting from the accidental overdose of $^{131}$I, physicians administered potassium iodide to children in Poland, and other countries, after the Chernobyl disaster. By offering a substitute for take-up by the thyroid gland, potassium iodide is intended to block the gland's uptake of $^{131}$I. The degree of effectiveness of this preventive treatment remains to be determined. In other accidentally exposed populations, thyroid cancer has occurred in some individuals at doses of 1 $Gy_t$ or less. The approximate time for the

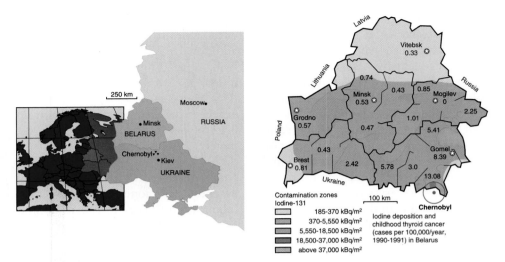

**FIGURE 9-11**    In the first 10 years after the Chernobyl nuclear accident, a dramatic increase in thyroid cancer was seen among children living in the regions of Belarus, Ukraine, and Russia, where the heaviest contamination occurred.

appearance of such radiation-induced thyroid malignancies is usually 10 to 20 years after exposure.

***Incidence of Thyroid Cancer and Breast Cancer since the Accident.*** During the first 10 years after the Chernobyl disaster, the incidence of thyroid cancer increased dramatically among children living in the regions of Belarus, Ukraine, and Russia (Fig. 9-11), where the heaviest radioactive iodine contamination occurred. Thyroid cancer has been the "most pronounced health effect" of the radiation accident.[18] As of April 1996, more than 700 cases of thyroid cancer were diagnosed in children residing in these areas. The number of new thyroid cancer cases identified since the Chernobyl incident is significantly higher than anticipated, and by 1998 a total of 1700 cases had been diagnosed.[19] Radiation scientists from the Western and Eastern Hemispheres are collaborating to determine the reason for this increase. Some possible explanations for the higher-than-expected number of thyroid cancers are as follows:

1. Chronic iodine deficiency during the years preceding the accident in the children living in the regions contaminated.

2. Genetic predisposition to developing thyroid malignancy after radiation exposure in some subgroups of the exposed population.[18]

If the first theory is valid, the thyroid glands of these individuals would have preferentially assimilated isotopes of the radioactive material inhaled from a cloud or ingested from contaminated milk supplies. If the second theory is valid, some of the exposed individuals may have a disorder that prevents the mechanism normally used by healthy cells to initiate repair and mend the genetic damage.

***Why Early Studies Did Not Demonstrate a Significant Increase in the Incidence of Leukemia after the Accident.*** From the earlier discussion of the Japanese atomic bomb survivors, we have learned that radiation causes leukemia and that the disease follows a linear, nonthreshold dose-response curve. However, early studies of the Chernobyl victims did not demonstrate a significant increase in the incidence of leukemia, possibly because the radioactive iodine and cesium expelled into the environment during the accident may produce damaging health effects in different ways.[20] For example, $^{131}I$ has a relatively short half-life (about 8 days) and is assimilated

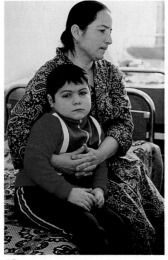

**FIGURE 9-12** Mother with son who has radiation-induced leukemia. The child is a victim of the 1986 nuclear power plant explosion at Chernobyl.

by the body and quickly distributed to the thyroid gland, thereby delivering an abrupt, acute dose to that organ. Radioactive cesium, conversely, has a much longer life (e.g., for Cs$^{137}$, T$_{1/2}$ = 30 years). It causes whole-body irradiation over a lengthy time span through its long-term presence in the environment and food supply lines. This probably increases the incidence of childhood leukemia (Fig. 9-12). However, this increase is difficult to detect without very sensitive and reliable monitoring procedures.

*Subsequent Findings.* As stated in Chapter 2, later studies began to demonstrate some of the expected effects. Reports indicated an approximately 50% increase in leukemia cases in children and adults in the Gomel region since the Chernobyl disaster.[21,22] Although the World Health Organization (WHO) reported that it found no increase in leukemia in the populations hit hardest by fallout from Chernobyl by 1993,[23] in 1995 the WHO reported that nearly 700 cases of thyroid cancer among children and adolescents had been linked to the Chernobyl accident.[24] In addition, in June 2001 at the Third International Conference, held in Kiev, a statistically significant rise in the number of leukemia

cases was reported in the Russian liquidators (cleanup workers) who worked during 1986 and 1987 at the Chernobyl power station complex.[25] Since the time of the Chernobyl accident, there has also been an increase in the incidence of breast cancer directly attributed to the radiation exposure.[26] If these findings continue to be substantiated, it will take many more years of observation and analysis before all the adverse health effects can be understood. Further investigation is indeed necessary.

Given that the actual levels of risk from the accident are still unknown, because of the limited data provided by the Russians, the risk for development of radiation-induced malignancies is difficult to determine.

*The ETHOS Project.* Since the accident at Chernobyl, the affected population continues to work toward reconstructing their overall quality of life. The rehabilitation process among those persons living in contaminated territories is ongoing. The goal of ventures such as the ETHOS Project (see Chapter 2) is to help the local population rebuild acceptable living conditions through their own active involvement in the reconstruction process.[27]

### Life Span Shortening

*Animal Studies.* Laboratory experiments on small animals have shown that the life span of animals that were exposed to nonlethal doses of ionizing radiation was shortened as a consequence of the exposure. When compared with a control group of unexposed small animals, the exposed animals died sooner. Radiation was then believed to have accelerated all causes of death. This reduction in the life cycle was termed *nonspecific life span shortening.* It was also believed that radiation accelerated the aging process, thus making the animals more susceptible to several diseases. In actuality, early demise of the experimental animals resulted from the induction of cancer.

### Human Studies

*American Radiologists.* In humans, studies of the life span of U.S. radiologists that were conducted by the Radiological Society of North America from 1945 to 1954 revealed that radiologists did have a shorter life span than nonradiologist physicians.[9] However, the process of evaluation of the information has been subject to considerable criticism, and the conclusions of the study are questionable. Further analysis of the epidemiologic studies showed that shortening of the life span in both animals and humans was the result of cancer and leukemia and not other "nonspecific" causes or accelerated aging.

*American Radiologic Technologists.* Initiated in 1982 and currently still in progress, as mentioned in Chapter 8, an extensive study of approximately 146,000 U.S. Radiologic Technologists (USRT) is continuing to evaluate potential radiation-related adverse health effects resulting from long-term, repeated exposures to low-dose ionizing radiation. These responses include cancer incidence and other work-related conditions. This occupational epidemiologic study is a collaborative effort among the University of Minnesota School of Public Health, the National Cancer Institute, and the American Registry of Radiologic Technologists. The study involves a series of mail surveys to all participating technologists and telephone interviews with approximately 1200 retired technologists who were in the field before 1950. The interviews provide important information about work practices that were common in the early years before personnel monitoring devices were routinely used.[28,29]

As reported in the Volume 2, Spring 2004 edition of the *USRT Newsletter,* among the 90,305 technologists who completed the first survey in the mid-1980s, there were 1283 deaths from cancer. A comparison was made between technologists who started working in the 1960s or later and those who began working before 1940. A slightly higher risk of dying from any type of cancer was found in technologists working before 1940. Technologists who began working after 1940 did not demonstrate any elevated risk. However, technologists entering the medical radiation industry before 1950 demonstrated a somewhat higher risk of dying from leukemia compared with individuals entering the workforce in 1950 or later. The risk of dying from

breast cancer has also been studied in technologists working in the field before 1940, in those working between 1940 and 1950, and in those entering the field in 1960 or later. Technologists who began working before 1940 had the greatest risk of dying of breast cancer, followed by those who worked up to 1950. When the risk of dying of breast cancer in women who began their careers in the 1950s is compared with that in women employed from 1960 or later, the risk is only slightly higher for the women first employed in the 1950s. Improvements in radiologic technology, medical imaging equipment, and radiation safety are factors in cancer risk reduction. Readers interested in obtaining more information about this ongoing study can visit the website at www.radtechstudy.org, or they can write to U.S. Radiologic Technologist Study, University of Minnesota, Health Science Section, MMC 807, 420 Delaware Street S.E., Minneapolis, MN 55455.

Compared with others who started working in the 1960s or later, technologists who began working before 1940 had a slightly higher risk of dying of any type of cancer. The risks were not elevated in technologists who began working in subsequent decades. Radiologic technologists who began working before 1950 had a somewhat higher risk of dying of leukemia compared with technologists who started working in 1950 or later.

**Cataractogenesis.** The lens of the eye contains transparent fibers that transmit light. The lens focuses light on the retina so that as the image forms, it may be transmitted through the optic nerve (Fig. 9-13, *B*). The probability that a single dose of ionizing radiation of approximately 2 $Gy_t$ will induce the formation of cataracts (opacity of the eye lens) (see Fig. 9-13, *A*) is high. Cataracts result in partial or complete loss of vision. Laboratory experiments with mice show that cataracts may be induced with doses as low as 0.1 $Gy_t$. Highly ionizing neutron radiation is extremely efficient in inducing cataracts. A neutron dose as low as 0.01 $Gy_t$ has been known to cause cataracts in mice. Radiation-induced cataracts in humans follow a threshold,

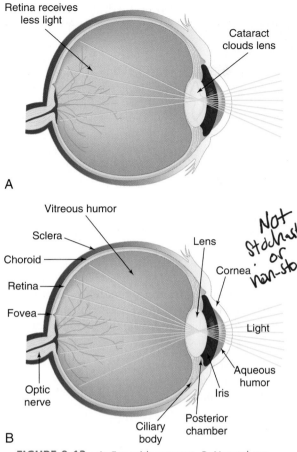

A

B

**FIGURE 9-13 A,** Eye with cataract. **B,** Normal eye.

nonlinear dose-response relationship. Evidence of human radiation cataractogenesis comes from the observation of small groups of people who accidentally received substantial doses to the eyes. These groups include:

- Japanese atomic bomb survivors
- Nuclear physicists working with cyclotrons (units that produce beams of high-energy particles such as 150-MeV proton beams) between 1932 and 1960
- Patients undergoing radiation therapy who received significant exposures to the eyes during treatment

The chance of radiation-induced cataracts occurring as a result of any diagnostic imaging procedure is very remote. However, in the realm of diagnostic radiology, fluoroscopic procedures do result in the highest radiation exposure to the lens of the eye. Occupational dose to this sensitive area can be substantially reduced when radiologists and radiographers wear protective eyewear while participating in the examination (see Chapter 13 for further information). In patients, exposure to the lens of the eye, and subsequent dose, can be decreased by also having them wear protective eye shields, provided the use of such shields does not compromise the diagnostic value of the fluoroscopic examination.

## Embryologic Effects (Birth Defects)

***Stages of Gestation in Humans.*** All life forms seem to be most vulnerable to radiation during the embryonic stage of development. The period of gestation during which the embryo-fetus is exposed to radiation governs the effects (death or congenital abnormality) of the radiation. Gestation in humans is divided into three stages:

1. Preimplantation, which corresponds to 0 to 9 days after conception
2. **Organogenesis**, which corresponds to approximately 10 days to 12 weeks after conception
3. The fetal stage, which corresponds to term (Fig. 9-14)

***Embryonic Cell Radiosensitivity during the First Trimester of Pregnancy.*** Because embryonic cells begin dividing and differentiating after conception, they are extremely radiosensitive and hence may easily be damaged by exposure to ionizing radiation. The first trimester is the most crucial period, with respect to adverse consequences from irradiation, because the embryo-fetus contains a large number of stem cells* during this period of gestation. Given that the central nervous system and related sensory organs of the embryo contain many stem cells,

---

*In fact, the use for medical research of these nonspecialized cells derived from embryos that would otherwise be discarded has become the focus of much controversy between those who perceive great potential for medical benefit and those who view these embryos as living entities that should not be used for research.

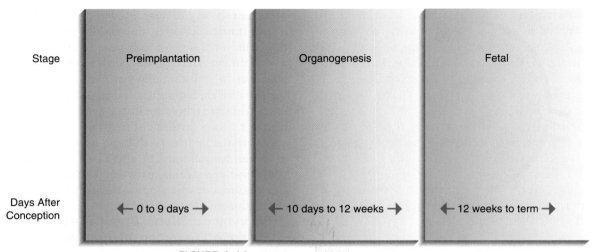

| Stage | Preimplantation | Organogenesis | Fetal |
|---|---|---|---|
| Days After Conception | ← 0 to 9 days → | ← 10 days to 12 weeks → | ← 12 weeks to term → |

**FIGURE 9-14    Division of Gestation in Humans.**

they are extremely radiosensitive and are thus very susceptible to radiation-induced damage. Irradiation of the embryo-fetus during the first 12 weeks of development to equivalent doses in excess of 200 mSv frequently results in death or severe congenital abnormalities. When a high dose of radiation is received by the embryo within approximately 2 weeks of fertilization (before the start of organogenesis), prenatal death is the most obvious adverse consequence of such an exposure. This usually results in a spontaneous abortion. If this does not occur, the pregnancy will simply continue to term without any adverse effect.[9]

During the preimplantation stage, the fertilized ovum divides and forms a ball-like structure containing undifferentiated cells. If this structure is irradiated with a dose in the range of 0.05 to 0.15 $Gy_t$, embryonic death will occur. Malformations resulting from radiation exposure do not occur at this stage. Because organogenesis occurs at approximately 10 days to 12 weeks after conception, the developing fetus is most susceptible to radiation-induced congenital abnormalities during this period. This is actually the time when the undifferentiated cells are beginning to differentiate into organs. The central nervous system in the growing human fetus, however, remains undifferentiated and does not normally complete

development until approximately the twelfth year of life. Abnormalities occurring as a consequence of irradiation during the period of organogenesis may include:

- Growth inhibition
- Mental retardation
- Microcephaly
- Genital deformities
- Sense organ damage

During the late stages of organogenesis, the presence of fatal abnormalities in the fetus will cause neonatal death (death at birth). Skeletal damage from radiation exposure occurs most frequently during the period from week 3 to week 20 of development. Cancer and functional disorders during childhood are other possible effects of irradiation during the fetal stage (a growth period).

***Embryonic Cell Radiosensitivity during the Second and Third Trimesters of Pregnancy.*** Fetal radiosensitivity decreases as gestation progresses. Hence, during the second and third trimesters, the developing fetus is less sensitive to ionizing radiation exposure. However, even in these later trimesters, congenital abnormalities and functional disorders such as sterility may be caused by radiation exposure. Much of the evidence for radiation-induced congenital abnormalities in humans comes from more than 4 decades of follow-up studies of children exposed in utero during the atomic bomb detonations in Hiroshima and Nagasaki. Although the risk of radiation-induced leukemia is greater when the embryo-fetus is irradiated during the first trimester, leukemia also may be induced by exposure to radiation during the second and third trimesters. Studies of the latter, however, have not demonstrated significant rates of cancer and leukemia deaths.[30]

**Embryonic Effects Resulting from the Chernobyl Nuclear Power Plant Accident.** Of the 135,000 evacuees from the 18-mile (30-km) radial zone of the Chernobyl nuclear power plant, approximately 2000 were pregnant women. Each received an average total-body equivalent dose of 0.43 Sv. No obvious abnormalities were observed in the 300 live babies born by August 1987. However, from after 1987 through 1990, the Ministry of Health in the Ukraine recorded an increased number of miscarriages, premature births, and stillbirths.[21,22] Also recorded by the Ministry was an increase, to three times the normal rate, of deformities and developmental abnormalities in newborns.[21,22]

***Review of Fetal Effects by UNSCEAR.*** Fetal effects such as mortality, induction of malformations, mental retardation, and childhood cancer were reviewed by the United Nations Scientific Committee on the Effects of Atomic Radiation (UNSCEAR).[31] This group proposed an upper-limit increased combined radiation risk for the aforementioned fetal effects of "3 chances per 1000 children (0.3%) for each rem of fetal dose."[32] If each effect was estimated individually, the estimate would be a little lower. Without radiation, these fetal effects have an estimated normal total risk of "60 chances per 1000 children (6%)."[32] In simple terms, this means that the radiation causes an increased risk of 3 per 1000 children over the existing risk of 60 per thousand so now there is a total risk of 63 per thousand.

***International Chernobyl Project.*** In 1990 the International Chernobyl Project was initiated in response to a request for assistance from the former Soviet Union. The Director of the Radiation Effects Research Foundation in Hiroshima, Japan, led this project. The study compared 7 contaminated Russian villages with 6 uncontaminated villages. By 1990, no significant increases in fetal and genetic abnormalities were seen in this population.[33] However, because of the relatively long latency period for radiogenic cancer, particularly solid tumors, researchers expect that more time will be required before the ultimate impact on the population of Russia is known. Estimates of as many as 500 excess cancers in the former Soviet Union during the next 50 to 60 years have been made.[34]

***Effects of Low-Level Ionizing Radiation on the Embryo-Fetus.*** The effects of low-level ionizing radiation on the embryo-fetus can only be poorly estimated. Documentation of the effects of low-level radiation on the unborn irradiated in utero is insufficient because some types of abnormalities occur in a small percentage (approximately 4%) of all live births in the United States. In addition, no birth abnormalities unique to high levels of radiation have appeared. Abnormalities in this context are the same as those that occur naturally; however, if the exposure occurs during a period of major organogenesis, the abnormality may be more pronounced. Assessment of radiation-induced birth abnormalities from low-level exposure also can be difficult because human genes vary naturally or as a consequence of the environment.

Because the embryo-fetus is very sensitive to radiation, radiation workers should exercise caution and employ appropriate safety measures when performing diagnostic radiographic procedures that result in any dose to the unborn. Most diagnostic procedures result in equivalent doses less than 0.01 Sv. Such doses are not usually considered dangerous to the unborn.

## GENETIC (HEREDITARY) EFFECTS

### Cause of Genetic (Hereditary) Mutations

Biologic effects of ionizing radiation on future generations are termed **genetic (hereditary) effects.**

These responses occur as a result of radiation-induced damage to the DNA molecule in the sperm or ova of an adult. When these germ cell mutations occur, faulty genetic information is transmitted to the offspring. This faulty hereditary information may manifest as various diseases or malformations.

## Natural Spontaneous Mutations

Normally, mutations in genetic material occur spontaneously, without a known cause. Mutations in genes and DNA that occur at random as a natural phenomenon are called *spontaneous mutations.* Because these genetic alterations are permanent and heritable, they can be transmitted from one generation to the next. Spontaneous mutations in human genetic material cause a wide variety of disorders or diseases, including:

- Hemophilia
- Huntington's chorea
- Down syndrome (mongolism)
- Duchenne's muscular dystrophy
- Sickle cell anemia
- Cystic fibrosis
- Hydrocephalus

A hereditary disorder is present in approximately 10% of all live births in the United States.

## Mutagens Responsible for Genetic Mutations

In each generation, some genetic mutations occur as part of a natural order of events. However, certain agents can increase the frequency of mutations. Some of these include:

- Elevated temperatures, which cause the speed of chemical reactions within the body to increase more rapidly, thereby damaging DNA molecules
- Ionizing radiation
- Viruses
- Absorption of certain chemicals

These agents are called *mutagens,* and ionizing radiation is one of the more effective mutagens

known. Any nonlethal radiation dose received by the germ cells can cause chromosome mutations that may be transmitted to successive generations.

## Radiation Interaction with DNA Macromolecules

When radiation interacts with DNA macromolecules, it can modify the structure of these molecules by causing breaks in the chromosomes or change the amount of DNA belonging to a cell by causing a deletion or an alteration in the sequence of nitrogen bases. Such modifications change the cell's hereditary information. A mutation of this type could eventually lead to genetic disease in subsequent generations.

## Cellular Damage Repair by Enzymes

Enzymes attempt to repair cellular damage by mending structural breaks in chromosomes that have been hit by ionizing radiation. If repair is successful, the cell will continue to function normally. If repair does not occur, the cell may undergo functional impairment or die.

## Incapacities of Mutant Genes

Mutant genes cannot properly govern the cell's normal chemical reactions or properly control the sequence of amino acids in the formation of specific proteins. These incapacities result in various genetic diseases. For example, sickle cell anemia arises from the defective synthesis of the protein hemoglobin. About 300 amino acids combine to form the hemoglobin molecule. Sickle cell anemia is caused by the omission of only a single vital amino acid.

## Dominant or Recessive Point Mutations

Point mutations (genetic mutations at the molecular level) may be either *dominant* (probably expressed in the offspring) or *recessive* (probably not expressed for several generations). Radiation is thought to cause primarily recessive mutations. For a recessive mutation to appear in the offspring, both parents must have the same genetic defect. This means that the defect must be located on the same part of a specific DNA base sequence in each parent.

Because this rarely occurs, the effects of recessive mutations are not likely to appear in a population. However, an increase in the number of individuals who receive radiation exposure raises the likelihood that two individuals having the same type of mutation will have children. Therefore, imaging professionals should limit not only the amount of radiation received by an individual but also the radiation exposure of the entire population. Damage from recessive mutations sometimes manifests more subtly and may appear as:

- Allergies
- A slight alteration in metabolism
- Decreased intelligence
- Predisposition to certain diseases

## Ionizing Radiation as a Cause of Genetic (Hereditary) Effects

The only concrete evidence showing that ionizing radiation causes genetic effects comes from extensive experimentation with fruit flies and mice at high radiation doses. The data on mice may be extrapolated to low doses and then applied to humans. The information obtained from the experiments indicates that hereditary effects do not have a threshold dose. Because this implies that even the smallest radiation dose could cause some hereditary damage, there is no such thing as a "100% safe" gonadal radiation dose.

Existing data on radiation-induced genetic effects in humans are both contradictory and inconclusive. Some of the data accumulated come from observation of test groups of children conceived after one or both parents had been exposed to radiation, as a result of the atomic bomb detonation in Hiroshima or Nagasaki. As of the third generation, no radiation-induced

genetic effects are known. However, this does not mean that they will not be seen in subsequent generations. J.F. Crow, a geneticist who spent many years experimenting with fruit flies, stated the following: "The most frequent mutations in man are not those leading to freaks or obvious hereditary diseases, but those causing minor impairments leading to higher embryonic death rates, lower life expectancy, increase in disease, or decreased fertility."[35]

In 2001 an UNSCEAR study on the hereditary effects of radiation concluded that no radiation-induced genetic diseases had so far been demonstrated in human populations exposed to ionizing radiation.[36] However, several other studies after the Chernobyl accident contradicted this conclusion. These studies indicated an increase in abnormalities, or at least in gene mutations, as a result of the accident.[22]

Currently, evidence of radiation-induced hereditary effects has not been observed in persons employed in diagnostic imaging or in patients undergoing radiologic examinations. To minimize the possibility of these adverse responses in those persons engaged in the practice of medical imaging and in patients, gonadal shielding must be effectively used, and all radiation exposure must be maintained ALARA (as low as reasonably achievable).

## Doubling Dose Concept

Animal studies of radiation-induced hereditary changes led to the development of the doubling dose concept. This dose measures the effectiveness of ionizing radiation in causing mutations. **Doubling dose** is the radiation dose that causes the number of spontaneous mutations occurring in a given generation to increase to two times their original number. For example, if 7% of the offspring in each generation are born with mutations in the absence of radiation other than background levels, the administration of the doubling dose to all members of the population would eventually increase the number of mutations to 14% (Box 9-3). The radiation doubling equivalent dose for humans, as determined from studies

| BOX 9-3 | Doubling Dose Concept | |
| --- | --- | --- |
| Percentage (%) of offspring born in each generation with mutations in the absence of radiation other than background | Estimated radiation dose in sieverts (Sv) received | Percentage (%) of offspring born with mutation after receiving a doubling equivalent dose |
| 7% | 1.56 Sv | 14% |

of the children of the atomic bomb survivors of Hiroshima and Nagasaki, is estimated to have a mean value of 1.56 Sv based on the hereditary indicators of untoward pregnancy outcome (e.g., stillbirths, major congenital abnormalities, death during the first postnatal week), childhood mortality, and sex chromosome aneuploidy (possession of an abnormal number of chromosomes). For this reason, the administration of even low doses of radiation to the gonads must be strictly controlled to reduce the risk of genetic damage in future generations. This precaution will help preserve the biologic fitness of the human race.

## SUMMARY

- Scientists use the information from epidemiologic studies to formulate dose-response estimates to predict the risk of cancer in human populations exposed to low doses of ionizing radiation.
- Information obtained from a radiation dose-response curve can be used to attempt to predict the risk of occurrence of malignancies in human populations exposed to low levels of ionizing radiation.
  - Curves that graphically demonstrate radiation dose-response relationships can be either linear or nonlinear and depict either a threshold or a nonthreshold dose.
  - A linear nonthreshold curve currently is used for most types of cancers.

- Risk associated with low-level radiation can be estimated with the linear-quadratic nonthreshold curve.
- Deterministic effects of significant radiation exposure may be demonstrated graphically through the use of a linear threshold curve of radiation dose response.
- High-dose cellular response may be demonstrated through the use of a sigmoid threshold curve.
- Late effects occur months or years after irradiation.
  - Late effects include carcinogenesis, cataractogenesis, and embryologic (birth) defects.
  - Cancer is the most important late stochastic somatic effect caused by exposure to ionizing radiation.
  - Effects directly related to dose received that occur months or years after radiation exposure are called *late deterministic somatic effects.*
  - Effects that have no threshold, occur arbitrarily, have a severity that does not depend on dose, and occur months or years after exposure are called *late stochastic effects.*
- Risk estimates are given in terms of *absolute risk* or *relative risk.*
  - The absolute risk model predicts that a specific number of excess cancers will occur as a result of radiation exposure.
  - The relative risk model predicts that the number of excess cancers rises as the natural incidence of cancer increases with advancing age in a population.
  - Linear and linear-quadratic models are used for extrapolation of risk from high-dose to low-dose data.
- The first trimester of pregnancy is the most critical period for radiation exposure of the embryo-fetus.
  - Radiation-induced congenital abnormalities can occur approximately 10 days to 12 weeks after conception.
  - Skeletal abnormalities most frequently occur from weeks 3 to 20.

- Radiation exposure in the second and third trimesters can cause congenital abnormalities, functional disorders, and a predisposition to the development of childhood cancer.
- Genetic (hereditary) effects of ionizing radiation are biologic effects on generations yet unborn.
  - Radiation-induced abnormalities are caused by unrepaired damage to DNA molecules in the sperm or ova of an adult.
  - There is no 100% safe gonadal radiation dose; even the smallest radiation dose could cause some hereditary damage.
  - Doubling dose measures the effectiveness of ionizing radiation in causing mutations; it is the radiation dose that causes the number of spontaneous mutations in a given generation to increase to two times their original number.
  - For humans, the doubling dose is estimated to have a mean value of 1.56 Sv.

# REFERENCES

1. Travis EL: *Primer of medical radiobiology*, ed 2, Chicago, 1989, Year Book.
2. Straume T, Dobson RL: Implications of new Hiroshima and Nagasaki dose estimates: cancer risks and neutron RBE. *Health Phys* 41:666, 1981.
3. Webster EW: *Critical issues in setting radiation dose limits*, Proceedings No. 3, Washington, DC, 1982, National Council on Radiation Protection and Measurements (NCRP).
4. Hendee WR, editor: *Health effects of low-level radiation*, Norwalk, Conn, 1984, Appleton-Century-Crofts.
5. *Doses from medical x-ray procedures*. Available at: http://hps.org/physicians/documents/Doses_from_Medical_X-Ray_Procedures.pdf. Accessed April 10, 2013.
6. International Commission on Radiological Protection (ICRP): Recommendations of the International Commission on Radiological Protection, ICRP Publication No. 60. *Ann ICRP* 21:1–3, 1991.
7. National Research Council, Commission of Life Sciences, Committee on Biological Effects on Ionizing Radiation (BEIR V), Board on Radiation Effects Research: *Health effects of exposure to low levels of ionizing radiations*, Washington, DC, 1989, National Academies Press.
8. Tilke B: Navajo miners battle long-term effects of radiation. *Adv Radiol Technol* 3:3, 1990.
9. Bushong SC: *Radiologic science for technologists: physics, biology and protection*, ed 10, St. Louis, 2013, Mosby.
10. Dowd SB, Tilson ER: *Practical radiation protection and applied radiobiology*, ed 2, Philadelphia, 1999, Saunders.
11. Hamilton TE, et al: Thyroid neoplasia in Marshall Islanders exposed to nuclear fallout. *JAMA* 258:629, 1987.
12. Lessard E, Miltenberger R, Conard R, et al: *Thyroid absorbed dose for people at Rongelap, Utrik, and Sifo on March 1, 1954*, U.S. Department of Energy publication (BNL) 51-882, Upton, NY, 1985, Brookhaven National Laboratory.
13. Sinclair WK: Radiation protection recommendations on dose limits: the role of the NCRP and the ICRP and future developments. *J Radiat Oncol Biol Phys* 131:387–392, 1995.
14. Hall EJ: *Radiobiology for the radiologist*, ed 5, Philadelphia, 2000, Lippincott Williams & Wilkins.
15. Gale RP: Immediate medical consequences of nuclear accidents: lessons from Chernobyl. *JAMA* 258:625, 1987.
16. Perry AR, Iglar AF: The accident at Chernobyl: radiation doses and effects. *Radiol Technol* 61:290, 1990.
17. WGBH Transcript: Back to Chernobyl, *Nova* No. 1604, Boston, 1989 (television program originally broadcast on PBS on February 14, 1989).
18. Balter M: Children become the first victims of fallout. *Science* 272:357, 1996.
19. United Nations Scientific Committee on the Effects of Atomic Radiation (UNSCEAR): *2000 report to the General Assembly, with Scientific Annexes, UNSCEAR 2000: sources and effects of ionizing radiation*, New York, 2000, United Nations.
20. Williams N: Leukemia studies continue to draw a blank. *Science* 272:358, 1996.
21. Otto Hug Strahleninstit: *Information*, Ausgabe 9/2001 K, 2001.
22. *Chernobyl: the facts—what you need to know—almost 20 years after the disaster*. Available at: http://www.chernobyl-international.org/documents/chernobylfacts2.pdf. Accessed April 15, 2013.
23. Walker SJ: *Permissible dose: a history of radiation protection in the twentieth century*, Berkeley, 2000, University of California Press.
24. *Chernobyl accident*. Available at: http://www.martinfrost.ws/htmlfiles/chernobyl1.html. Accessed April 15, 2013.
25. Conclusions of 3rd International Conference: Health effects of the Chernobyl accident. *Int J Radiat Med* 3:3–4, 2001.

26. *Fifteen years after the Chernobyl accident: lessons learned*, International Conference Executive Summary, Kiev, 2001.
27. Dubreuil GH, Lochard J, Girard P, et al: Chernobyl post-accident management: the ETHOS Project. *Health Phys* 77:361–372, 1999.
28. University of Minnesota, Health Studies Section: *U.S. Radiologic Technologists Study*, vol 2, Minneapolis, 2004.
29. University of Minnesota, Health Studies Section: *U.S. Radiologic Technologists Study*. Available at: www.radtechstudy.org. Accessed March 17, 2005.
30. Stewart A, et al: A survey of childhood malignancies. *Br Med J* 1:1495, 1958.
31. United Nations Scientific Committee on the Effects of Atomic Radiation (UNSCEAR): *Biological effects of pre-natal irradiation*, 35th Session of UNSCEAR, Vienna, April 1986, New York, 1986, United Nations.
32. Webster EW, the Biological Effects Committee of the American Association of Physicists in Medicine (AAPM): *A primer on low-level ionizing radiation and its biological effects*, AAPM Report No. 18, New York, 1986, American Institute of Physics (published for the American Association of Physicists in Medicine).
33. Eijgenraam F: Chernobyl's cloud: a lighter shade of gray. *Science* 252:1245, 1991.
34. Goss LB: International team examines health in zones contaminated by Chernobyl. *Phys Today* 40:20, 1991.
35. Crow JF: Genetic effects of radiation. *Bull At Sci* 14:19, 1958.
36. United Nations Scientific Committee on the Effects of Atomic Radiation (UNSCEAR): *Hereditary effects of radiation*, New York, 2001, United Nations.

## GENERAL DISCUSSION QUESTIONS

1. How can the information obtained from a radiation dose-response curve be used?
2. What did the BEIR Committee's 1990 revised risk estimates for the atomic bomb survivors of Hiroshima and Nagasaki indicate?
3. What rationale is used when regulatory agencies establish radiation protection standards?
4. What is the difference between late deterministic somatic effects and late stochastic (probabilistic) effects of ionizing radiation?
5. What is the difference between the absolute risk model and the relative risk model used for estimating risk caused by a specific exposure to ionizing radiation?
6. Name five groups of humans exposed to high doses of ionizing radiation that demonstrate proof that radiation induces cancer, and explain the circumstances that led to the exposure received by each group.
7. What is organogenesis, and what are the consequences to the developing fetus, if irradiated during this period?
8. Describe the concept of doubling dose.
9. Describe the importance of epidemiologic studies as they related to radiation-induced cancer.
10. Name two groups of individuals who have demonstrated an increase in the incidence of breast cancer after radiation exposure.

## REVIEW QUESTIONS

1. Cancer and genetic defects are examples of _____ effects.
   A. Stochastic
   B. Nonstochastic
   C. Birth
   D. Deterministic
2. Some examples of measurable late biologic damage are:
   1. Cataracts.
   2. Leukemia.
   3. Nausea and vomiting.
   4. Genetic mutations.
   A. 1 and 2 only
   B. 2 and 3 only
   C. 1, 2, and 3 only
   D. 1, 2, and 4 only

3. Which of the following provide the foundation for the sigmoid or S-shaped (nonlinear) threshold curve of radiation dose response?
   1. Data from human populations observed after acute high doses of radiation
   2. Data from human populations observed after chronic low doses of radiation
   3. Laboratory experiments on animals
   A. 1 only
   B. 2 only
   C. 3 only
   D. 1, 2, and 3

4. The linear nonthreshold curve implies that biologic response is:
   A. Directly proportional to the dose.
   B. Inversely proportional to the dose.
   C. Insignificant in relation to dose.
   D. Not able to be plotted on a dose-response curve.

5. Reevaluation of the quantity and type of radiation that was released in the atomic bombing of the cities of Hiroshima and Nagasaki has led to revised atomic bomb data in which radiation-induced leukemia and solid tumors may now be attributed predominantly to:
   A. Alpha radiation exposure.
   B. Gamma radiation exposure.
   C. Neutron radiation exposure.
   D. X-radiation exposure.

6. The radiation dose-response relationship is demonstrated graphically through the use of a curve that maps the observed effects of radiation exposure in relation to the dose of radiation received. Which of the following curves expresses a linear-quadratic nonthreshold dose response?
   A. ⌁
   B. ⌁
   C. ⌁
   D. ⌁

7. During the 10 years immediately after the 1986 Chernobyl nuclear power station accident, which of the following was the *most pronounced* health effect observed?
   1. Dramatic increase in the incidence of childhood leukemia
   2. Dramatic increase in thyroid cancer in children living in the regions where the heaviest radioactive contamination occurred
   3. Major increase in the number of solid tumors in the general population of the former Soviet Union
   A. 1, 2, and 3
   B. 1 only
   C. 2 only
   D. 3 only

8. The early demise of experimental animals exposed to nonlethal doses of ionizing radiation actually resulted from:
   A. Accelerated aging.
   B. Hemorrhage.
   C. Induction of cancer.
   D. Respiratory distress.

9. According to data from studies performed on U.S. Radiologic Technologists, individuals who began working before 1950 had a somewhat higher risk of dying of _____ when compared with technologists who started working in 1950 and later.
   A. Darkroom disease
   B. Leukemia
   C. Pancreatic cancer
   D. Thyroid cancer

10. Most diagnostic procedures result in equivalent doses:
    A. Above 0.01 Sv, but less than 1.56 Sv
    B. Less than 0.01 Sv.
    C. Above 1.56 Sv.
    D. Between 0.01 Sv and 1.56 Sv.

## CHAPTER 10

# Dose Limits for Exposure to Ionizing Radiation

**OBJECTIVES**

*After completing this chapter, the reader will be able to perform the following:*

- List and describe the function of the four major organizations that share the responsibility for evaluating the relationship between radiation equivalent dose and induced biologic effects and five U.S. regulatory agencies responsible for enforcing established radiation effective dose limiting standards.
- Explain the function of the radiation safety committee (RSC) in a medical facility, and describe the role of the radiation safety officer (RSO) by listing the various responsibilities he or she must fulfill.
- Explain the purpose of the Radiation Control for Health and Safety Act of 1968 and the Consumer Patient Health and Safety Act of 1981.
- List the important provisions of the code of standards for diagnostic x-ray equipment that began on August 1, 1974.
- Explain the ALARA concept.
- Describe the current radiation protection philosophy, and state the goal and objectives of radiation protection.
- Identify radiation-induced responses that warrant serious concern for radiation protection.
- Explain the concept of risk as it relates to the medical imaging industry.
- Describe the effective dose limit and the effective dose limiting system.
- Identify the risk from exposure to ionizing radiation at low absorbed doses.

- Discuss current National Council on Radiation Protection and Measurements recommendations.
- Given appropriate data, calculate the cumulative effective dose for the whole body for a radiation worker.
- Explain the function of collective effective dose, and list the unit used to express this quantity.
- Discuss the significance of action limits in health care facilities.
- Explain the concept of radiation hormesis.
- State the following in terms of International System (SI) units:
  - Annual occupational effective dose limit and cumulative effective dose (CumEfD) limit for whole-body exposure excluding medical and natural background exposure, which are based on stochastic effects
  - Annual occupational equivalent dose limits for tissues and organs such as lens of the eye, skin, hands, and feet, which are based on deterministic effects
  - Annual effective dose limits for continuous (or frequent) exposure and for infrequent exposure of the general public from manmade sources other than medical and natural background, which are based on stochastic effects
  - Annual equivalent dose limits for tissues and organs such as lens of the eye, skin, hands, and feet of members of the general public, which are based on deterministic effects

Copyright © 2014, Elsevier Inc.

- Annual effective dose limit for an occupationally exposed student under the age of 18 years (excluding medical and natural background radiation exposure)

- Occupational monthly equivalent dose limit to the embryo-fetus (excluding medical and natural background radiation) once the pregnancy is known

## CHAPTER OUTLINE

## KEY TERMS

| | | |
|---|---|---|
| and Measurements (NCRP) | optimization | radiation safety officer (RSO) |
| negligible individual dose (NID) | person-sievert | risk |
| | radiation hormesis | stochastic effects |
| Nuclear Regulatory Commission (NRC) | radiation-induced malignancy | tissue weighting factor ($W_T$) |
| | radiation safety committee (RSC) | |

Exposure of the general public, patients, and radiation workers to ionizing radiation must be limited to minimize the risk of harmful biologic effects. To this end, scientists have developed occupational and nonoccupational **effective dose (EfD)** limits and **equivalent dose (EqD)** limits for tissues and organs such as the lens of the eye, skin, hands, and feet. An **effective dose (EfD) limiting system** (i.e., a set of numeric dose limits that are based on calculations of the various risks of cancer and genetic [hereditary] effects to tissues or organs exposed to radiation) has been incorporated into Title 10 of the Code of Federal Regulations, Part 20, a document prepared and distributed by the U.S. Office of the Federal Register. The rules and regulations of the Nuclear Regulatory Commission (NRC) and fundamental radiation protection standards governing occupational radiation exposure are included in this document.

## BASIS OF EFFECTIVE DOSE LIMITING SYSTEM

The concept of radiation exposure and of the associated risk of **radiation-induced malignancy** is the basis of the effective dose limiting system. Information contained in Report No. 116 of the National Council on Radiation Protection and Measurement (NCRP) and Publication No. 60 of the International Commission on Radiological Protection (ICRP) serves as a resource for the revised recommendations. Future radiation protection standards are expected to continue to be based on *risk*.

Because medical imaging professionals share the responsibility for patient safety from radiation exposure and also are subject themselves to such exposure in the performance of their duties, they must be familiar with previous, existing, and new guidelines. By keeping informed, they will be more conscious of good radiation safety practices. A radiographer may obtain the required knowledge by becoming familiar with the functions of the various advisory groups and regulatory agencies discussed in this chapter (Fig. 10-1).

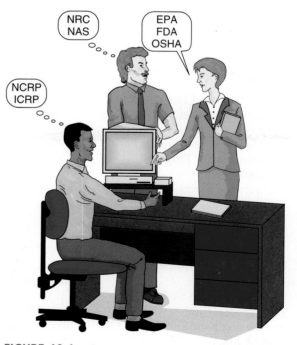

**FIGURE 10-1**  The various advisory groups and regulatory agencies, usually referred to by abbreviations and acronyms, may be extremely confusing.

# RADIATION PROTECTION STANDARDS ORGANIZATIONS

The discussion that follows concerns the four major organizations responsible for evaluating the relationship between radiation EqD and induced biologic effects. In addition, the following organizations are concerned with formulating risk estimates of somatic and genetic effects of irradiation:

1. International Commission on Radiological Protection (ICRP)
2. National Council on Radiation Protection and Measurements (NCRP)
3. United Nations Scientific Committee on the Effects of Atomic Radiation (UNSCEAR)
4. National Academy of Sciences/National Research Council Committee on the Biological Effects of Ionizing Radiation (NAS/NRC-BEIR)

A summary of radiation standards organizations is presented in Table 10-1.

## International Commission on Radiological Protection

The **International Commission on Radiological Protection (ICRP)** is considered the international authority on the safe use of sources of ionizing radiation. It is composed of a main commission with 12 active members, a chairman, and 4 standing committees, which include committees on radiation effects, radiation exposure, protection in medicine, and the application of ICRP recommendations.[1] Since its inception in 1928, the ICRP has been the leading international organization responsible for providing clear and consistent radiation protection guidance through its recommendations for:

- Occupational dose limits
- Public dose limits

Originally, these recommendations were published as reports in selected scholarly journals. Since 1959 the ICRP has had its own series of publications, and from 1977 onward the scientific journal *Annals of the ICRP* has published ICRP information. The information that serves as a basis for the recommendations is supplied by scientific articles published in scholarly journals and by organizations such as UNSCEAR and NAS/NRC-BEIR, which are discussed later in this chapter. The ICRP only makes recommendations; it does not function as an enforcement agency. Each nation must develop and enforce its own specific regulations.

| TABLE 10-1 | Summary of Radiation Protection Standards Organizations |
|---|---|
| **Organization** | **Function** |
| International Commission on Radiological Protection (ICRP) | Evaluates information on biologic effects of radiation and provides radiation protection guidance through general recommendations on occupational and public dose limits |
| National Council on Radiation Protection and Measurements (NCRP) | Reviews regulations formulated by the ICRP and decides ways to include those recommendations in U.S. radiation protection criteria |
| United Nations Scientific Committee on the Effects of Atomic Radiation (UNSCEAR) | Evaluates human and environmental ionizing radiation exposure and derives radiation risk assessments from epidemiologic data and research conclusions; provides information to organizations such as the ICRP for evaluation |
| National Academy of Sciences/National Research Council Committee on the Biological Effects of Ionizing Radiation (NAS/NRC-BEIR) | Reviews studies of biologic effects of ionizing radiation and risk assessment and provides the information to organizations such as the ICRP for evaluation |

## National Council on Radiation Protection and Measurements

In the United States a nongovernmental, non-profit, private corporation known as the **National Council on Radiation Protection and Measurements (NCRP)**, chartered by Congress in 1964, reviews the recommendations formulated by the ICRP. The NCRP determines the way ICRP recommendations are incorporated into U.S. radiation protection criteria. The council implements this task by:

- Formulating general recommendations
- Publishing their recommendations in the form of various NCRP reports

These reports may be purchased from NCRP Publications in Bethesda, Maryland. A listing of current NCRP reports available for purchase at cost may be found at www.ncrp.com.

Because the NCRP is not an enforcement agency, enactment of its recommendations lies with federal and state agencies that have the power to enforce such standards after they have been established. To facilitate understanding of the function of the NCRP, the council's objectives are identified in Box 10-1. Governmental organizations (e.g., the NRC, the Environmental Protection Agency [EPA], and state governments) use the recommendations of the NCRP as the scientific basis for their radiation protection activities.[2] Nongovernmental groups desiring to improve their radiation safety practices and their promotion and disbursement of pertinent radiation protection materials look to this public service organization for direction.

## United Nations Scientific Committee on the Effects of Atomic Radiation

UNSCEAR, which was established in 1955, is another group that plays a prominent role in the formulation of radiation protection guidelines. This group evaluates human and environmental ionizing radiation exposures from a variety of sources, including:

| BOX 10-1 | Objectives of the National Council on Radiation Protection and Measurements |
|---|---|

Objectives 4 to 7 are identified in the "charter" of the council (Public Law 88-376) as follows:
"To:
4. Collect, analyze, develop and disseminate in the public interest information and recommendations about (a) protection against radiation (b) radiation measurements, quantities and units, particularly those concerned with radiation protection.
5. Provide a means by which organizations concerned with the scientific and related aspects of radiation protection and of radiation quantities, units, and measurements may cooperate for effective utilization of their combined resources, and to stimulate the work of such organizations.
6. Develop basic concepts about radiation quantities, units, and measurements, about the application of these concepts, and about radiation protection.
7. Cooperate with the International Commission on Radiological Protection, the International Commission on Radiation Units and Measurements, and other national and international organizations, government and private, concerned with radiation quantities, units, and measurements and with radiation protection."

From National Council on Radiation Protection and Measurements (NCRP): *Limitation of exposure to ionizing radiation,* Report No. 116, Bethesda, Md, 1993, NCRP.

- Radioactive materials
- Radiation-producing machines
- Radiation accidents

UNSCEAR uses epidemiologic data (e.g., information from follow-up studies of Japanese atomic bomb survivors), information acquired from the Radiation Effects Research Foundation (a group run by the government of Japan primarily for the purpose of studying the survivors), and research conclusions to derive radiation risk assessments for radiation-induced cancer and for genetic (hereditary) effects.

## National Academy of Sciences/National Research Council Committee on the Biological Effects of Ionizing Radiation

NAS/NRC-BEIR is another advisory group that reviews studies of biologic effects of ionizing radiation and risk assessment. This group formulated the 1990 BEIR V Report, *Health Effects of Exposure to Low Levels of Ionizing Radiation.* BEIR V supersedes four earlier BEIR reports that listed studies of biologic effects and the associated risk of groups of people who were either routinely or accidentally exposed to ionizing radiation. Such groups include:

• Early radiation workers
• Atomic bomb victims of Hiroshima and Nagasaki
• Evacuees from the Chernobyl nuclear power station disaster

As previously noted, recommendations for EfD limits and EqD limits are made by the ICRP, NCRP, UNSCEAR, and NAS/NRC-BEIR. Based on these recommendations, limits on radiation exposure are established by congressional act or state mandates. National and state agencies are charged with the responsibility of enforcing standards after they have been established.

## U.S. REGULATORY AGENCIES

After radiation protection standards have been determined, responsible agencies must enforce them for the protection of the general public, patients, and occupationally exposed personnel.

Regulatory agencies include the following:

1. Nuclear Regulatory Commission (NRC)
2. Agreement states
3. Environmental Protection Agency (EPA)
4. U.S. Food and Drug Administration (FDA)
5. Occupational Safety and Health Administration (OSHA)

A summary of the U.S. regulatory agencies is presented in Table 10-2.

## Nuclear Regulatory Commission

The **Nuclear Regulatory Commission (NRC)**, formerly known as the *Atomic Energy Commission (AEC),* is a federal agency that has the authority to control the possession, use, and production of atomic energy in the interest

| TABLE 10-2 | Summary of U.S. Regulatory Agencies | |
|---|---|
| **Agency** | **Function** |
| Nuclear Regulatory Commission (NRC) | Oversees the nuclear energy industry, enforces radiation protection standards, publishes its rules and regulations in Title 10 of the U.S. Code of Federal Regulations, and enters into written agreements with state governments that permit the state to license and regulate the use of radioisotopes and certain other material within that state |
| Agreement states | Enforce radiation protection regulations through their respective health departments |
| Environmental Protection Agency (EPA) | Facilitates the development and enforcement of regulations pertaining to the control of radiation in the environment |
| U.S. Food and Drug Administration (FDA) | Conducts an ongoing product radiation control program, regulating the design and manufacture of electronic products, including x-ray equipment |
| Occupational Safety and Health Administration (OSHA) | Functions as a monitoring agency in places of employment, predominantly in industry |

of national security. This agency also has the power to enforce radiation protection standards. However, the NRC does not regulate or inspect x-ray imaging facilities. The main function of the NRC is to oversee the nuclear energy industry. This agency supervises the:

- Design and working mechanics of nuclear power stations
- Production of nuclear fuel
- Handling of expended fuel
- Supervision of hazardous radioactive waste material

In addition, the NRC controls the manufacture and use of radioactive substances formed in nuclear reactors and used in:

- Research
- Nuclear medicine imaging procedures
- Therapeutic treatment (e.g., most commonly, prostate cancer radioactive seed implants and iodine-131 ($^{131}$I) used for the treatment of thyroid carcinoma)
- Industry

The NRC also licenses users of such radioactive materials and periodically makes unannounced inspections to determine whether these users are in compliance with the provisions of their licenses. Up until 2008 the NRC did not regulate the use of radioactive substances that either are naturally occurring or are produced outside of a reactor by high-energy particle accelerators such as cyclotrons. These materials are given the word designation *NARM*. It stands for "naturally occurring and/or accelerator produced materials." Two common examples of cyclotron-produced isotopes are:

- Thallium-201 ($^{201}$Tl) used in nuclear medicine for heart stress tests
- Palladium-103 ($^{103}$Pd) used for therapeutic prostate seed implants

NARM materials were formerly solely regulated by State Bureaus of Radiation Protection. In 2008 the NRC expanded its definition of by-product substances to include NARM materials. This meant, by a certain specified date, all facilities in nonagreement states (i.e., those states that have decided to maintain their own designed independent radiation protection program for radioactive materials) in order to be in compliance, would have to amend their NRC radioactive materials licenses to include all NARM materials that they are currently using.

The NRC writes standards that are presented as rules and regulations. The agency publishes these rules and regulations in Title 10 of the U.S. Code of Federal Regulations. The U.S. Office of the Federal Register prepares and distributes this document. Fundamental radiation protection standards governing occupational radiation exposure may be found in Part 20 of Title 10. Therefore the abbreviation 10 CFR 20 is used.

The NRC has the authority to enter into written contracts with state governments. These agreements permit the contracting state to undertake the responsibility of licensing and regulating the use of radioisotopes and certain other radioactive materials within that state.

## Agreement States

Most states in the United States have entered into "agreements" with the NRC to assume responsibility for enforcing radiation protection regulations through their respective health departments. These states are known as **agreement states.** In *nonagreement states*, both the state and the NRC enforce radiation protection regulations by sending agents to health care facilities. Hospitals that use x-rays and radioactive materials are evaluated to determine whether they are in compliance with existing radiation safety regulations. Individual states also may legislate their own regulations regarding radiation safety. Inspection of nuclear reactors and assurance of adherence to federal radiation safety regulations in agreement or nonagreement states fall solely under the jurisdiction of the NRC.

## Environmental Protection Agency

The EPA was established on December 2, 1970. It was created through the reorganization plan of former U.S. president Richard M. Nixon. The agency was created to bring several departments under one organization that would be responsible for protecting the health of humans and for safeguarding the natural environment.

The EPA, as part of its general overseer responsibilities, facilitates the development and enforcement of regulations pertaining to the control of radiation in the environment. It:

• Directs federal agencies
• Oversees the general area of environmental monitoring
• Has the authority for specific areas such as determining the action level for radon

## U.S. Food and Drug Administration

Under Public Law 90-602, the Radiation Control for Health and Safety Act of 1968, the FDA:

• Conducts an ongoing product radiation control program, regulating the design and manufacturing of electronic products, including diagnostic x-ray equipment

A more detailed explanation of the Radiation Control for Health and Safety Act of 1968 is given later in this chapter.

To determine the level of compliance with standards in a given x-ray facility, the FDA conducts on-site inspections of x-ray equipment, especially mammography units. Compliance with FDA standards ensures the protection of occupationally and nonoccupationally exposed persons from faulty manufacturing.

## Occupational Safety and Health Administration

OSHA functions as a monitoring agency in places of employment, predominantly in industry. OSHA regulates occupational exposure to radiation through Part 1910 of Title 29 of the U.S. Code of Federal Regulations (*29 CFR 1910*). It is responsible for regulations concerning an employee's "right to know" with regard to hazards that may be present in the workplace. A series of statutes passed by the individual states

requires that employees be made aware of the hazards in the workplace. The act covers:

• Hazardous substances
• Infectious agents
• Ionizing radiation
• Nonionizing radiation

The act requires employers to evaluate their workplaces for hazardous agents and to provide training and written information to their employees. OSHA also regulates training programs in the workplace.

## RADIATION SAFETY PROGRAM

### Requirement

Facilities providing imaging services must have an effective and detailed radiation safety program to ensure adequate safety of patients and radiation workers. The implementation of an effective program begins with the administration of the facility. Individuals in executive positions must provide the resources necessary for creating and maintaining such a program. They can:

• Delegate operational funds in the budget
• Oversee the development of policies and procedures
• Provide the equipment necessary for starting and for continuing the program

### Radiation Safety Committee and Radiation Safety Officer

The NRC mandates that a **radiation safety committee (RSC)** be established for the facility. This committee provides guidance for the program and facilitates its ongoing operation. A **radiation safety officer (RSO)** should also be selected to:

• Oversee the program's daily operation
• Provide for formal review of the program each year

An RSO is normally a medical physicist, health physicist, radiologist, or other individual qualified through adequate training and experience.

This person has been designated by a health care facility and approved by the NRC and the state.

**Responsibilities of the Radiation Safety Officer.** The RSO is specifically responsible for developing an appropriate radiation safety program for the facility that follows internationally accepted guidelines for radiation protection. He or she is charged with ensuring that the facility's operational radiation practices are such that all persons, especially those who are or could be pregnant, are adequately protected from unnecessary exposure. To fulfill this responsibility, management of the facility must grant the RSO the authority necessary to:

- Implement and enforce the policies of the radiation safety program

The RSO also must review and maintain radiation-monitoring records for all personnel and be available to provide counseling for individuals (e.g., those who receive monitor readings in excess of allowable limits).

**Required Training and Experience for a Radiation Safety Officer.** The necessary training and experience for an RSO are described in sections 10 CFR 35.50 and 10 CFR 35.900 of the Code of Federal Regulations. The NRC publishes regulatory guides to accompany its rules. Although on a legal level health care facilities do not need to comply with the guide, they frequently choose to do so to facilitate the chances of a successful outcome of an NRC inspection or approval of license changes because the guide is actually the NRC's interpretation of how to implement its own rules.

The training and experience requirements for the RSO allow for three training pathways. These pathways are identified in Box 10-2.

**Authority of the Radiation Safety Officer.** 10 CFR 35.24 requires that the licensee provide the RSO:

- Sufficient authority
- Organizational freedom
- Management prerogative to perform certain duties

**BOX 10-2**   **Allowable Pathways for a Radiation Safety Officer to Meet Training and Experience Requirements as Described in 10 CFR 35.50 and 10 CFR 35.900**

1. Certification by one of the professional boards approved by the Nuclear Regulatory Commission (NRC)
2. Didactic and work experience as described in detail in the regulations
3. Identification as an authorized user, authorized medical physicist, or authorized nuclear physicist on the license, with experience in the types of uses for which the individual has radiation safety officer (RSO) responsibilities

**BOX 10-3**   **Duties That 10 CFR 35.24 Requires the Licensee to Freely Provide the Radiation Safety Officer to Perform**

1. Identify radiation safety problems.
2. Initiate, recommend, or provide corrective action.
3. Stop unsafe operations involving by-product material.
4. Verify implementation of corrective actions.

These duties are identified in Box 10-3. The licensee must establish, in writing, the authority, duties, and responsibilities of the RSO. Because the RSO is responsible for the day-to-day supervision of the facility's radiation safety program, he or she must have independent authority to stop operations that are considered unsafe. In addition, this individual must be given adequate time and resources and have a sufficient commitment from management to ensure that radioactive materials are used in a safe manner. The NRC requires the name of the RSO on the facility's radioactive materials license to ensure that licensee management has always identified a responsible, qualified person who can directly interact with the NRC during inspections and also concerning any inquiries about the facility's safety program. Usually, the RSO is a full-time employee of the licensed facility; however, the NRC has authorized individuals who are not employed by the licensee (e.g., a consultant) to fill the role of an RSO or to provide support to the facility's RSO. Training for this role is covered in 10 CFR 35. A list of these requirements may be found in Appendix H.

## RADIATION CONTROL FOR HEALTH AND SAFETY ACT OF 1968

In 1968 the U.S. Congress passed the Radiation Control for Health and Safety Act (Public Law 90-602) to protect the public from the hazards of unnecessary radiation exposure resulting from electronic products such as microwave ovens and color televisions. Diagnostic x-ray equipment also was included. The act permitted the establishment of the Center for Devices and Radiological Health (CDRH). Until 1982 this organization was known as the *Bureau of Radiological Health* (BRH). The CDRH falls under the jurisdiction of the FDA. Essentially, it is responsible for conducting an ongoing electronic product radiation control program. This includes setting up standards for the manufacture, installation, assembly, and maintenance of machines for radiologic procedures. Further responsibilities include:

- Assessing the biologic effects of ionizing radiation
- Evaluating radiation emissions from electronic products in general
- Conducting research to reduce radiation exposure

## Code of Standards for Diagnostic X-Ray Equipment

The code of standards for diagnostic x-ray equipment went into effect on August 1, 1974. This code applies to complete systems and major components manufactured after that date. Equipment in use before August 1, 1974, does not need to be modified or discarded. Some important

provisions of the standards for diagnostic x-ray equipment are listed in Box 10-4.

Public Law 90-602 does not regulate the diagnostic x-ray user. It is strictly an equipment performance standard.

---

| BOX 10-4 | Provisions Included in the Standards for Diagnostic X-Ray Equipment |
| --- | --- |

1. Automatic limitation of the radiographic beam to the image receptor regardless of image receptor size, a condition known as *positive beam limitation.*
2. Appropriate minimal permanent filtration of the x-ray beam to ensure an acceptable level of beam quality. Filtration provides significant reduction in the intensity of very "soft" x-rays that contribute only to the added patient absorbed dose.
3. Ability of x-ray units to duplicate certain radiation exposures for any given combination of kilovolts at peak value (kVp), milliamperes (mA), and time to ensure both exposure reproducibility and linearity. *Reproducibility* is defined as consistency in output in radiation intensity for identical generator settings from one individual exposure to subsequent exposures.* A variance of 5% or less is acceptable. *Exposure linearity* is defined as consistency in output radiation intensity at a selected kVp setting when changing from one milliamperage and time combination (mAs = mA × exposure time) to another. *Linearity,* which is defined as the ratio of the difference in mR/mAs values between two successive generator stations to the sum of those mR/mAs values, must be less than 0.1).
4. Inclusion of beam limitation devices for spot films taken during fluoroscopy. Such devices should be located between the x-ray source and the patient.
5. Presence of "beam on" indicators to give visible warnings when x-ray exposures are in progress and both visual and audible signals when exposure has terminated.
6. Inclusion of manual backup timers for automatic (photo-timed) exposure control to ensure the termination of the exposure if the automatic timer fails.

---

*Mathematically, reproducibility is described by the coefficient of variation $C$, which is equal to the standard deviation of at least five successive output measurements employing the same technique factors divided by the average, or mean value, of those measurements. The regulation requires that $C$ must not exceed 0.05.

## ALARA CONCEPT

In 1954 the National Committee on Radiation Protection (later known as the *National Council on Radiation Protection and Measurements*) put forth the principle that radiation exposures should be kept "as low as reasonably achievable" (ALARA) with consideration for economic and societal factors. According to NCRP Report No. 160, "The protection from radiation exposure is as low as reasonably achievable when the expenditure of further resources would be unwarranted by the reduction in exposure that would be achieved."[3]

This principle, known as the **ALARA concept,** is accepted by all regulatory agencies. In 1987, the NCRP described the ALARA concept as "the continuation of good radiation protection programs and practices which traditionally have been effective in keeping the average and individual exposures for monitored workers well below the limit."[4] It also may be referred to as **optimization** in accordance with ICRP Publication No. 37 and Publication No. 55. Medical imaging personnel and radiologists share the responsibility to:

- Keep occupational and nonoccupational dose limits ALARA

In practice this translates into EfDs and EqDs well below maximal allowable levels. This goal can usually be simply achieved through the employment of proper safety procedures performed by qualified personnel. Such procedures should be clearly described in a facility's radiation safety program. To define ALARA, health care facilities usually adopt *investigation levels*, defined as level I and level II. In the United States, these levels are traditionally one tenth to three tenths the applicable regulatory limits.

## Model for the ALARA Concept

The ALARA concept presents an extremely conservative model with respect to the relationship between ionizing radiation and potential risk.

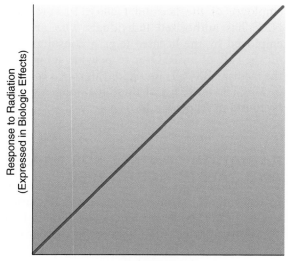

**FIGURE 10-2** **Dose-Response Curve.** Hypothetical linear (straight-line) nonthreshold curve for radiation dose-response relationship. The straight-line curve passing through the origin in this graph indicates both that the response to radiation (in terms of biologic effects) is directly proportional to the dose of radiation and that no known level of radiation dose exists below which absolutely no chance of sustaining biologic damage is evident.

The relationship is assumed to be completely linear (i.e., biologic effect and radiation dose are directly proportional) and without any threshold (Fig. 10-2). In the interest of safety, risk of injury should be overestimated rather than underestimated.

## FOOD AND DRUG ADMINISTRATION WHITE PAPER

The U.S. Food and Drug Administration (FDA) supports the premise that "each patient should get the right imaging exam, at the right time, with the right radiation dose."[5] This declaration is clearly stated in the FDA document known as the "White Paper," published in February 2010, in which they announce "the launch of a cooperative *Initiative to Reduce Unnecessary Radiation Exposure from Medical Imaging*."[5] Working in conjunction with their partners, the FDA intends to take action to:

1. "Promote safe use of medical imaging devices"[5]
2. "Support informed clinical decision"[5]
3. "Increase patient awareness"[5]

By coordinating these efforts, the FDA will be able to "optimize patient exposure to radiation from certain types of medical exams, and thereby reduce related risks while maximizing the benefits of these studies."[5] For those desiring more information about this document, a link to the website is provided in reference 5 at the end of this chapter.

## CONSUMER-PATIENT RADIATION HEALTH AND SAFETY ACT OF 1981

The Consumer-Patient Radiation Health and Safety Act of 1981 (Title IX of Public Law 97-35) (see Appendix I) provides federal legislation requiring the establishment of minimal standards for the accreditation of education programs for persons who perform radiologic procedures and the certification of such persons. The purpose of this federal act, which is under the directorship of the secretary of Health and Human Services, is to ensure that standard medical and dental radiologic procedures adhere to rigorous safety precautions and standards. Individual states are encouraged to enact similar statutes and administer certification and accreditation programs based on the standards established therein. Because no legal penalty exists for noncompliance, many states, unfortunately, have not responded with appropriate legislation.

## GOAL FOR RADIATION PROTECTION

NCRP Report No. 116, *Limitation of Exposure to Ionizing Radiation,* provides the most recent guidance on radiation protection. This report enunciates the goal of radiation protection, which reads as follows: "to prevent the occurrence of serious radiation-induced conditions (acute and chronic deterministic effects) in exposed persons and to reduce stochastic effects in exposed persons to a degree that is acceptable in relation to the benefits to the individual and to society from the activities that generate such exposures."[4] The essence of radiation protection is contained in the preceding statement.

## RADIATION-INDUCED RESPONSES OF CONCERN IN RADIATION PROTECTION

### Categories for Radiation-Induced Responses

Two all-inclusive categories encompass the radiation-induced responses of serious concern in radiation protection programs:

1. Deterministic effects
2. Stochastic (probabilistic) effects

**Deterministic Effects.** As described in the preceding chapters, **deterministic effects** are biologic somatic effects of ionizing radiation that can be directly related to the dose received. They exhibit a threshold dose below which the response does not normally occur and above which the severity of the biologic damage increases as the dose increases. For example, if a certain dose of radiation produces a skin burn, a higher dose of radiation will cause the skin burn to be more severe; however, a dose below the threshold level for skin burn will not demonstrate the effect. When radiation-induced biologic damage escalates, it does so because greater numbers of cells interact with the increased number of x-ray photons that are present at higher radiation exposures. As mentioned in Chapter 9, in general, deterministic effects typically occur only after large doses of radiation. However, they could also result from long-term individual low doses of radiation sustained over several years. In either instance the cumulative amounts of such radiation doses are usually much greater than those typically encountered by a patient in diagnostic radiology.*

***Early and Late Deterministic Effects.*** Deterministic effects may be early, such as:

- Diffuse redness over an area of skin after irradiation (erythema)
- A decrease in the white blood cell count
- Epilation, or loss of hair

Other, far more serious early consequences of radiation sickness can also arise, such as:

- Hematopoietic syndrome
- Gastrointestinal syndrome
- Cerebrovascular syndrome

These effects usually occur within a few hours or days after a very high-level radiation exposure to a significant portion of the body. The aforementioned syndromes are collectively referred to as the *acute radiation syndrome.* (Early deterministic effects, including radiation syndromes, are discussed in detail in Chapter 8.) Late deterministic somatic effects, as discussed in Chapter 9, also may occur months or years after high-level radiation exposure. They include:

- Cataract formation
- Fibrosis
- Organ atrophy
- Loss of parenchymal cells
- Reduced fertility
- Sterility caused by a decrease in reproductive cells

Early deterministic somatic effects such as erythema and late deterministic somatic effects such as cataract formation have a high probability of occurring when entrance radiation doses exceed 2 $Gy_t$. The frequency of occurrence of high-dose deterministic effects is not proportional to the dose but rather follows a nonlinear, threshold curve that is sigmoidal (S-shaped) with a threshold (see Fig. 9-1, *B*).

**Stochastic Effects.** As described in Chapter 9, **stochastic effects** are mutational, nonthreshold, randomly occurring biologic somatic changes. Mutational refers to changes to somatic cells that would affect the individual when the cells divide as opposed to genetic which refers to changes to germ cells that would affect future generations. Their chances of occurrence increase with each radiation exposure. Examples of stochastic effects are:

- Cancer
- Genetic alterations

Stochastic responses may be demonstrated with the use of both the linear (see Fig. 9-2) and the linear-quadratic dose-response curves (see Fig. 9-3). Because a stochastic event is an all-or-none, random effect, ionizing radiation could induce cancers within a general large population, but determining beforehand which members of that population will develop cancer is not possible. Injury may result from exposure of a single cell or from damage in a sensitive substructure, such as a gene. The assumption is that no minimal safe dose exists. The frequency of an occurrence in a population, however, does increase in proportion to the magnitude of the absorbed dose of ionizing radiation delivered to the entire population. Therefore, the net effect on the population group depends not only on the number of individuals irradiated but also on the mean dose that each individual receives.

A summary of both early and late deterministic and stochastic (probabilistic) effects is presented in Box 10-5.

## OBJECTIVES OF RADIATION PROTECTION

Radiation protection has two explicit objectives:

1. To prevent any clinically important radiation-induced deterministic effect from occurring by adhering to dose limits that are beneath the threshold levels

---

*A significant exception to this is high–dose-rate fluoroscopic procedures. For these studies, entrance dose rates as great as 200 $mGy_a$/min are possible. A fluoroscopic exposure of 15 minutes then, at this level, results in a patient entrance dose of approximately 3 $Gy_a$. This represents a therapeutic dose level.

BOX 10-5

## BOX 10-5 | Summary of Serious Radiation-Induced Responses of Concern

**Deterministic Effects**
**Early Effects**
Erythema (diffuse redness over an area of skin after irradiation)
Blood changes (decrease of lymphocytes and platelets)
Epilation (loss of hair)
Acute radiation syndrome
Hematopoietic syndrome
Gastrointestinal syndrome
Cerebrovascular syndrome

**Late Effects**
Cataract formation
Fibrosis
Organ atrophy
Loss of parenchymal cells
Reduced fertility
Sterility

**Stochastic (Probabilistic) Effects**
Cancer

**Genetic (Hereditary) Effects**
Mutagenesis (irradiation of DNA of somatic cells leading to abnormalities in new cells as they divide in that individual)

2. To limit the risk of stochastic responses to a conservative level as weighted against societal needs, values, benefits acquired, and economic considerations

## CURRENT RADIATION PROTECTION PHILOSOPHY

Both genetic and somatic responses to ionizing radiation were considered in developing the present EfD limiting recommendations. Current radiation protection philosophy is based on the assumption that a linear nonthreshold relationship exists between radiation dose and biologic response. Thus, even the most minuscule dose of radiation has a non-zero potential to cause some harm. The current philosophy also acknowledges that ionizing radiation possesses a beneficial and

a destructive potential. It proposes that, when employed in the healing arts for the welfare of the patient:

- The potential benefits of exposing the patient to ionizing radiation must far outweigh any potential risk

## RISK

### Risk in the Medical Imaging Industry

In general terms, *risk* may be defined as the probability of injury, ailment, or death resulting from an activity. In the medical imaging industry, **risk** after irradiation is viewed as the possibility of inducing a:

- Radiogenic cancer
- Genetic defect

The way people look at probability and severity affects the perception of risk. As stated previously, no conclusive proof exists that low-level ionizing radiation causes a statistically significant increase in the threat of a malignancy. Although this risk may in fact be negligible, the subject is still highly controversial. (A discussion of risk estimates for both stochastic and deterministic effects is presented in Chapter 9.)

### Effective Dose Limiting System

The EfD limiting system is the current method for assessing radiation exposure and associated risk of biologic damage to radiation workers and the general public (Fig. 10-3). The **effective dose limit** concerns the upper boundary dose of ionizing radiation that results in a negligible risk of:

- Bodily injury
- Hereditary damage

These limits may be expressed for whole-body exposure, partial-body exposure, and exposure of individual organs. Separate limits are set for occupationally exposed individuals and for the general public. The sum of both the external

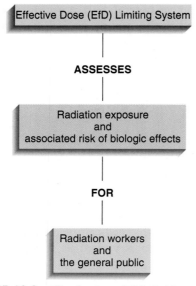

**FIGURE 10-3**   **Effective Dose (EfD) Limiting System.**

and internal whole-body exposures is considered when EfD limits are established. These upper limits are designed to minimize the risk to humans in terms of deterministic and stochastic effects, and they do not include natural background and medical exposure. Deterministic and stochastic effects are discussed earlier in this chapter and also in Chapters 8 and 9.

Upper boundary radiation exposure limits for occupationally exposed persons are associated with risks that are similar to those encountered by employees in other industries that are generally considered to be reasonably safe. These industries include:

- Manufacturing
- Trade
- Government

Radiation risks are derived from the complete injury caused by radiation exposure. The potential for terminal cancer, hereditary imperfections induced by reproductive cell mutations, shortening of life span because of the induction of cancer, or other abnormalities and the overall poorer quality of life are taken into account.

## Revised Concepts of Radiation Exposure and Risk

Revised concepts of radiation exposure and risk have brought about more recent changes in NCRP recommendations for limits on exposure to ionizing radiation. Because many conflicting views exist on assessing the risk of cancer induction from low-level radiation exposure, the trend has been to:

- Create more rigorous radiation protection standards

The adoption of the EfD limiting system is a direct consequence of this conservatism. The benefit obtained from any diagnostic imaging procedure must always be weighed against the risk that is taken. (Methods for assessing risk estimates for cancer induction are discussed in Chapter 9.)

## Occupational Risk

Occupational risk associated with radiation exposure may be equated with occupational risk in other industries that are generally considered reasonably safe (see Chapter 13). That risk is generally estimated to be a 2.5% chance of fatal accident over an entire career. The lifetime fatal risk in hazardous occupations is many times greater. These occupations include:

- Logging
- Deep sea fishing

To ensure that the hazard to radiation workers is no greater than the hazard to the general working public, the NCRP proposes that radiation protection programs for radiation workers be designed to prevent individual workers from having a total external plus internal cumulative EfD in excess of their age in years times 10 mSv.[4] Consider the following situation: A worker at age 40 years has been employed at a nuclear power plant for 10 years. He had previously been employed as a radiation worker in another industry, during the course of which he received a cumulative EfD of 100 mSv. Therefore, the radiation protection program for his current position should have ensured that he has not accumulated a total EfD greater than 300 mSv during his 10 years of employment.

## Vulnerability of the Embryo-Fetus to Radiation Exposure

The embryo-fetus in utero is particularly sensitive to radiation exposure. Epidemiologic studies of atomic bomb survivors exposed in utero provided conclusive evidence of a dose-dependent increase in the incidence of severe mental retardation for fetal doses greater than approximately 0.4 Sv. The greatest risk for radiation-induced mental retardation occurred when the embryo-fetus was exposed 8 to 15 weeks after conception.

## BASIS FOR THE EFFECTIVE DOSE LIMITING SYSTEM

### Concept Underlying Radiation Protection

The essential concept underlying radiation protection is that any organ in the human body is vulnerable to damage from exposure to ionizing radiation. Even though some organs are known to be more sensitive to radiation than others, every organ is at some risk because of the assumed random nature of somatic or hereditary radiation-induced effects.

The EfD limiting system includes, for the determination of EqD for tissues and organs, all radiation-vulnerable human organs that can contribute to potential risk, rather than only those human organs considered critical. In earlier recommendations such as NCRP Report No. 39 (released in 1971), critical organs such as the gonads, blood-forming organs such as bone marrow, and lung tissue were identified.[6]

### Tissue Weighting Factor

Although this factor is discussed in Chapter 4, a brief description follows to reinforce greater understanding of its importance as it relates to

the EfD limiting system. The EfD limiting system is an attempt to equate the various risks of cancer and hereditary effects to the tissues or organs that were exposed to radiation. Because various tissues and organs do not have the same degree of sensitivity to these effects, the system employed must compensate for the differences in risk from one organ to another. Therefore, a **tissue weighting factor** ($W_T$) is used. This factor "indicates the ratio of the risk of stochastic effects attributable to irradiation of a given organ or tissue ($T$) to the total risk when the whole body is uniformly irradiated."[7] Organ or tissue weighting factors ($W_T$) recommended by the ICRP in Report No. 60 (released in 1991) and adopted by the NCRP in Report No. 116 (released in 1993) are reproduced in Box 10-6.

| BOX 10-6 | Organ or Tissue Weighting Factors for Calculating Effective Dose |
|---|---|
| **0.01** | **0.12** |
| Bone surface | Red bone marrow |
| Skin | Colon |
| | Lung |
| **0.05** | Stomach |
| Bladder | |
| Breast | **0.20** |
| Liver | Gonads |
| Esophagus | |
| Thyroid | |
| Remainder*† | |

From National Council on Radiation Protection and Measurements (NCRP): *Limitation of exposure to ionizing radiation,* Report No. 116, Bethesda, Md, 1993, NCRP.
*The remainder takes into account the following additional tissues and organs: adrenals, brain, small intestine, large intestine, kidney, muscle, pancreas, spleen, thymus, and uterus.
†In extraordinary circumstances in which one of the remainder tissues or organs receives an equivalent dose in excess of the highest dose in any of the 12 organs for which a weighting factor ($W_T$) is specified, a $W_T$ of 0.025 should be applied to that tissue or organ and a $W_T$ of 0.025 to the average dose in the other remainder tissues or organs.

# CURRENT NATIONAL COUNCIL ON RADIATION PROTECTION AND MEASUREMENTS RECOMMENDATIONS

## National Council on Radiation Protection and Measurements Reports

The NCRP reiterates and updates its position on radiation protection standards and publishes recommendations on these standards in the form of reports. Recommendations contained in NCRP Report No. 116 now supersede those contained in NCRP Reports No. 91 and No. 39. A summary of some important issues and changes follows.

**Annual Occupational Effective Dose Limit.** An **annual occupational effective dose limit** of 50 mSv (not including medical and natural background exposure) has been established for the whole body, with an added recommendation that the lifetime EfD in mSv should not exceed 10 times the occupationally exposed person's age in years.

**Cumulative Effective Dose (CumEfD) Limit.** A radiation worker's **lifetime effective dose** must be limited to his or her age in years times 10 mSv. This is called the **cumulative effective dose (CumEfD) limit** and pertains to the whole body. Adhering to this limit ensures that the lifetime risk for these workers remains acceptable. EfD limits, however, do not include:

- Radiation exposure from natural background radiation
- Exposure acquired as a consequence of a worker's undergoing medical imaging procedures

The limits do include the possibility of both:

- Internal exposure
- External exposure

The effective dose is therefore the sum or total of both the internal and external EqDs. The example in Box 10-7 demonstrates the application of the CumEfD limit for the whole body.

---

| BOX 10-7 | Application of Cumulative Effective Dose Limit for the Whole Body |
|---|---|

In the example, EqD represents the cumulative effective dose (CumEfD).

EXAMPLE: Determine the CumEfD limit to the whole body of an occupationally exposed person who is 37 years old.

ANSWER: In International System (SI) units:

$$EqD = 10\,mSv \times age\ (in\ years)$$

$$EqD = 10\,mSv \times 37$$

$$EqD = 370\,mSv$$

This represents the CumEfD for the whole body that the occupationally exposed person may receive as a consequence of age.

---

Medical imaging personnel hardly ever receive EqDs that are close to the annual EfD limit. If a radiation safety program is well structured and properly maintained, occupational exposure will not remotely approach 50 mSv in any given year.

**Collective Effective Dose.** The **collective effective dose (ColEfD)** has been designated for use in the description of population or group exposure from low doses of different sources of ionizing radiation. ColEfD is determined as the product of the average EfD for an individual belonging to the exposed population or group and the number of persons exposed. The **person-sievert** (previously referred to as *man-rem)* is the unit of choice to express this quantity. If 1000 people are exposed to low doses of different sources of ionizing radiation and receive an average EfD of 0.5 mSv, the ColEfD is 500 person-mSv, which equals 0.5 person-Sv.

**International Commission on Radiological Protection Recommendation for Downward Revision of the Annual Effective Dose Limit.** Levels of ionizing radiation formerly considered acceptable by the ICRP have been revised downward. In 1991 the ICRP recommended the reduction of the annual EfD limit for occupationally exposed persons from 50 mSv to 20 mSv as a result of newer information obtained regarding the Japanese atomic bomb survivors in whom the risk of radiation from the atomic bomb detonations was estimated to be approximately three to four times greater (more damaging) than previously estimated.[8] The NCRP is still considering the possibility of reducing exposure standards because of the:

1. Revised risk estimates derived from the more recent reevaluations of dosimetric studies on the atomic bomb survivors of Hiroshima and Nagasaki[6]
2. Appearance, as a result of longer follow-up time, of increased numbers of solid tumors in the survivor population

In the future, the annual whole-body EfD limit for occupationally exposed persons in the United States may be limited to 10 to 20 mSv per year.* Of course, such a change will necessitate further evaluation of actual risk for persons employed in radiation industries. In the United States, lowering of the current limits is the responsibility of the NRC, individual states, and the FDA.

**Limits for Nonoccupationally Exposed Individuals.** In addition to limits for occupationally exposed individuals, the NCRP also sets limits for nonoccupationally exposed individuals who are not undergoing medical imaging procedures. An example would be a person accompanying a patient to the imaging department such as a:

- Spouse
- Parent
- Guardian

A limit also has been set for individual members of the general public not occupationally exposed. The NCRP-recommended annual EfD limit is 1 mSv for continuous or frequent exposures from artificial sources other than

medical irradiation and natural background and a limit of 5 mSv annually for infrequent exposure.[4] The annual EfD nonoccupational limit set for individual members of the general public is designed to limit that exposure "to reasonable levels of risk comparable with risks from other common sources, i.e., about $10^{-4}$ to $10^{-6}$ annually."[4] The 5-mSv annual limit for infrequent exposure is made because "annual exposures in excess of the 1 mSv recommendation, usually to a small group of people, need not be regarded as especially significant to the group as a whole provided it does not occur often to the same groups and that the average exposure to individuals in these groups does not exceed an average annual EfD of about 1 mSv."[4]

**Limits for Pregnant Radiation Workers.** To reduce exposure for pregnant radiation workers and control the exposure to the unborn during potentially sensitive periods of gestation, the NCRP now "recommends" a monthly EqD limit not exceeding 0.5 mSv per month to the embryo-fetus and a limit during the entire pregnancy not to exceed 5.0 mSv after declaration of the pregnancy. The recommended monthly limit is more stringent. Nevertheless, both limits are proposed to reflect the fact that not all pregnant workers are monitored monthly and that personnel dosimetry does not result in exact measures of EqD, just approximations based on the personnel dosimeter readings. This 9-month EqD value excludes both medical and natural background radiation. It is designed to restrict significantly the total lifetime risk of leukemia and other malignancies in persons exposed in utero.[4] The occurrence of deterministic effects is expected to be statistically negligible if the EqD remains at or below the recommended limit. These effects include:

- Small head size
- Mental retardation

**Limits for Education and Training Purposes.** For education and training purposes, the same dose limits should apply to students of radiography in general and to those individuals under 18 years of age. The dose limit is the same

---

*Manual 60 of the ICRP* (Oxford, 1991, Pergamon Press) contains a recommendation for lowering the allowable occupational level of exposure to ionizing radiation from 50 mSv/year to 20 mSv/year averaged over defined periods of 5 years. This lower limit is not enforced in the United States.

for kindergarten through twelfth-grade students attending science demonstrations involving ionizing radiation as it is for student radiologic technologists who begin their education before they are 18 years old. The limit for any education and training exposures of individuals under the age of 18 years is an EfD of 1 mSv annually. Occasional exposure for the purpose of education and training is permitted, provided special care is taken to ensure that the annual EfD limit of 1 mSv is not exceeded.

**Limits for Tissues and Organs Exposed Selectively or Together with Other Organs.** Annual occupational dose limits for deterministic effects, for tissues and organs exposed selectively or together with other organs, have been set to prevent excessive doses to those organs and tissues. They include 150 mSv to the crystalline lens of the eyes and 500 mSv for localized areas of the skin, the hands, and the feet.[4] Even though the established annual dose limit for localized areas of skin provides adequate protection for that organ against stochastic effects, it will actually be necessary to specify an additional limit to prevent deterministic effects.

**Negligible Individual Dose.** To provide a low-exposure cutoff level so that regulatory agencies may dismiss a level of effective dose as being of negligible risk, an annual **negligible individual dose (NID)** of 0.01 mSv/year per source or practice has been set. This means that below this EfD level, a reduction of individual exposure is unnecessary.

## ACTION LIMITS

Health care facilities go to great lengths to avoid having personnel even "approach" EfD limits. In a well-designed and well-run facility, radiologic technologists' personnel dosimeter readings should be well below a tenth of the maximum EfD limits, even for those technologists who receive the most exposure. Health care facilities, such as hospitals, establish their own internal **action limits.** These limits are set at levels far below the actual limits, typically a tenth of the limit, but at levels that are not routinely exceeded by

personnel. They are meant to trigger an investigation that should uncover the reason for any unusually high exposure. A prime reason for an unusual reading is that a personnel dosimeter was left in an x-ray room when exposures were made because a technologist accidentally lost the monitor without realizing that it had fallen off his or her uniform. Sometimes work habits, such as where the technologist stands during interventional radiography or computed tomography procedures, can be modified, if the extra radiation exposure was a result of the position of the exposed individual. In any case, the RSO must be an active participant along with the imaging department manager in an ongoing program that is designed to prevent personnel from receiving anywhere near the maximum allowed exposures.

## RADIATION HORMESIS

In Report No. 5 of the National Academy of Science on the Biological Effects of Ionizing Radiation (BEIR V), conclusions regarding the adverse effects on health of low levels of ionizing radiation are based on extrapolations from radiation EqDs greater than 0.5 Sv. Such radiation levels are more than a factor of 1000 greater than ordinary background radiation levels (3.3 mSv/year). BEIR V espouses the linear "no threshold" view of the Japanese atomic bomb lifetime survival study (LSS) data. However, studies from the Radiation Effects Research Council in Hiroshima have indicated an apparent threshold dosage in the atomic bomb LSS data that is approximately 0.2 to 0.5 Sv. This lower value corresponds to the amount of natural radiation that average U.S. residents receive in their lifetimes. What is curious is that the lifetime survival data possibly appear to indicate that Japanese atomic bomb survivors with moderate radiation exposure of 5 mSv to 50 mSv, the equivalent of 1.5 to 15 years of natural radiation, have a reduced cancer death rate compared with a normally exposed control population. These data contradict the predictions of the BEIR V report and, if substantiated, seem to cast doubt on the BEIR V conclusion that any amount of radiation is potentially harmful. The reverse could actually be true, at least for very moderate amounts of radiation exposure. More specifically, in seven Western states with background radiation levels higher than other states by approximately 1 mSv per year, residents experience approximately 15% fewer cancer deaths per 1000 individuals than the U.S. average.

A study was conducted in China from 1972 to 1975 of 2 stable populations of approximately 70,000 persons; each of whose annual background radiation levels differed by approximately 2 mSv. This study disclosed a cancer rate in the more exposed population of only approximately 50% of that of the other group. Other intriguing studies exist. These suggest a potential **radiation hormesis** effect, which is a beneficial consequence of radiation for populations continuously exposed to moderately higher levels of radiation. During the course of human evolution over millions of years, advantageous genetic mutations caused by radiation exposure may have occurred, resembling those that allow lower animals today to demonstrate radiation hormesis. Therefore, to assume risk from very small amounts of radiation exposure (two or three times normal background levels) may be incorrect. However, until the radiation hormesis theory is proven, the medical radiation industry will continue to follow the principle of ALARA for radiation protection purposes.

## OCCUPATIONAL AND NONOCCUPATIONAL DOSE LIMITS

### Effective Dose Limits for Radiation Workers and the Population as a Whole

For the protection of radiation workers and the population as a whole, EfD limits have been established as guidelines (Table 10-3). All medical imaging personnel should be familiar with current NCRP recommendations. For this group the most important item is the:

- 50-mSv/year whole-body occupational dose limit

This annual upper boundary is designed to limit the stochastic (probabilistic) effects of radiation. It takes into account the EqD in all radiation-sensitive organs found in the body.

## Special Limits for Selected Areas

Because the tissue weighting factors (see Box 10-6) used for calculating EfD are so small for some organs, an organ that is associated with a low weighting factor may receive an unreasonably large dose, whereas the EfD remains within the allowable total limit. Therefore, special limits are set for the crystalline lens of the eye and localized areas of the skin, hands, and feet to prevent deterministic effects. These special limits may be found in Table 10-3.

## SUMMARY

- Effective dose (EfD) limiting system:
  - Adherence to occupational and nonoccupational EfD limits helps prevent harmful biologic effects of radiation exposure.
  - The concept of radiation exposure and the associated risk of radiation-induced malignancy is the basis of the EfD limiting system.
  - The sum of both external and internal whole-body exposures is considered when establishing the EfD limit.
  - Accounting for tissue weighting factors is important because various tissues and organs do not have the same degree of sensitivity.
  - Different biologic threats posed by different types of ionizing radiation must be taken into consideration even when the absorbed dose is the same.
- Radiation hormesis is the hypothesis that a positive effect exists for certain populations that are continuously exposed to moderately higher levels of radiation.

| TABLE 10-3 | Summary of the National Council on Radiation Protection and Measurements (NCRP) Recommendations*[†] (NCRP Report No. 116) | |
|---|---|---|
| A. Occupational exposures[‡] | | |
|   1. Effective dose limits | | |
|     a. Annual | 50 mSv | |
|     b. Cumulative | 10 mSv $\times$ age | |
|   2. Equivalent dose annual limits for tissues and organs | | |
|     a. Lens of eye | 150 mSv | |
|     b. Localized areas of the skin, hands, and feet | 500 mSv | |
| B. Guidance for emergency occupational exposure[‡] (see Section 14, NCRP No. 116) | | |
| C. Public exposures (annual) | | |
|   1. Effective dose limit, continuous or frequent exposure[‡] | 1 mSv | |
|   2. Effective dose limit, infrequent exposure[‡] | 5 mSv | |
|   3. Equivalent dose limits for tissues and organs[‡] | | |
|     a. Lens of eye | 15 mSv | |
|     b. Localized areas of the skin, hands, and feet | 50 mSv | |
|   4. Remedial action for natural sources | | |
|     a. Effective dose (excluding radon) | >5 mSv | |
|     b. Exposure to radon and its decay products[§] | >26 J/(sm$^{-3}$)[‖] | |
| D. Education and training exposures (annual)[‡] | | |
|   1. Effective dose limit | 1 mSv | |
|   2. Equivalent dose limit for tissues and organs | | |
|     a. Lens of eye | 15 mSv | |
|     b. Localized areas of the skin, hands, and feet | 50 mSv | |
| E. Embryo and fetus exposures[‡] | | |
|   1. Equivalent dose limit | | |
|     a. Monthly | 0.5 mSv | |
|     b. Entire gestation | 5.0 mSv | |
| F. Negligible individual dose (annual)[‡] | 0.01 mSv | |

*Excluding medical exposures.

[†]See Tables 4.2 and 5.1 in NCRP Report No. 116 for recommendations on radiation weighting factors and tissue weighting factors, respectively.

[‡]Sum of external and internal exposures, excluding doses from natural sources.

[§]WLM stands for working level month and refers to a cumulative exposure for a working month (170 hours). As applied to radon and its daughter products, 1 WLM represents the cumulative exposure experienced in a 170-hour period resulting from a radon concentration of 100 pCi/L. The occupational limit for miners is 4 WLM per year, which results in an equivalent dose of approximately 0.15 Sv per year.

[‖]A measure of the rate of release of energy (joules per second) by radon and its decay products per unit volume of air (cubic meters).

- Major organizations involved in regulating radiation exposure include the following:
  - The United Nations Scientific Committee on the Effects of Atomic Radiation (UNSCEAR) and the National Academy of Sciences/National Research Council Committee on the Biological Effects of Ionizing Radiation (NAS/NRC-BEIR) supply information to the International Commission on Radiological Protection (ICRP).
  - The ICRP makes recommendations on occupational and public dose limits.

- The National Council on Radiation Protection and Measurements (NCRP) reviews ICRP recommendations and implements them into U.S. radiation protection policy.
- The Nuclear Regulatory Commission (NRC) is the watchdog of the nuclear energy industry; it controls the manufacture and use of radioactive substances.
- The Environmental Protection Agency (EPA) develops and enforces regulations pertaining to the control of environmental radiation.
- The U.S. Food and Drug Administration (FDA) regulates the design and manufacture of products used in the radiation industry.
- The Occupational Safety and Health Administration (OSHA) monitors the workplace and regulates occupational exposure to radiation.
- Individual health care facilities establish a radiation safety committee (RSC) and designate a radiation safety officer (RSO).
  - The RSO is responsible for developing a radiation safety program for the health care facility; he or she maintains personnel radiation-monitoring records and provides counseling in radiation safety.
- The ALARA concept (optimization) states that radiation exposure should be kept "as low as reasonably achievable."
- Serious radiation-induced responses may be classified as having either deterministic or stochastic effects.
  - Deterministic effects are those biologic somatic effects of ionizing radiation that exhibit a threshold dose below which the effect does not normally occur and above which the severity of the biologic damage increases as the dose increases.
  - Stochastic effects are nonthreshold, randomly occurring biologic somatic changes in which the chance of occurrence of the effect rather than the severity of the effect is proportional to the dose of ionizing radiation.

- EfD limit:
  - The NCRP has established an annual occupational EfD limit of 50 mSv and a lifetime EfD that does not exceed 10 times the occupationally exposed person's age in years.
  - Collective effective dose (ColEfD) is used in the description of population or group exposure from low doses of different sources of ionizing radiation.
  - Internal action limits are established by health care facilities to trigger an investigation to uncover the reasons for any unusual high exposures received by individual staff members.

## REFERENCES

1. International Commission on Radiological Protection (ICRP): ICRP: structure and organization. Available at: http://www.icrp.org/. Accessed April 11, 2013.
2. National Council on Radiation Protection and Measurements (NCRP): Background information. Available at: www.ncrp.com/info.html. Accessed April 11, 2013.
3. National Council on Radiation Protection and Measurements (NCRP): *Ionizing radiation exposure of the population of the United States*, Report No. 160, Bethesda, Md, 2009, NCRP.
4. National Council on Radiation Protection and Measurements (NCRP): *Limitation of exposure to ionizing radiation*, Report No. 116, Bethesda, Md, 1993, NCRP.
5. FDA White Paper: *Initiative to reduce unnecessary radiation exposure from medical imaging*. 2010, Center for Devices and Radiological Health, U.S. Food and Drug Administration. Available at: http://www.fda.gov/Radiation-EmittingProducts/RadiationSafety/RadiationDoseReduction/ucm199994.htm. Accessed April 11, 2013.
6. National Council on Radiation Protection and Measurements (NCRP): *Basic radiation protection criteria*, Report No. 39, Washington, DC, 1971, NCRP.
7. National Council on Radiation Protection and Measurements (NCRP): *Recommendations on limits for exposure to ionizing radiation*, Report No. 91, Bethesda, Md, 1987, NCRP.
8. Committee on Biological Effects of Ionizing Radiation, National Research Council, Commission of Life Sciences, Board of Radiation Research: *Health effects of exposure to low levels of ionizing radiation (BEIR V Report)*, Washington, DC, 1989, National Academies Press.

## GENERAL DISCUSSION QUESTIONS

1. Why must radiation exposure of the general public, patients, and radiation workers be limited?
2. What is the basis of the effective dose limiting system?
3. Why must health care facilities have an effective and detailed radiation safety program?
4. Describe the responsibilities of a radiation safety officer.
5. What authority must a radiation safety officer have?
6. What responsibilities does the Center for Devices and Radiological Health (CDRH) fulfill?
7. What is the goal of radiation protection according to NCRP Report No. 116?
8. What is the difference between the deterministic and stochastic effects of ionizing radiation?
9. Describe the effective dose limiting system.
10. Describe current NCRP dose limiting recommendations.

## REVIEW QUESTIONS

1. Which of the following agencies is responsible for enforcing radiation safety standards?
   A. ICRP
   B. NRC
   C. NCRP
   D. UNSCEAR
2. Determine the cumulative effective dose (CumEfD) to the whole body of an occupationally exposed person who is 27 years old.
   A. 2700 mSv
   B. 270 mSv
   C. 27 mSv
   D. 2.7 mSv
3. Biologic effects such as cataracts that result from exposure to ionizing radiation appear to have which of the following?
   A. Circular dose-response threshold relationship
   B. Linear nonthreshold dose pattern
   C. Sigmoid threshold dose-response curve
   D. Sigmoid nonthreshold dose-response relationship
4. For radiation workers, such as medical imaging personnel, occupational risk may be equated with occupational risk in which of the following?
   A. Other industries that are generally considered reasonably safe
   B. Somewhat hazardous industries
   C. Hazardous industries
   D. Extremely hazardous industries
5. Revised estimates derived from more recent reevaluations of dosimetric studies on the atomic bomb survivors of Hiroshima and Nagasaki indicates which of the following?
   A. A decrease in the number of solid tumors in the survivor population
   B. An increase in the number of solid tumors in the survivor population
   C. That low-level radiation causes cancer
   D. That the risk of radiation-induced cancer is nonexistent
6. When exposed to radiation as part of their educational experience, 18-year-old students should *not* exceed an effective dose limit of _____ annually.
   A. 0.5 mSv
   B. 1 mSv
   C. 5 mSv
   D. 50 mSv

7. Which of the following groups has provided sufficient evidence of the induction of stochastic effects in humans resulting from high radiation absorbed doses?
   A. Japanese atomic bomb survivors
   B. General population of the United States
   C. Population of occupationally exposed radiographers in the United States
   D. The 2 million people living within 50 miles of the Three Mile Island nuclear power plant after the accident on March 28, 1979

8. Responsibilities of a medical facility's radiation safety officer (RSO) include which of the following?
   1. Developing an appropriate radiation safety program
   2. Maintaining radiation monitoring records for all personnel
   3. Repairing all broken or defective imaging equipment
   A. 1 and 2 only
   B. 1 and 3 only
   C. 2 and 3 only
   D. 1, 2, and 3

9. To reduce exposure for pregnant imaging professionals and to control the exposure of the unborn during potentially sensitive periods of gestation, the NCRP now recommends a monthly equivalent dose limit not exceeding _____ per month to the embryo-fetus and a limit during the entire pregnancy not to exceed _____ after declaration of a pregnancy.
   A. 0.5 mSv, 5.0 mSv
   B. 5 mSv, 7.0 mSv
   C. 150 mSv, 300 mSv
   D. 250 mSv, 500 mSv

10. Which of the following is the annual occupational effective dose that applies to radiographers during routine operations?
   A. 5 mSv
   B. 50 mSv
   C. 250 mSv
   D. 750 mSv

# Equipment Design for Radiation Protection

OBJECTIVES

*After completing this chapter, the reader will be able to perform the following:*

- Explain the requirements for a diagnostic-type protective tube housing, x-ray control panel, or console, radiographic examination table, and source-to-image distance indicator and discuss their purpose.
- List the various x-ray beam limiting devices, and describe each.
- Explain the importance of luminance of the collimator light source, state the requirements for good coincidence between the radiographic beam and the localizing light beam when a variable rectangular collimator is used, and explain the function of the collimator's positive beam limitation (PBL) feature.
- Explain the function of x-ray beam filtration in diagnostic radiology, list two types of filtration used to filter the beam adequately, describe half-value layer (HVL), and give examples of HVLs required for selective peak kilovoltages.
- Explain the function of a compensating filter in radiography of a body part that varies in thickness, and list two types of such filters.
- Explain the significance of exposure reproducibility and exposure linearity.

- Explain how the use of high-speed screen-film combinations reduces radiographic exposure for the patient when film is the image receptor of choice.
- Explain how radiographic grids increase patient dose.
- Identify the minimal source-skin distance (SSD) that must be used for mobile radiography to ensure patient safety, and state the reason for this minimal SSD requirement.
- Explain the process of digital radiography and computed radiography, and discuss why it is imperative that patients undergoing digital imaging procedures not be overexposed initially.
- Explain how patient exposure may be reduced during routine fluoroscopic procedures, C-arm fluoroscopic procedures, high-dose (high-level-control [HLC]) fluoroscopy interventional procedures, cineradiographic procedures, and digital fluoroscopic procedures.
- Discuss the use of fluoroscopic equipment by nonradiologist physicians who perform interventional procedures or other potentially lengthy tasks, and identify the responsibilities of the radiographer during such procedures.

Copyright © 2014, Elsevier Inc.

## KEY TERMS

computed radiography (CR)
control panel, or console
cumulative timer
diagnostic-type protective tube
  housing
digital radiography (DR)
digital fluoroscopy (DF)
entrance skin exposure rates
exposure linearity
exposure reproducibility
filtration

half-value layer (HVL)
high-level-control fluoroscopy
  (HLCF)
image matrix
light-localizing variable-
  aperture rectangular
  collimator
off-focus, or stem, radiation
positive beam limitation
  (PBL)
primary protective barrier

quantum mottle
radiographic examination
  table
radiographic grid
rare-earth screens
scattered radiation
source-to–image receptor
  distance (SID)
source-to-skin distance (SSD)
useful, or primary, beam
x-ray beam limitation device

State-of-the-art diagnostic radiographic and fluoroscopic equipment has been designed with many devices that radiologists and technologists can use to optimize the quality of the image while also reducing radiation exposure for patients undergoing various imaging procedures. Although many safety features have been built into x-ray-producing machines by the manufacturers to ensure radiation safety, some features have also been included to meet federal regulations. In addition to newer designs for imaging equipment, many accessories are also available to lower the radiation dose for the patient. This chapter provides an overview of equipment components and accessories that imaging professionals can use to minimize exposure of patients.

In this chapter, the learner also will experience greater use of metric units for measurements. For example, if the distance from the focal spot of the anode of the x-ray tube to the radiographic image receptor was stated in inches in previous editions of this text, with the exact equivalent metric unit in parenthesis, it will now be given in metric units first, with the equivalent English text in parenthesis, where applicable, since these traditional units are still used in regulatory statements physics reports, and are still used on x-ray equipment. In addition, for purposes of standardization, when any distance is identified in metric units, the effective equivalent metric unit will be given. Thus, if a source-to–image receptor distance (SID) of 40 inches is converted to metric units, it equals exactly 101.6 cm. The effective metric equivalent,* however, used in practical applications will be 100 cm.

## RADIATION SAFETY FEATURES OF RADIOGRAPHIC EQUIPMENT, DEVICES, AND ACCESSORIES

Measures must be taken to ensure that radiographic equipment operates safely. Every diagnostic imaging system must have a protective tube housing and a correctly functioning control panel. The radiographic examination table and other devices and accessories must also be designed to reduce the patient's radiation dose.

## Diagnostic-Type Protective Tube Housing

**Requirements.** A lead-lined metal **diagnostic-type protective tube housing** (Fig. 11-1) is required to protect the patient and imaging personnel from off-focus, or leakage, radiation by restricting the emission of x-rays to the area of the **useful, or primary, beam** (those x-rays emitted through the x-ray port tube window, or port).

**X-Ray Tube Housing Construction.** The housing enclosing the x-ray tube must be constructed so that the leakage radiation measured at a distance of 1 m from the x-ray source does not exceed 1 mGy$_a$/hr (100 mR/hr) when the tube is operated at its highest voltage at the highest

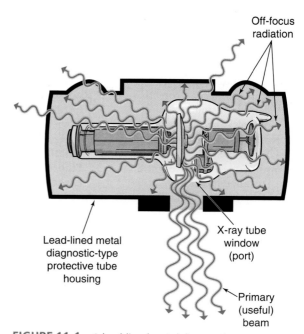

FIGURE 11-1   A lead-lined metal diagnostic-type protective tube housing protects patients and imaging personnel from off-focus, or leakage, radiation by restricting x-ray emission to the area of the primary (useful) beam.

current that allows continuous operation. The protective tube housing also confines the high voltage entering the x-ray tube, thus preventing electric shock. Additionally, it also makes cooling of the x-ray tube possible. Because the x-ray tube and housing assembly are relatively heavy, the housing is designed to give needed mechanical support. It is robust enough to minimize the potential for damage of the x-ray tube in the event that rough handling occurs.

## Control Panel, or Console

The **control panel**, or **console**, is where technical exposure factors such as milliamperes (mA) and peak kilovoltage (kVp) are selected and visually displayed. It must be located behind a suitable protective barrier that has a radiation-absorbent window that permits observation of the patient during any procedure. This panel must indicate the conditions of exposure and provide a positive

---

*Conversion of English units of measure to effective metric equivalent units.

| English unit | Effective Metric Equivalent Unit |
| --- | --- |
| 40 inches | 100 cm |
| 48 inches | 120 cm |
| 72 inches | 180 cm |

indication when the x-ray tube is energized.[1] The visible mA and kVp digital readouts permit the operator to assess exposure conditions. For state-of-the-art operating consoles, digital controls and meters are available on a touch screen, where radiographic exposure factors may be selected by the equipment operator. Generally, when an x-ray exposure begins, a tone is emitted. When the exposure terminates, the sound stops. For the operator of the equipment, this audible sound clearly indicates that the x-ray tube is energized and ionizing radiation is being emitted.

## Radiographic Examination Table

The **radiographic examination table** must be strong and must adequately support the patient. Frequently, this piece of equipment has a floating tabletop that makes it easier to maneuver the patient during an imaging procedure. The thickness of the tabletop must be uniform, and for undertable x-ray tubes as used in fluoroscopy, the patient support surface also should be as radiolucent as possible so that it will absorb only a minimal amount of radiation, thereby reducing the patient's radiation dose. A carbon fiber material is commonly used in the tabletop to meet this requirement.

## Source-to–Image Receptor Distance Indicator

When radiographing a patient, radiographers must have a means to measure the distance from the anode focal spot to the image receptor to ensure that the correct **source-to–image receptor distance (SID)** is maintained. To meet this need, radiographic equipment comes with an indicator that will perform this function. Frequently, a simple device such as a tape measure is attached to the collimator or tube housing so that the radiographer can manually measure the SID. Lasers are also sometimes used to accomplish the same task. SID accuracy is essential. "Distance and centering indicators must be accurate to within 2% and 1% of the source-to–image receptor distance (SID), respectively."[2]

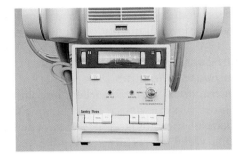

**FIGURE 11-2** Light-Localizing Variable-Aperture Rectangular Collimator.

## X-Ray Beam Limitation Devices

The primary x-ray beam shall be adequately collimated so that it is no larger than the size of the image receptor being used for the examination. With modern equipment, this is accomplished by providing the unit with a **light-localizing variable-aperture rectangular collimator** to adjust the size and shape of the x-ray beam either automatically or manually (Fig. 11-2). The collimator is currently the most popular x-**ray beam limitation device** in use at the time of this publication.

**Types of X-Ray Beam Limitation Devices.** In addition to the light-localizing variable-aperture rectangular collimator, earlier x-ray beam limitation devices include:

* Aperture diaphragms
* Cones
* Cylinders

All these devices confine the useful, or primary, beam before it enters the area of clinical interest and thereby limit the quantity of body tissue irradiated. This also reduces the amount of scattered radiation in the tissue and prevents unnecessary exposure to tissues not under examination.

**Scattered radiation** is all the radiation that arises from the interaction of an x-ray beam with the atoms of a patient or any other object in the path of the beam. When the size of the x-ray field is restricted to include only the anatomic structures of clinical interest, the patient's dose is significantly reduced because a smaller field size produces less scatter radiation. This improves the overall quality of the radiographic image.

### Light-Localizing Variable-Aperture Rectangular Collimators

*Construction.* As stated earlier, the collimator is the most versatile device for defining the size and shape of the radiographic beam. The light-localizing variable-aperture rectangular collimator is the type of collimator most often used with multipurpose x-ray units. It is box shaped and contains the radiographic beam–defining system (Fig. 11-3). This system consists of:

- Two sets of adjustable lead shutters mounted within the device at different levels
- A light source to illuminate the x-ray field and permit it to be centered over the area of clinical interest

- A mirror to deflect the light beam toward the patient to be radiographed

The first set of shutters, the upper shutters, are mounted as close as possible to the tube window to reduce the amount of **off-focus, or stem, radiation** (x-rays emitted from parts of the tube other than the focal spot) coming from the primary beam and exiting at various angles from the x-ray tube window. This radiation can never be completely eliminated because the metal shutters cannot be placed immediately beneath the actual focal spot of the x-ray tube, but placing the first set, or upper, shutters as close as possible to the tube window can reduce it significantly. This practice reduces the patient's exposure resulting from off-focus radiation.

The second set of collimator shutters, the lower shutters, are mounted below the level of

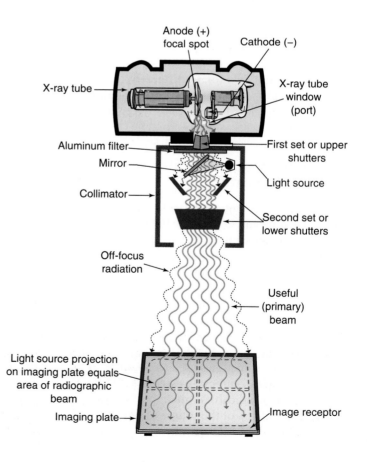

**FIGURE 11-3** Diagram of a typical collimator demonstrating radiographic beam-defining system: 1, anode focal spot; 2, x-ray tube window; 3, first set of shutters, or upper shutters; 4, aluminum filter; 5, mirror; 6, light source; 7, second set of shutters, or lower shutters. The metal shutters collimate the radiographic beam so that it is no larger than the image receptor.

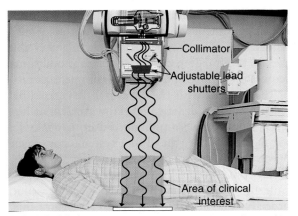

**FIGURE 11-4** Collimator containing the radiographic beam-defining system, which establishes the parameters (margins) of the beam. Adjustable lead shutters limit the cross-sectional area of the beam and confine it to the area of clinical interest.

the light source and mirror and function to further confine the radiographic beam to the area of clinical interest (see Fig. 11-3; Fig. 11-4). This set of shutters consists of two pairs of lead plates oriented at right angles to each other. Each set may be adjusted independently so that an extensive variety of rectangular shapes can be selected. In this way, the field is not limited to the circular or fixed square shapes that sometimes cause areas of the patient not requiring imaging to receive radiation.

*Skin Sparing.* To minimize skin exposure to electrons produced by photon interaction with the collimator, the patient's skin surface should be at least 15 cm below the collimator. Some collimator housings contain "spacer bars," which project down from the housing to prevent the collimators from being closer than 15 cm to the patient.

*Luminance.* Luminance is a scientific term referring to the brightness of a surface. Specifically, luminance quantifies the intensity of a light source (i.e., the amount of light per unit area coming from its surface). Luminance is determined by measuring the concentration of light over a particular field of view. This may be understood by examining the units used to describe luminance. The primary unit is the

*candela per square meter,* known more simply as the *nit.* One candela corresponds to 3.8 million billion photons per second being emitted from a light source through a conelike field of view. A good analogy is the sound intensity emerging from a drill sergeant with a megaphone held to his lips. With appropriate dimensions, the megaphone's larger opening corresponds to the conelike field of view associated with the candela. The luminance of the collimator light source must be sufficient to permit the localizing light beam to outline the margins of the radiographic beam adequately on the patient's anatomy. Because the light field and the x-ray field are designed to coincide, if the light field were not sufficiently bright, a radiographer could improperly position the x-ray field on a patient or, at the very least, have great difficulty accurately centering the x-ray beam. This would be especially true in the case of a patient with dark skin coloration. With insufficient brightness, the x-ray unit may fail a state inspection. The luminance must be high enough so that a calibrated light meter reading taken at a distance of 100 cm will be at least 15 foot-candles when averaged over the four quadrants of a 25 × 25 cm field size. A foot-candle is approximately equivalent to 10.76 nit (the unit of luminance). Therefore, a reading of 15 foot-candles corresponds to a collimator light source with a luminance of approximately 161 nit or 161 candela per square meter.

In summary, if the luminance of the collimator light source is adequate, the localizing light beam will adequately outline the margins of the radiographic beam on the area of clinical interest on all patients.

*Coincidence between the Radiographic Beam and the Localizing Light Beam.* When a light-localizing variable-aperture rectangular collimator is used, good coincidence (i.e., both physical size and alignment) between the radiographic beam and the localizing light beam is essential to eliminate collimator cutoff of the body structures being irradiated. The sum of the cross-table and along-the-table alignment differences between the x-ray and light beams must not exceed 2% of the SID. This condition is also imposed on the relative "sizing" differences between the x-ray and light beams. These coincidence requirements are collectively known as:

- Alignment
- Congruence

As an example, 100 cm (40 inches) is a commonly used SID in radiography. For this the maximal allowable total difference in length and width alignments of the projected light field with the radiographic beam at the level of the image receptor must be no more than 2% of approximately 100 cm (40 inches), which equals 2 cm (0.8 inch). Acceptable congruence at 100-cm (40-inch) SID requires that the sum of the dimensions of the x-ray field should also differ from the length and width span of the light field by no more than 2 cm (0.8 inch).

The SID used in radiography actually depends on the individual radiographic projection. For example, a 180-cm (72 inches) SID is normally used for routine chest x-ray examinations performed on ambulatory patients. In some imaging departments, the use of 120-cm (48-inch) SID for many projections has become standard instead of using 100-cm (40-inch) SID because increasing the SID from 100 cm (40 inches) to 120 cm (48 inches) causes less geometric divergence of the x-ray beam within the patient's body. This will improve the sharpness, or recorded detail, of the radiographic image. The extended SID can also decrease the patient's dose.[3-5]

*Positive Beam Limitation.* In some earlier collimation systems the radiographer could inadvertently use an image receptor size much smaller than the size of the radiation field. Thus, areas of the patient would be irradiated that would not be recorded on the image receptor. Either the radiation field size should be smaller (if the additional anatomy is not of diagnostic interest) or the image receptor should be larger (if the anatomy is indeed of diagnostic interest). To prevent such a mismatch, radiographic collimators that are part of fixed radiographic equipment manufactured in the United States generally include a feature called **positive beam limitation** (**PBL**). The PBL feature consists of electronic sensors in an image receptor holder that sends

signals to the collimator housing. When PBL is activated, the collimators are automatically adjusted so that the radiation field matches the size of the image receptor. If special conditions require the radiographer to have complete control of the system, with the turn of a key, the PBL feature may be deactivated. However, in such a circumstance a warning light is automatically lit to indicate that the PBL system has been deactivated.

The PBL system illustrates an important principle of patient protection during radiographic procedures. The radiographer must ensure that collimation is adequate by collimating the radiographic beam so that it is no larger than the image receptor (Fig. 11-5). In most states, regulatory standards require accuracy of 2% of the SID with PBL. However, in some states, regulatory standards may require only an accuracy of 3% of the SID with PBL.

*Alignment of the X-Ray Beam.* It is imperative that the x-ray beam and the image receptor be correctly aligned with each other. Every radiographic tube must have a device in place to ensure accurate beam alignment.

**Aperture Diaphragm.** An aperture diaphragm is the simplest of all beam limitation devices. It consists of a flat piece of lead with a hole of designated size and shape cut in its center. The dimensions of the hole determine the size and shape of the radiographic beam. Different image receptor sizes and different SIDs require aperture diaphragms of various sizes to accommodate them. Diaphragm openings are:

- Rectangular
- Square
- Round

The rectangular shape is the most common. Aperture diaphragms are used in:

- Trauma radiographic imaging systems
- X-ray units designed specifically for chest radiography
- Dental radiographic units

Placed directly below the window of the x-ray tube, the aperture diaphragm confines the primary radiographic beam to dimensions

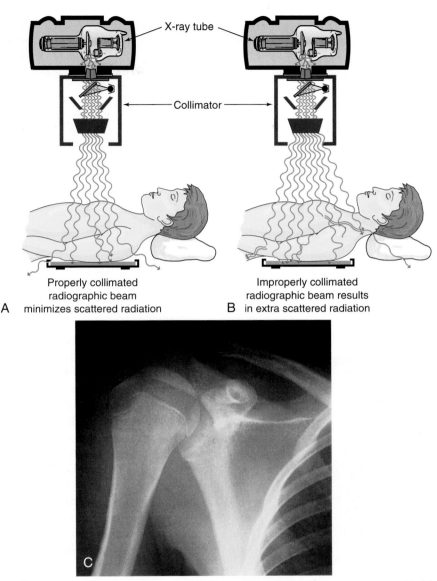

**FIGURE 11-5** Collimate the radiographic beam so that it is no larger than the image receptor. Limiting the beam to the area of clinical interest decreases the amount of tissue irradiated and minimizes patient exposure by reducing the amount of scattered and absorbed radiation. **A,** Good collimation. **B,** Poor collimation. **C,** Anteroposterior radiograph of the shoulder demonstrating good collimation.

suitable for covering a given size image receptor at a specified SID (Fig. 11-6). Because an aperture diaphragm limits field size, and thus the area of the body irradiated, the amount of scattered radiation produced decreases.

**Cones.** Light-localizing variable-aperture rectangular collimators have replaced cones for most radiographic examinations. However, cones are still sometimes used for radiographic examinations of specific areas such as the:

- Head (e.g., coned-down lateral projection of the sella turcica [Fig. 11-7], projections of the paranasal sinuses [Fig. 11-8])
- Vertebral column
- Chest

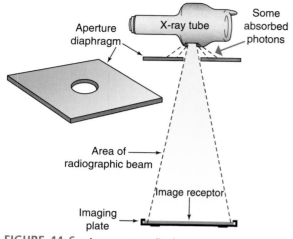

**FIGURE 11-6**  An aperture diaphragm, a flat piece of lead with a hole of designated size and shape cut in its center, is placed directly below the window of the x-ray tube to confine the primary radiographic beam dimensions suitable to cover a given size of an image receptor at a specified source-to-image receptor distance.

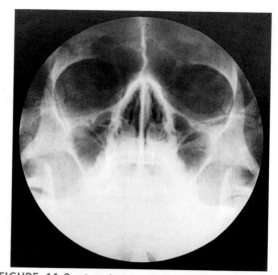

**FIGURE 11-8    Coned-Down Parietoacanthial Projection of the Maxillary Sinuses.**

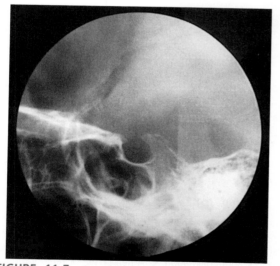

**FIGURE 11-7    Coned-Down Lateral Projection of the Sella Turcica.**

### Flared Metal Tubes and Straight Cylinders.

Radiographic cones are circular metal tubes that attach to the x-ray tube housing or variable rectangular collimator to limit the x-ray beam to a predetermined size and shape. The design of this collimating device is simple, consisting of either a flared metal tube with the diameter of the upper end smaller than the diameter of the lower end or a straight cylinder with the diameter the same at both the upper and lower ends (Fig. 11-9). Although the length and diameter of the cones vary, it is primarily the lower rim of the cone that governs beam limitation. Sharper size restriction is achieved when the cone or cylinder is longer. Field size at selected SIDs should be indicated on the cone.

*Beam-Defining Cones Used in Dental Radiography.*  Beam-defining cones are widely used in dental radiography. Because dental x-ray equipment is usually less bulky than general-purpose equipment, a one-piece beam limitation device, such as a cone made of plastic, is convenient. Some dental cones are lined with lead. By using lead-lined cones instead of the conventional plastic cones, dentists reduce the patient's exposure by eliminating the source of secondary radiation (the plastic cone itself).[6]

## Filtration

### Purpose of Radiographic Beam Filtration.

**Filtration** of the radiographic beam reduces exposure to the patient's skin and superficial

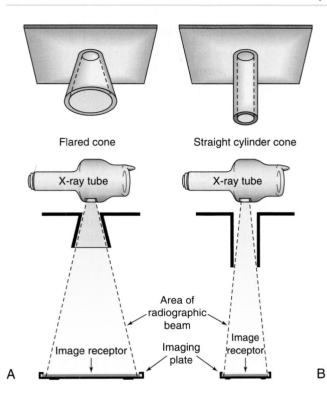

**FIGURE 11-9** Radiographic cones are circular metal tubes that attach to the x-ray tube housing or variable rectangular collimator to limit the radiographic beam to a predetermined size and shape. **A,** Cone fashioned in the form of a flared metal tube. **B,** Cone fashioned in the form of a straight cylinder.

tissue by absorbing most of the lower-energy photons (long-wavelength or soft x-rays) from the heterogeneous beam (Fig. 11-10). This increases the mean energy, or "quality," of the x-ray beam. This change is also referred to as "hardening" the beam.

**Effect of Filtration on the Absorbed Dose to the Patient.** Because filtration absorbs some of the photons in a radiographic beam, it decreases the overall intensity (quantity, or amount) of incident radiation. The remaining photons, however, are, as a whole, more penetrating and therefore less likely to be absorbed in body tissue. Hence, the absorbed dose to the patient decreases when the correct amount and type of filtration are placed in the path of the radiographic beam. If adequate filtration were not present, very low-energy photons (20 keV or lower) would enter the patient and be almost totally absorbed in the body, thus increasing the patient's radiation dose, especially near or at the surface, but contributing

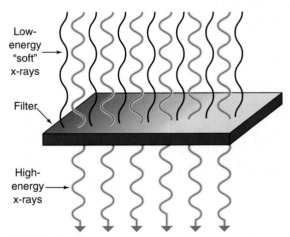

**FIGURE 11-10** Filtration removes low-energy photons (long-wavelength or "soft" x-rays) from the beam by absorbing them and permits higher energy photons to pass through. This reduces the amount of radiation that the patient receives.

nothing to the image process. The low-energy photons should be removed from the radiographic beam through filtration. Filter material used for this purpose includes elements that are built in or added to the x-ray tube.

**Types of Filtration.** The following two types of filtration are available:

- Inherent filtration
- Added filtration

Inherent filtration includes the:

- Glass envelope encasing the x-ray tube
- Insulating oil surrounding the tube
- Glass window in the tube housing

This inherent material amounts to approximately 0.5 mm aluminum equivalent, meaning that the built-in material provides the same amount of filtration as a 0.5-mm thickness of aluminum. The light-localizing variable-aperture rectangular collimator provides an additional 1 mm aluminum equivalent. The reflective surface of the collimator mirror provides most of this aluminum equivalent.

*Added filtration* usually consists of:

- Sheets of aluminum (or the equivalent) of appropriate thickness

This extra filtration is located outside the glass window of the tube housing above the collimator shutters. It is readily accessible to service personnel and may be changed as the x-ray tube ages. The inherent filtration and added filtration combine to equal the required amount necessary to filter the useful beam adequately (Box 11-1).

**Requirement for Total Filtration.** The kVp of a given x-ray unit determines the amount of attenuation required. *Total filtration* of 2.5 mm aluminum equivalent for fixed x-ray units operating above 70 kVp is the regulatory standard (Fig. 11-11).[7] Because each x-ray tube and collimator system typically has a total inherent

**BOX 11-1 | Total Filtration**

Total filtration = Inherent filtration plus added filtration

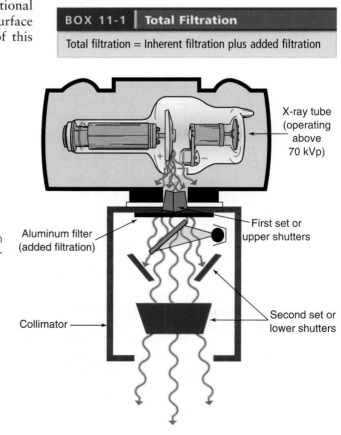

FIGURE 11-11 A minimum of 2.5 mm aluminum equivalent total filtration is required for fixed radiographic units operating at above 70 kVp.

filtration of 1.5 mm aluminum equivalent, the manufacturer needs only to place an additional 1-mm aluminum equivalent filter between the tube housing and collimator to meet the minimum regulatory requirement.

Stationary (fixed) radiographic equipment requires total filtration of 1.5 mm aluminum equivalent for x-ray units operating at 50 to 70 kVp, whereas fixed units operating at below 50 kVp require only 0.5 mm aluminum equivalent.[7] Mobile diagnostic units and fluoroscopic equipment require a minimum of 2.5 mm aluminum equivalent. A summary of required minimum total filtration may be found in Box 11-2.

**Filtration for Mammographic Equipment.** Appropriate attenuation also is necessary for mammographic equipment, which produces photons with an energy range of 17 to 20 keV. Metallic elements such as molybdenum (Z = 42) and rhodium (Z = 45) are commonly employed as filters. When the x-ray tube target is made of molybdenum, either a 0.03-mm molybdenum filter or a 0.025-mm rhodium filter may be

selected.[3] For rhodium x-ray tube targets, rhodium filters are used. These filtration materials facilitate adequate contrast in the radiographic image over the clinical extent of compressed breast thickness by preferentially selecting a particular range or window of energies from the x-ray spectrum emerging from the x-ray tube target. Molybdenum filters allow a lower energy window (17 to 20 keV) than rhodium filters (20 to 23 keV) (Fig. 11-12). Molybdenum filters are therefore suitable for small and average breast thickness, whereas rhodium filters used with a molybdenum or rhodium anode are better for larger or dense breasts[7] (i.e., compression thickness of 6 cm and greater) because they will produce an x-ray beam with higher energy. Systemic use of such materials has the effect of reducing the mean glandular dose in firm breast tissue. Maintaining and enhancing subject contrast are important in mammography. Beryllium (Z = 4) takes the place of the glass in the window of the low-kVp–producing mammographic x-ray tube to accommodate this need. This light, strong metal permits the relatively soft characteristic radiation important for enhancing contrast to exit the tube without undergoing any significant attenuation.

**Filtration for General Diagnostic Radiology.** In general diagnostic radiology, aluminum (Z = 13) is the metal most widely selected as a filter material because it effectively removes low-energy (soft) x-rays from a polyenergetic (heterogeneous) x-ray beam without severely decreasing the x-ray beam intensity. In addition, aluminum is:

- Lightweight
- Sturdy
- Relatively inexpensive
- Readily available

In compliance with the Radiation Control for Health and Safety Act of 1968, a diagnostic x-ray beam must always be adequately filtered. This means that a sufficient quantity of low-energy photons has been removed from a beam produced at a given kVp. The **half-value layer** (**HVL**) of the beam must be measured to verify

| BOX 11-2 | Summary of Required Minimum Total Filtration |
|---|---|

**Stationary (Fixed) Radiographic Equipment**

| Tube Potential Minimum Total Filtration Required (kVp) | Minimum Total Filtration Required (Specified in mm Al Eq)* |
|---|---|
| Above 70 | 2.5 |
| 50-70 | 1.5 |
| Below 50 | 0.5 |

**Mobile Diagnostic Units and Fluoroscopic Equipment**
Mobile diagnostic units and fluoroscopic equipment require a minimum of 2.5 mm Al Eq total permanent filtration.

*Al Eq,* Aluminum equivalent.
*Modified from National Council on Radiation Protection and Measurements (NCRP): *Medical x-ray, electron beam and gamma-ray protection for energies up to 50 MeV (equipment design, performance, and use),* Report No. 102, Bethesda, Md, 1989, NCRP.

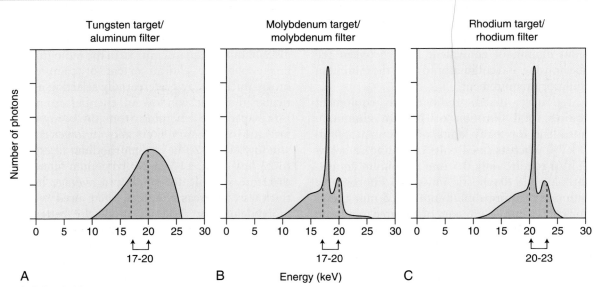

**FIGURE 11-12  A** and **B,** X-ray emission spectra for tungsten and molybdenum anodes. Note that tungsten produces a high volume of x-ray photons above the 17- to 20-keV range considered ideal for mammography. These photons merely degrade the quality of the recorded image. The molybdenum anode produces few x-ray photons above the ideal energy range, initiating a higher-contrast image on the finished image. **C,** A rhodium anode produces a higher average energy x-ray beam than does the molybdenum anode. The energy range for rhodium-produced photons is 20 to 23 keV. Photons from this energy range can provide better penetration of larger, denser breasts.

this. HVL is defined as the thickness of a designated absorber (customarily a metal such as aluminum) required to decrease the intensity of the primary beam by 50% of its initial value. A radiologic physicist should obtain this measurement at least once a year and also after an x-ray tube is replaced or repairs have been made on the diagnostic x-ray tube housing or collimation system. For diagnostic x-ray beams, the HVL is expressed in millimeters of aluminum. Because HVL is a measure of beam quality, or effective energy of the x-ray beam, a certain minimal HVL is required at a given kVp. Examples of required HVLs for selected kVp values are listed in Table 11-1.

## Compensating Filters

Dose reduction and uniform radiographic imaging of body parts that vary considerably in

| TABLE 11-1 | Half-Value Layer Required by the Radiation Control for Health and Safety Act of 1968 and Detailed by the Bureau of Radiological Health* in 1980 |
|---|---|
| **Peak Kilovoltage** | **Minimum Required HVL in Millimeters of Aluminum** |
| 30 | 0.3 |
| 40 | 0.4 |
| 50 | 1.2 |
| 60 | 1.3 |
| 70 | 1.5 |
| 80 | 2.3 |
| 90 | 2.5 |
| 100 | 2.7 |
| 110 | 3.0 |
| 120 | 3.2 |

*HVL,* Half-value layer.
*The Bureau of Radiological Health changed its name to the Center for Devices and Radiological Health in 1982.

thickness or tissue composition may be accomplished by use of compensating filters constructed of:

- Aluminum
- Lead-acrylic
- Other suitable materials

These devices partially attenuate x-rays that are directed toward the thinner, or less dense, area while permitting more x-radiation to strike the thicker, or denser, area. For example, the *wedge filter* (Fig. 11-13) is used to provide uniform density when the foot is undergoing radiography in the dorsoplantar projection. For this examination, the wedge is attached to the lower rim of the collimator and positioned with its thickest part toward the toes and thinnest part toward the heel. The *trough, or bilateral, wedge filter,* which is used in some dedicated chest radiographic units, is another example of a compensating filter. This filter is thin in the center to permit adequate x-ray penetration of the mediastinum and thick laterally to reduce exposure of the aerated lungs. With this device, a radiographic image with uniform average density is obtained.

## Exposure Reproducibility

In Chapter 10, Box 10-4 describes some important provisions included in the code of standards for diagnostic x-ray equipment that went into effect on August 1, 1974. **Exposure reproducibility** is defined, in that chapter, as consistency in output in radiation intensity for identical generator settings from one individual exposure to subsequent exposures. This means that the x-ray unit must be able to duplicate certain radiographic exposures for any given combination of kilovolts at peak (kVp), milliamperes (mA), and time. A variance of 5% or less is acceptable. Reproducibility may be verified by using the same technical exposure factors to make a series of repeated radiation exposures and then,

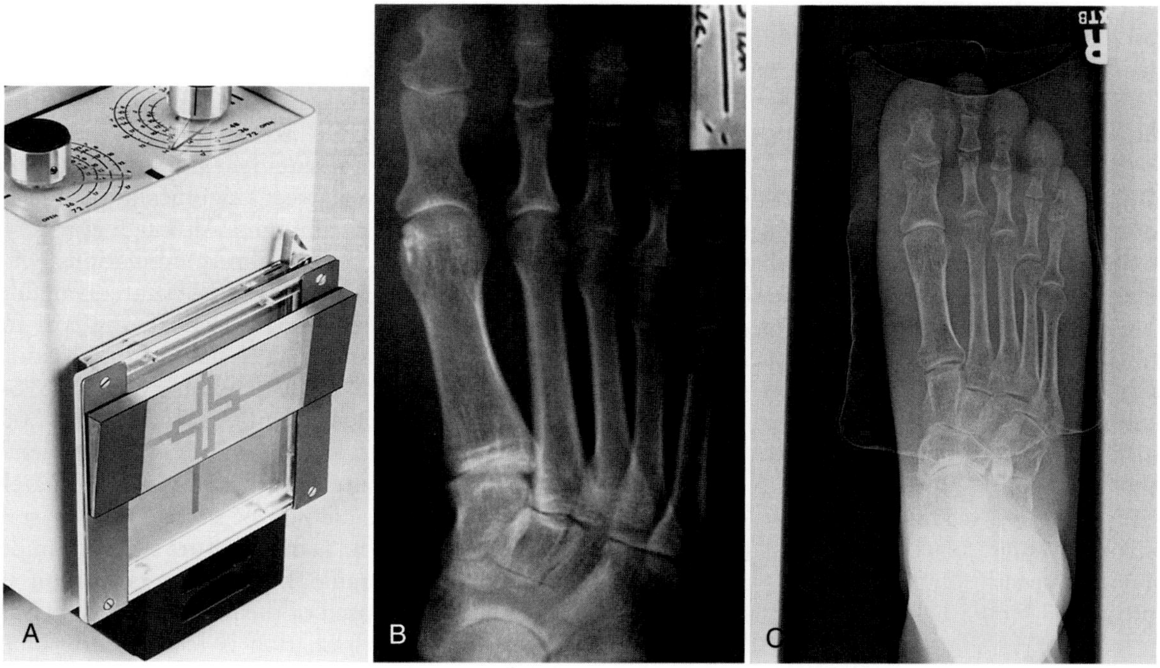

FIGURE 11-13 **A,** Wedged-shaped lead-acrylic compensating filter used to provide uniform density for (**B**) a dorsoplantar projection of the foot without a compensating filter. (**C**) A dorsoplantar projection of the foot with a wedge-shaped lead-acrylic compensating filter.

observing with a calibrated ion chamber, how radiation intensity typically varies.

## Exposure Linearity

**Exposure linearity** (see Chapter 10, Box 10-4) refers to a consistency in output radiation intensity at any selected kVp settings when generator settings are changed from one milliamperage and time combination (mAs = mA × exposure time) to another. *Linearity (L)* has been mathematically defined as the ratio of the difference in mR/mAs values between two successive generator stations to the sum of those mR/mAs values. It must be less than 0.1 (i.e., L cannot exceed 10%).

## Screen-Film Combinations

With advances in technology, many health care facilities are now using image receptors other than radiographic film. These newer technologies, which include digital radiography (DR) and computed radiography (CR), are discussed later in this chapter. Because some health care providers have continued to use film as an image receptor, the following discussion concerning screen-film combinations continues to be of significant value.

**Value of Intensifying Screens in Patient Dose Reduction.** X-ray film, most of which is double-emulsion x-ray film (i.e., emulsion coated on both sides of the film), responds strongly to the light emitted by intensifying screens. By amplifying the effects of the exit, or image formation, radiation reaching the radiographic film, intensifying screens enhance the action of x-rays on the film and thereby convert x-ray energy into visible light to produce radiographic density on the film. Approximately 95% of the radiographic density of the recorded image results from the visible light photons that are emitted by the intensifying screens. Because a single x-ray photon can produce 80 to 95 light photons, this conversion:

- Dramatically enhances the film exposure process
- Permits radiographic exposure time to be substantially reduced

The latter leads to a sizable reduction in patient dose. At the time of this writing, when screen-film image receptors are still used in some health care facilities, the intensifying screens used in conjunction with matching radiographic film are predominantly **rare-earth screens**. These screens are made with phosphors of the following elements:

- Gadolinium
- Lanthanum
- Yttrium

These are nonabundant, or rare, elements that have atomic numbers ranging from 57 to 71. Consequently, because of their high atomic numbers, the screens facilitate higher x-ray absorption of the incident x-ray beam, can convert the x-ray energy to light more efficiently (by 15% to 20%), and are therefore noticeably faster than the calcium tungstate screens that were used until the 1970s. Rare-earth screens also place less thermal stress on the x-ray tube, thus increasing its life span. In addition, when these screens are used, radiation shielding requirements for the x-ray room are decreased because of a general reduction of x-radiation in the environment.

**Effect of Faster Screen-Film Systems on Patient Dose.** To reiterate, film speed and the use of intensifying screens significantly influence radiographic exposure time. Although rare-earth screens and matching film combinations with relative speeds from 200 to 1200 are available, 400-speed systems are considered standard for general radiography at the time of this writing. When the speed of screen-film systems (SFSs) doubles (e.g., when a change is made from a 200-speed system to a 400-speed system), the patient's radiation exposure is reduced by approximately 50%. When the amount of silver halide crystals (approximately 95% of which are silver bromide) contained in radiographic film emulsion is increased, the speed of the film is increased. This means that less radiation is required to obtain an image. As radiographic exposure decreases, patient dose decreases. One manufacturer has developed an 800-speed medical film that can be used with regular intensifying screens. The use of such a film can reduce the patient's radiation exposure by as much as 50%.[8]

It is essential that SFSs be matched correctly. If they are not correctly matched or compatible, patient dose can increase.

**Effect of Kilovoltage on Screen Speed and Patient Dose.** Kilovoltage also affects screen speed. As kilovoltage increases, effective screen speed increases for rare earth screens, which reduces the patient dose. The higher atomic numbers of the materials used in rare earth screens increase the probability for photoelectric interaction between the incident x-rays and the rare earth atoms in the screens. The selection of kVp and the screen-film combination are two of the most important technical considerations in the amount of patient dose.

**Selection of Film-Based Image Receptor Systems.** Although the high-speed screen-film image receptor systems with calcium tungstate intensifying screens that were used until the 1970s significantly reduced patient dose, a loss of radiographic quality was also possible because the recorded image may have had poorer resolution. As a result, the use of these image receptor systems was not practical for all radiography. In addition, when compared with slower rare-earth screen-film image receptor systems, faster rare-earth screen-film image receptor systems can demonstrate an effect referred to as **quantum mottle.** These faint blotches (image noise) can degrade the radiographic image and be annoying to the radiologist interpreting the image. Therefore, higher-speed rare-earth systems may not be suitable for all radiography, either. To be able to select the appropriate film-based image receptor system for a given radiographic examination, the radiographer must be aware of the capabilities and limitations of the different systems available. Manufacturers or distributors supply product information about the various film-based image receptor systems, which can be obtained by contacting the appropriate source.

**Summary of Benefits of Rare-Earth Intensifying Screens.** As mentioned previously, rare-earth intensifying screens are more efficient than their predecessors, calcium tungstate intensifying screens, in converting x-ray energy into light photons. These screens absorb approximately five times more x-ray energy than do calcium tungstate screens and hence they emit considerably more light. This significantly reduces the radiographic exposure required to obtain an image of acceptable quality. An additional benefit of rare-earth screens is that high resolution (the ability of a system to make two adjacent objects visually distinguishable) of the recorded image remains constant. This ensures radiographic quality. Higher-speed rare-earth systems do, however, produce quantum mottle in the recorded image that causes some degradation of image quality. Because required x-ray radiation intensity is reduced when rare-earth screens are used, x-ray tube life span is increased, and radiation shielding requirements for the room decrease.

**Use of Carbon Fiber as a Front Material in a Radiographic Cassette.** The use of carbon fiber as a front material in a cassette that holds radiographic film and intensifying screens is a technologic advancement over previously used cassette front materials. When compared with the traditional cassette front materials such as aluminum or cardboard, the cassette front containing the carbon fiber absorbs approximately half as much radiation. This lowers the patient dose because lower radiographic techniques are required to produce the recorded image. In addition, because lower radiographic techniques are employed, the life of the x-ray tube may also be prolonged.

**Use of Asymmetric Film Emulsion and Intensifying Screen Combinations.** Another technologic advance that is still in use comprises asymmetric film emulsion and intensifying screen combinations. With this system, the front screen and film emulsion (the side that faces the x-ray tube) is slower than the back screen and film emulsion, which contains a faster system. This screen-film combination results in a recorded image with greater uniformity and a decrease in patient exposure.

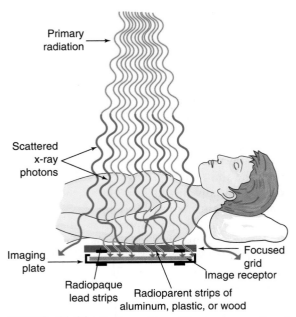

Primary radiation

Scattered x-ray photons

Imaging plate

Focused grid

Image receptor

Radiopaque lead strips

Radioparent strips of aluminum, plastic, or wood

**FIGURE 11-14** Radiographic grids remove scattered x-ray photons that emerge from the patient being radiographed before this scattered radiation reaches the image receptor and decreases radiographic quality.

## Radiographic Grids

**Construction, Purpose, Technical Value, and Impact of a Radiographic Grid on Patient Dose.** A **radiographic grid** (Fig. 11-14) is a device made of parallel radiopaque strips alternately separated with low-attenuation strips of:

- Aluminum
- Plastic
- Wood

It is placed between the patient and the radiographic image receptor to remove scattered x-ray photons that emerge from the patient before they reach the film or other image receptor. This significantly improves:

- Radiographic contrast
- Visibility of detail

Generally, this device is used when the thickness of the body part to be radiographed is greater than 10 cm. Although the use of a grid increases patient dose, the benefit obtained in terms of the improved quality of the recorded image, making available a greater quantity of diagnostic information, is a fair compromise. Because several different types of grids and grids with different ratios are available, care must be taken to ensure that the correct type and grid ratio* are used for a particular examination, or else a repeat examination may be necessary, which would additionally increase patient dose.

**Summarizing the Function of a Radiographic Grid.** To summarize, when x-rays pass through an object, some of the photons are scattered away from their original path as a result of coherent and Compton scattering processes. Radiographic quality is highest when these scattered photons are not recorded on the image. If scattered photons are recorded, a general darkening of the image occurs, which detracts from the viewer's ability to distinguish among the different structures of the object being radiographed. Ideally, only those photons that have passed through matter with no deviation from their original geometric path should be recorded. To minimize the influence of scattered photons, a grid is inserted between the patient and the image receptor. It is designed to act as a sieve to block the passage of photons that have been scattered beyond some maximum angle from their original path (Fig. 11-15).

**Grid Ratio and Patient Dose.** As previously noted, grids are made of parallel radiopaque lead strips alternately separated with low-attenuation strips of aluminum, plastic, or wood. Therefore, because some fraction of the image receptor is covered with lead, more mAs must be used to compensate. Thus, patient dose increases whenever a grid is inserted, and because extra lead is contained in higher-ratio grids (e.g., 16:1), patient dose increases as grid ratio increases.

---

*Grid ratio* is defined as the ratio of the height of the lead strips in the grid to the distance between them. High-ratio grids reduce scatter radiation more effectively than do low-ratio grids. However, high-ratio grids require more radiation exposure.

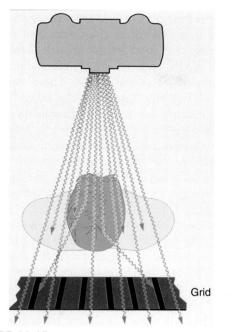

**FIGURE 11-15** The radiographic grid acts as a sieve to block the passage of photons that have been scattered at some angle from their original path.

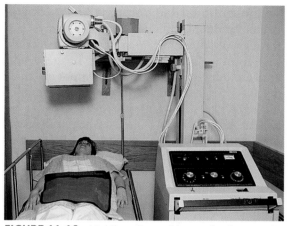

**FIGURE 11-16** Mobile radiographic examinations require a minimal source-skin distance of 30 cm (12 inches). The 30 cm distance limits the effects of inverse square falloff of radiation intensity with distance.

## Minimal Source-Skin Distance for Mobile Radiography

**Requirement.** Mobile radiographic units require special precautions to ensure patient safety. When operating the unit, the radiographer must use a source-skin distance (SSD) of at least 30 cm (12 inches) (Fig. 11-16). The 30-cm (12-inch) distance limits the effects of the inverse square falloff of radiation intensity with distance. This falloff is more pronounced the shorter the SSD. In practice, much longer distances (e.g., 100 cm (40 inches) from x-ray source to image receptor or even 120 cm (48 inches)) are generally used.

**Effect of Source-Skin Distance on Patient Entrance Exposure.** When the SSD is small, the patient's entrance exposure is significantly greater than the exit exposure. By increasing SSD, the radiographer maintains a more uniform distribution of exposure throughout the patient.

**Use of Mobile Units.** Mobile (portable) units should be used to perform radiographic procedures only on patients who cannot be transported to a fixed radiographic installation (an x-ray room). Mobile units are not designed to replace specially designated imaging rooms.

## RADIATION SAFETY FEATURES OF DIGITAL IMAGING EQUIPMENT, DEVICES, AND ACCESSORIES

### Digital Imaging

**Use of the Computer.** The computer is capable of rapidly processing vast amounts of independent groups of information. Since the 1970s, the use of computers has virtually revolutionized the medical industry. In particular, computers have had a major impact on imaging. They are now used extensively in almost all imaging modalities. The primary examples of this are:

* Computed tomography (CT)
* Computed radiography (CR)
* Digital radiography (DR)
* Digital fluoroscopy (DF)
* Nuclear medicine (NM) imaging
* Magnetic resonance imaging (MRI)
* Ultrasound (US)
* Digital mammography

**Conventional Radiography: Analog Image.** In conventional radiography, after x-rays pass through an anatomic area of clinical interest, they form an invisible, or latent, image of that area on radiographic film. This temporary image produced conventionally by ionizing radiation must then be chemically processed to make the unseen image visible. The finished radiograph that results from this process is an "analog image." Conventional radiography permits the production of optimal-quality images that make possible adequate visualization and demonstration of various anatomic structures. However, the use of this technology has some disadvantages in addition to the waiting time it takes for the chemical processing of these film-based images. Radiographic film must be physically handled by authorized personnel and then stored in a centralized file. Manually retrieving radiographs is often time-consuming and requires adequate personnel power. As a consequence of human error, film jackets containing patients' radiographs may be misfiled or misplaced, thus making these records unavailable at a time when a physician may need them for patient care.

**Digital Radiography.** The information contained in a conventional radiograph consists of various shades of gray that represent the amount of x-ray penetration through various biologic tissues. With **digital radiography (DR)**, the latent image, formed by x-ray photons on a radiation detector, is actually an electronic latent image.[9] Because this anatomic information is subsequently collected by a computer and shown on its display, it is called a *digital image*.[10] The familiar radiographic densities then appear as levels of brightness associated with shades of gray. "**Brightness** is defined as the amount of luminance (light emission) of a display monitor. The shades of gray that are displayed constitute the contrast in the image. The number of different shades of gray that can be stored in memory and displayed on a computer monitor is termed grayscale. Digital images are composed of numerical data that can be easily manipulated by a computer."[11]

The numeric values of the digital image are aligned in a fixed number of rows and columns (an array) that form many individual miniature square boxes, each of which corresponds to a particular place in the image. These individual boxes collectively constitute the **image matrix.** Each miniature square box in this matrix is called a picture element, or *pixel*. The pixels collectively produce a two-dimensional representation of the information contained in a volume of tissue.[12] The size of the pixels determines the sharpness of the image. Resolution is sharper when pixels are smaller. Common matrix sizes are $512 \times 512$ and $1024 \times 1024$. The latter corresponds to a much higher resolution because it has four times as many elements distributed over the same area. The pixels are therefore smaller, which leads to improved image detail.

When compared with the resolution of an optimal-quality image produced on radiographic film, the resolution of the digital image is actually somewhat lower. However, the digital image is still diagnostic, permitting adequate visualization of anatomic structures because it has better image contrast. This is so, because unlike in a developed film, the contrast in the digital image can be enhanced by computer manipulation.

The image receptors used in direct radiography convert the energy of x-rays into electrical signals. The image receptor is divided into small detector elements that make up the picture elements, or pixels, of the digital image. There are various types of digital radiography image receptors. Some use a scintillator, such as amorphous silicon,* to convert the x-ray energy into visible light. The visible light is then converted into electrical signals by an array of transistors or an array of charge-coupled devices (CCDs), such as those found in video cameras. Other systems use a photoconductor, such as amorphous selenium, to convert the x-ray energy directly into electrical signals that are then read by an array of transistors. In all these systems, the number

---

*A noncrystalline grouping of silicon atoms in which, rather than in a regular geometric pattern, the silicon atoms are distributed in a continuous random fashion.

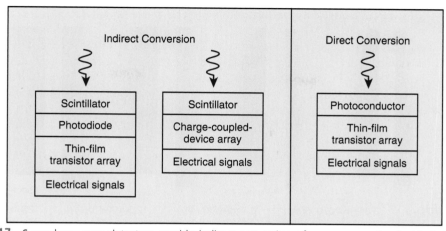

**FIGURE 11-17** Some large area detectors provide indirect conversion of x-ray energy to electrical charge through intermediate steps involving photodiodes or charge-coupled devices. Other area detectors provide direct conversion of x-ray energy to electrical charge through the use of a photoconductor.

and size of small transistors or CCDs determine the number and size of pixels in the digital image. Advances in materials technology have resulted in pixel sizes as small as 50 micrometers, which approaches the resolution of screen-film imaging systems (Fig. 11-17).

DR images can be accessed at several workstations at the same time, thus making image viewing very convenient for physicians providing patient care. Patient information and reports can be included in the patient's DR imaging file, along with records from other imaging modalities.[13]

**Repeat Rates in Digital Radiography.** Because the image contrast and overall brightness may be manipulated after image acquisition, DR eliminates the need for almost all retakes required as a result of improper technique selection (Fig. 11-18). However, repeat rates for reasons of mispositioning are not lowered. Because the image receptor is part of the imaging equipment and does not need to be removed for processing, the technologist can simply view the image on a monitor in the room. This raises a concern about knowing the number of repeats required because of mispositioning. There is no "penalty" for a quality control technologist viewing the image and monitoring repeats required because of mispositioning, so the examination may be repeated without the knowledge of supervisors. Therefore,

either each image should be monitored by an independent quality control technologist at a separate monitor or a quality control system should be used whereby the number of images per examination is compared with the number ordered for each technologist.

### Computed Radiography

***Process.*** Computed radiography (CR) involves the use of conventional radiographic equipment, traditional patient positioning performed by a radiographer, and the selection and use of standard technical exposure factors. The unseen radiographic image is actually produced in a rectangular, closed cassette containing a photostimulable phosphor (europium-activated barium fluorohalide is the most commonly employed phosphor[2]) imaging plate as the image receptor. This reusable device is inserted in place of radiographic film into a light-tight, closed cassette that resembles that found in conventional radiography. The CR cassette may be referred to as a *filmless cassette*.

When the enclosed phosphor is exposed to x-rays, it becomes energized. An image reading unit is used to scan the photostimulable phosphor imaging plate with a helium-neon laser beam. This results in the emission of violet light that is changed into an electronic signal by a device called a *photomultiplier tube*.

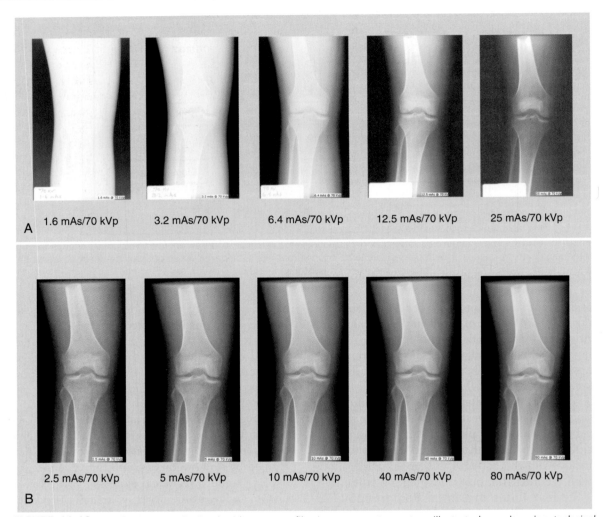

**FIGURE 11-18** **A,** The images obtained with a screen-film image receptor system illustrate how changing technical exposure factors greatly affect film image quality. **B,** Computed radiography (CR) images obtained through the same technique ranges as those used for **A** have much less effect on image quality because "CR image contrast is constant, regardless of radiation exposure."

A computer then converts the electronic signal into a digitized image of the anatomic area or part and stores the digital image for visual display on a monitor. If desired, the image can be printed on a laser film when hard copy is needed. While the digital image is displayed on a monitor, the radiographer, by manipulating the computer mouse[4] (Fig. 11-19), can adjust it to the correct:

- Size
- Brightness (radiographic density)
- Contrast

After adjustments have been completed, the image can be electronically sent for reading.

***Avoiding Overexposure of the Patient.*** Although the radiographer can manipulate the

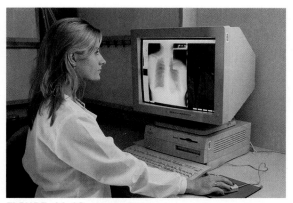

FIGURE 11-19 The radiographer at the monitor uses the mouse to adjust the computed radiography image of the body part to the proper size, density, and contrast before electronically sending the image for reading.

CR image of the patient's anatomy of interest to adjust image size, brightness, and contrast, this technologic flexibility does not excuse overexposing the patient. Even with sophisticated digital technology, it is still the radiographer's responsibility to determine and use correct technical exposure factors the first time a patient is x-rayed to minimize radiation exposure. If patients are overexposed by radiographers who claim the rationale that computerized images can be manipulated later on to produce a diagnostic-quality image, thereby avoiding the possibility of repeat exposures, patients are actually receiving higher radiation doses than are necessary to produce those initial images. This type of practice leads to a phenomenon known in many facilities as "dose creep." Therefore, the routine practice of overexposing patients to avoid possible repeat radiographic exposures is unethical and unacceptable. For this reason, radiographers must exercise good judgment in selecting correct technical exposure factors the first time. This good practice conforms with ALARA (as low as reasonably achievable) protection guidelines.

***Computed Radiography Phosphor Sensitivity.*** The sensitivity of the phosphor used in CR has been described as approximately equal to a 200-speed screen-film combination.[9] What this implies is that CR technique factors are generally somewhat greater than those used in conventional radiography, in which 400-speed screen-film combinations are typically employed.

***Kilovoltage.*** As in conventional radiography, kilovoltage controls radiographic contrast. However, CR imaging has greater kilovoltage flexibility than does conventional screen-film radiography. Therefore, a radiographer can select an appropriate kVp setting from a broader range of settings than are usually suitable for a particular radiographic projection.[4] An acceptable range of kVp that is adequate for penetration of the anatomy of interest should, however, always be used. Kilovoltage above or below this acceptable range should not be used. Technique charts indicating optimal kVp for all CR projections must be available in the x-ray room near the operating console for the radiographer.

***X-Ray Beam Collimation.*** For the computer to form a CR image correctly, the body area or part being radiographed must be positioned in or near the center of the CR image receptor. In practical application, only one projection per image is taken on a CR imaging plate.

***Use of Radiographic Grids.*** When compared with conventional SFSs in which radiographic film becomes more sensitive to scatter radiation after it is initially exposed to x-rays but before it is processed, the photostimulable phosphor in a CR imaging plate can absorb more low-energy scattered photons than rare-earth phosphor and film combinations initially. Therefore, it is much more sensitive to scatter radiation both before and after it is sensitized by exposure to a radiographic beam.[14] Because of this increased sensitivity, a radiographic grid should probably be used more frequently during CR imaging than during screen-film imaging. For chest radiography, Carlton and Adler advocated the use of a grid for optimum images when chest measurements exceed 24 to 26 cm.[14] Some CR imaging manufacturers recommend the use of a grid for certain radiographic projections that require relatively high-kVp settings. Grid selection depends on several factors: size of the anatomic features to be radiographed, kVp selected, amount of scatter removal preferred, and grid frequency (lines per centimeter or inch), for example.[14]

With SFSs, it is customary and, for the best image quality, necessary to use a grid for anatomy sections more than 10 cm thick or for techniques that exceed 70 kVp. This need remains true with both CR and DR. The problem one faces with CR is that the mAs required and consequently the patient dose received are significantly higher than delivered with screen-film imaging. The addition of a grid will only further increase that dose. Many quality assurance teams, however, are now realizing that CR, because of its higher exposure latitude, makes grid use on the pediatric population less necessary than was previously believed. As a result, satisfactory nongrid pediatric protocols have been developed and used.

DR systems offer several advantages over both CR and conventional SFSs. Some of these include:

- Lower dose
- Ease of use
- Immediate imaging results
- Manipulation of the image

One potential disadvantage, however, is that most fixed DR systems either do not allow the user to change the grid to accommodate the imaging task or have a preinstalled grid that is not easily accessible to the user.

These conditions result in the use of grids used for pediatric imaging, thereby unnecessarily giving these patients a higher dose of radiation. Facilities will now need to work with their radiation safety officer (RSO) and physics group more than ever before to ensure the highest quality imaging for the smallest patients. As a technologist, one must find out whether grids are truly not removable from the digital imaging equipment or whether they are being used merely because it is the manufacturer's recommendation.

## RADIATION SAFETY FEATURES OF FLUOROSCOPIC EQUIPMENT, DEVICES, AND ACCESSORIES

### Fluoroscopic Procedures

**Patient Radiation Exposure Rate.** Fluoroscopy is the process in which an x-ray examination

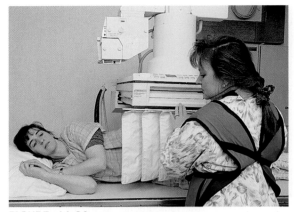

**FIGURE 11-20** Fluoroscopic procedures produce the largest patient radiation exposure rate in diagnostic radiology.

is performed that demonstrates dynamic, or active, motion of selected anatomic structures (e.g., a stomach filled with barium sulfate and air during an upper gastrointestinal series) by producing a real-time image of those structures on a television monitor that works in conjunction with an image intensification system under low-light conditions. Fluoroscopic procedures (Fig. 11-20) produce the greatest patient radiation exposure rate in diagnostic radiology. Therefore, the physician should carefully evaluate the need for a fluoroscopic examination to ascertain whether the potential benefit to the patient, in terms of information gained, outweighs any adverse somatic or genetic (hereditary) effects of the examination. If the fluoroscopic procedure is necessary, every precaution must be taken to minimize patient exposure time.

**Fluoroscopic Imaging Systems.** Traditionally, fluoroscopic imaging systems have the x-ray tube positioned under the x-ray examination table and the image intensifier and spot film system mounted on a C-arm and centered and suspended over the x-ray examination table. The C-arm design keeps the x-ray tube and the image receptor in constant alignment. Other equipment configurations are possible; for example, the unit can be arranged so that the x-ray tube can be placed over the x-ray examination table while the image receptor lies beneath the x-ray

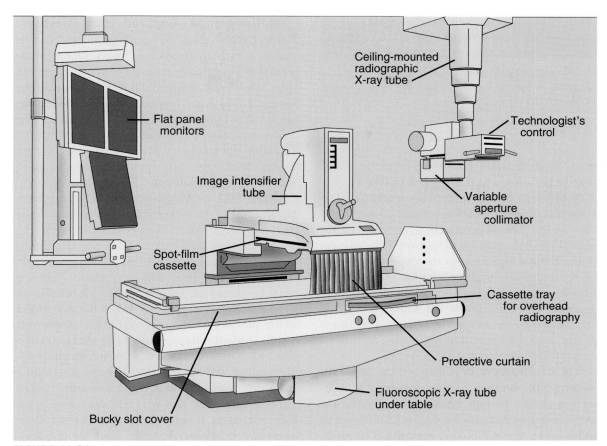

**FIGURE 11-21** Image intensification fluoroscopy unit. The x-ray tube used in this unit is mounted beneath the unit's radiographic table, which supports the patient. The image intensifier and other image detection devices are then drawn forward and placed over the patient on the table to perform the examination. Other fluoroscopic equipment arrangements are possible.

examination table. A fluoroscopic imaging system can also be set up as a remote control facility, thus permitting the equipment operator to remain outside the fluoroscopic room. In the interest of patient and personnel safety, radiologists and assisting radiologic technologists have a responsibility to become fully knowledgeable regarding the safe operation of the equipment they use.

### Image Intensification Fluoroscopy

***Benefits.*** Image intensification fluoroscopy (Fig. 11-21) involves the use of an image intensifier tube (Fig. 11-22) to increase the brightness of the real-time image produced on a fluorescent screen during fluoroscopy. It, or a digital device that performs the same function, is used in virtually all state-of-the-art fluoroscopic equipment.

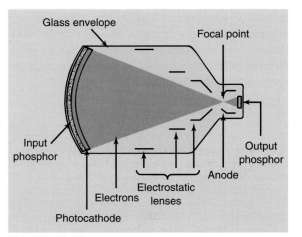

**FIGURE 11-22** **Basic Components of an Image Intensifier Tube.**

---

| BOX 11-3 | Benefits of Image Intensification Fluoroscopy |
|---|---|

1. Increased image brightness
2. Saving of time for the radiologist
3. Patient dose reduction

---

Image intensification fluoroscopy has three significant benefits, which are listed in Box 11-3.

**Brightness of the Fluoroscopic Image.** The x-ray image intensification system converts the x-ray image pattern into a corresponding amplified visible light pattern. The overall brightness of the fluoroscopic image increases to roughly 10,000 times the brightness of the image on the discontinued non–image intensifier fluoroscopic systems* operating under the same conditions. This dramatic increase in image brightness greatly improved the radiologist's perception of the fluoroscopic image.

**Use of Photopic or Cone Vision to View Fluoroscopic Image.** Because an image intensification system permits observing of the fluoroscopic image at ordinary brightness levels (regular white light), the radiologist makes use of photopic, or cone, vision (daytime vision) when viewing the image through this system. With cone vision, the radiologist no longer needs to adapt to the darkness by wearing of red goggles for up to 30 minutes, as was required to enable the use of scotopic, or rod, vision (night vision) to view the dim fluoroscopic image. Cone vision also significantly improves visual acuity and thereby permits the radiologist to discriminate better among small structures.

**Milliamperage Required and Effect on Patient Dose.** Because an image intensification system greatly increases brightness, image intensification fluoroscopy requires less milliamperage than does old-fashioned fluoroscopy (approximately 1.5 to 2 mA is used for many procedures with image intensification systems, whereas 3 to 5 mA was usually required for pre–image intensification fluoroscopy). The consequent decrease in exposure rate can result in a sizable dose reduction for the patient.

**Multifield, or Magnification, Image Intensifier Tubes.** An image intensifier tube is basically an "electronic device that receives the image-forming x-ray beam and converts it into a visible-light image of high intensity."[2] A simple diagram of this tube with components labeled may be found in Figure 11-22. Multifield, or magnification, image intensifier tubes are found in the majority of image intensifiers. They are also found in **digital fluoroscopy (DF)** units (see the discussion on DF presented later in this chapter). Depending on their manufacturer and geographic location, multifield image intensification tubes vary in size, but the 25/17/12 cm (10/6.8/4.8 inch) diameter trifield model may be the most common commercial tube used in general-purpose fluoroscopic units. However, other sizes and magnification modes are available.

When the normal viewing mode of 25 cm (10 inches) is used, photoelectrons from the entire surface of a cesium iodide (CsI) input phosphor (i.e., when the x-ray photons passing through the patient first strike the image intensifier assembly) are accelerated to a zinc–cadmium sulfide output phosphor. However, when magnification in the fluoroscopic image is needed and the viewing mode is changed to the 17-cm mode (6.8 inches) or even less (e.g., 12 cm (4.8 inches) in many new systems), the voltage on the electrostatic focusing lenses increases, thereby causing the focal point of the electrons to move to a greater distance away from the output phosphor.[2] As a result, only electrons from the central 17-cm diameter portion of the input phosphor actually reach the output phosphor of the image intensifier. The change in the focal point of the

---

*A pre–image intensification fluoroscopic operating system is an earlier system in which the fluoroscopic tube, mounted beneath the radiographic table as with most modern fluoroscopic systems, produces x-rays that pass through the tabletop and the patient before striking a zinc-cadmium sulfide (ZnCdS) fluoroscopic screen that phosphoresces and produces a very dim image of the anatomy of interest, thus yielding poor visibility of detail of those structures by the radiologist.

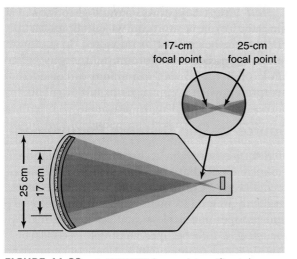

**FIGURE 11-23** A 25/17/12 image intensifier tube produces a magnified image in 17-cm mode, whereas the 12-cm mode produces an image that is even more highly magnified.

electrons decreases the field of view, with a corresponding increase in magnification of the image (Fig. 11-23). The quality of the magnified image, if there are no other changes, as viewed on a monitor, is somewhat degraded. This decrease in image clarity occurs because of a reduction in minification gain (i.e., increase in brightness resulting from minification of the image) caused when fewer photoelectrons are available to strike the output phosphor on the image intensifier. Therefore, the resultant image is dimmer. Because it is necessary and desirable to maintain a constant level of brightness on the monitor, fluoroscopic mA increases automatically. However, this increase in tube mA raises the dose to the patient. Although the use of smaller-diameter modes results in increased patient dose, the overall quality of the image is improved when compared with the use of larger-diameter modes because in smaller-diameter modes a greater number of x-ray photons is needed to form the image. This image will have a more even appearance (less noise), and it will be possible to distinguish among similar tissues more easily because of improved contrast.

## Intermittent, or Pulsed, Fluoroscopy

**Effect on Patient Dose.** Intermittent, or pulsed, fluoroscopy involves manual or automatic periodic activation of the fluoroscopic tube by the fluoroscopist, rather than lengthy continuous activation. This practice:

- Significantly decreases patient dose, especially in long procedures
- Helps extend the life of the tube

Many systems include a last-image-hold feature that allows the fluoroscopist to see the most recent image without exposing the patient to another pulse of radiation. This feature also reduces patient dose.

### Limiting Fluoroscopic Field Size
*Benefit of Fluoroscopic Field Size Limitation.* The radiologist must limit the size of the fluoroscopic field to include only the area of clinical interest by adequately collimating the x-ray beam. Adequate collimation involves adjusting the lead shutters placed between the fluoroscopic tube and the patient. When fluoroscopic field size is limited, patient area or integral dose decreases substantially.

*Fluoroscopic Beam Length and Width Limitation.* Primary beam length and width must be confined within the image receptor boundary. Regardless of the distance from the x-ray source to the image receptor, the useful beam ideally should not extend outside the image receptor. Visible borders should appear on the image monitor.

### Technical Exposure Factors
*Selection of Technical Exposure Factors for Adult Patients.* The fluoroscopist must select technical exposure factors that will minimize patient dose during manual fluoroscopic procedures. Increases in kVp and filtration reduce the patient radiation exposure rate. Most fluoroscopic examinations performed with image intensification systems employ a range of 75 to 110 kVp for adult patients, depending on the body area being examined. This kVp range produces the correct level of fluoroscopic image brightness. Lower kVp, when used for greater diameter regions, increases patient dose because

use of a lesser penetrating x-ray beam necessitates the use of a higher milliamperage (a larger quantity of x-ray photons in the beam) to obtain adequate image brightness. Besides using the correct kilovoltage, the operator can further limit excessive entrance exposure of the patient by ensuring that the x-ray **source-to-skin distance** (SSD) is not less than 38 cm (15 inches) for stationary (fixed) fluoroscopes and not less than 30 cm (12 inches) for mobile fluoroscopes. A 30-cm (12-inch) minimal distance is required, but a 38-cm (15-inch) minimal distance is preferred for all image intensification systems. On the other hand, the position of the input phosphor surface of the image intensifier should be maintained as close as is practical to the patient to reduce the patient's entrance exposure rate as well.

### Selection of Technical Exposure Factors for Children.
Technical exposure factors for fluoroscopic procedures for children necessitate a decrease in kVp by as much as 25%. The kVp chosen should depend on part thickness, just as it does in radiography. In addition to decreasing technical exposure factors, maintaining SSD and minimizing the height of the image intensifier entrance surface above the patient further limit excessive entrance exposure of the pediatric patient.

### Filtration
#### Purpose and Requirements.
The function of a filter in fluoroscopy, as in radiographic procedures, is to reduce the patient's skin dose from soft x-rays. Adequate layers of aluminum equivalent material placed in the path of the useful beam remove the more harmful lower-energy photons from the beam by absorbing them. A minimum of 2.5 mm total aluminum equivalent filtration must be permanently installed in the path of the useful beam of the fluoroscopic unit. With image intensification systems, a total aluminum equivalent filtration of 3.0 mm or greater may be preferred. Patient dose decreases by one fourth during fluoroscopic procedures when aluminum filtration increases from 1 to 3 mm aluminum. Although this increase in filtration causes a slight loss of fluoroscopic image brightness, increasing kVp somewhat may compensate.

#### Half-Value Layer.
As in radiography, when filtration of the x-ray beam is questionable, the HVL of the beam must be measured. In standard image intensification fluoroscopy, an x-ray beam HVL of 3 to 4.5 mm aluminum is considered acceptable when kVp ranges from 80 to 100.

## Source-to-Skin Distance Requirement

#### Requirement.
In accordance with National Council on Radiation Protection and Measurements (NCRP) regulations, the SSD must be no less than 38 cm (15 inches) for stationary (fixed) fluoroscopes and no less than 30 cm (12 inches) for mobile fluoroscopes.[7] As discussed earlier, this standard ensures that the patient's entrance surface is not excessively exposed. Maintaining an appropriate SSD reduces the radiographer's exposure as well.

#### Cumulative Timing Device.
A **cumulative timer** must be provided and used with each fluoroscopic unit. This resettable device times the x-ray beam-on time and sounds an audible alarm or temporarily interrupts the exposure after the fluoroscope has been activated for 5 minutes. It makes the radiologist aware of how long the patient receives exposure for each fluoroscopic examination. When the fluoroscope is activated for shorter periods, the patient, radiologist, and radiographer receive less exposure. Total fluoroscopic beam-on time should be documented for every fluoroscopic procedure.

#### Exposure Rate Limitation.
Current federal standards limit **entrance skin exposure rates** of general-purpose intensified fluoroscopic units to a maximum of 100 $mGy_a$ per minute (10 R/min). Measured at tabletop with the image intensifier entrance surface at a prescribed 30 cm (12 inches) above, this standard has been imposed to give consideration to the cumulative small doses of radiation the patient receives over a lifetime. Fluoroscopic units equipped with high-level control (HLC) may produce a skin entrance exposure rate as great as 200 $mGy_a$ per minute (20 R/min). Because special fluoroscopic procedures can result in the largest patient doses in diagnostic x-ray imaging, sometimes reaching the level of

therapeutic doses, a concerted effort must be made to keep fluoroscopic exposure rates and exposure times within established limits.

**Primary Protective Barrier.** A primary protective barrier of 2 mm lead equivalent is required for a fluoroscopic unit. The image intensifier assembly or a digital detector provides this barrier to direct radiation. The assembly must be physically joined with the x-ray tube and interlocked so that the fluoroscopic x-ray tube cannot be activated when the image intensifier is in the parked position.

**Fluoroscopic Exposure Control Switch.** The fluoroscopic exposure control switch (e.g., the foot pedal) must be of the dead-man type (i.e., only continuous pressure applied by the operator [usually a radiologist] can keep the switch activated and the fluoroscopic tube emitting x-radiation). This means that the exposure automatically terminates if the person operating the switch becomes incapacitated (e.g., has a heart attack).

# RADIATION SAFETY FEATURES OF MOBILE C-ARM FLUOROSCOPY EQUIPMENT, DEVICES, AND ACCESSORIES

## Mobile C-Arm Fluoroscopy

A mobile C-arm fluoroscopic unit is a portable x-ray unit that is C-shaped. It has an x-ray tube attached to one end of its arm and an image intensifier attached to the other end. C-arm fluoroscopes (Fig. 11-24) are frequently used in the operating room for orthopedic procedures (e.g., pinning of a fractured hip). They are also used for:

- Cardiac imaging
- Interventional procedures

The use of C-arm fluoroscopy in procedures such as these carries the potential for a relatively large patient radiation dose. C-arm fluoroscope operators, if standing close to the patient, could also receive a significant increase in occupational

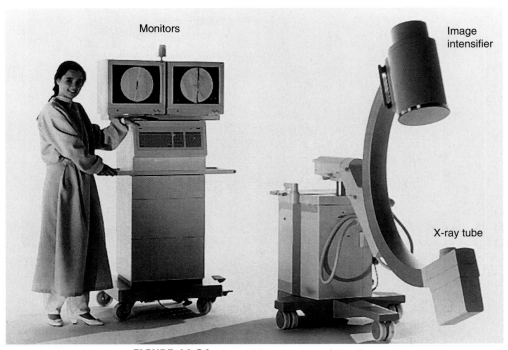

**FIGURE 11-24** C-Arm Fluoroscope and Monitor.

exposure from patient scatter radiation during such cases (see Chapter 13 for a discussion of C-arm operator protection). For this reason, equipment operators, including attending physicians, must have appropriate education and training to ensure that they will be able to follow guidelines for safe C-arm operation and also meet radiation safety protocols essential to patient and personnel safety.

Mobile fluoroscopic units are required to have a minimal source-to–end of collimator assembly distance of 30 cm (12 inches). Some type of spacer, or collimator, extension is usually installed to prevent any part of the patient from coming closer than 30 cm (12 inches) to the tube target. During C-arm fluoroscopic procedures, the patient–image intensifier distance should be as short as possible (Fig. 11-25). This reduces patient entrance dose. In addition, for dose-reduction purposes it is preferable to position the C-arm so that the x-ray tube is under the patient. With the x-ray tube in this position, scatter radiation is less intense (Fig. 11-26). When the x-ray tube is positioned over the patient, scatter radiation

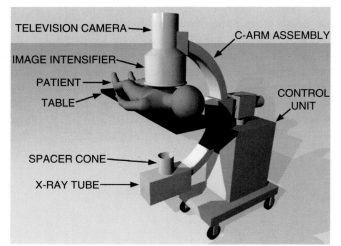

**FIGURE 11-25** To reduce the patient's entrance dose during C-arm fluoroscopy, the patient-image intensifier distance should be as short as possible.

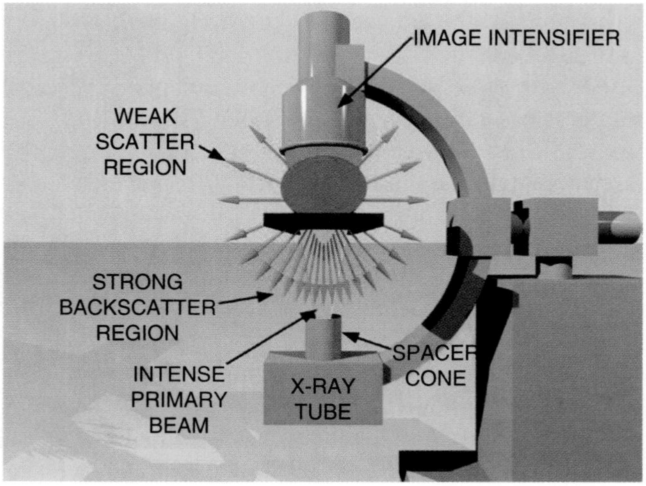

**FIGURE 11-26** To reduce scatter radiation during C-arm fluoroscopy, position the C-arm so that the x-ray tube is under the patient whenever possible.

becomes more intense, and radiation exposure of personnel increases correspondingly.

## RADIATION SAFETY FEATURES OF CINEFLUOROSCOPY EQUIPMENT, DEVICES, AND ACCESSORIES

### Cinefluorography

**Film Size.** The techniques to reduce patient dose during fluoroscopy also apply to dose reduction during cinefluorography. In cinefluorography, or cine, a movie camera that uses either 16- or 35-mm film is used to record the image from the output phosphor of the image intensifier. In the United States, 35-mm film is most frequently used because image quality is better. However, this format does result in an increased radiation dose for the patient. Cine is also rapidly being replaced by digital imaging.

**High–Dose-Rate Procedures.** Dose-reduction techniques are especially important in cine because cine procedures can result in the highest patient doses of all diagnostic procedures. The high dose resulting from cine studies is caused by:

- A relatively high inherent dose rate
- The potential duration of the procedure, particularly in cardiology, which often involves extensive dynamic imaging sequences such as in heart catheterization

Therefore, producing a percentage decrease in cine dose will yield a greater actual dose reduction than the same percentage decrease in noncine procedures.

**Filming Frame Rate.** Cinematic, or cine, cameras have filming frame rates of 7.5, 15, 30, and 60 frames per second.[9] Digital recording systems offer a similar range of image recording rates. Filming frame rate significantly affects patient radiation dose. When the frame rate is higher, so is the radiation dose. Swallow function studies and cardiac imaging procedures require higher frame rates because they are dynamic function studies. When compared with patients undergoing procedures that use lower frame rates, patients undergoing more rapid dynamic function studies, such as heart catheterization, receive noticeably higher radiation doses.

**Effect of Viewing Mode Size on Patient Dose.** In image intensified systems, patient exposure increases when a smaller viewing mode (15 cm (6 inches), compared with 23 cm (9 inches)) or a lower speed cine film is used. For example, switching from a 23-cm (9-inch) to a 15-cm (6-inch) field of view approximately doubles the tabletop exposure rate. Increasing the frame rate from 30 to 60 frames per second doubles the exposure rate as well. If both adjustments are made at the same time, the resulting exposure rate goes up by a factor of 4. Other characteristics play a role in determining the typical dose levels for a system. They include:

- Image intensifier input phosphor exposure level set by the vendor
- Grid factor
- SSD

**Collimation.** Collimating to the anatomic area of interest has the same effect in cine as in ordinary fluoroscopy. Collimation decreases the integral dose (product of dose and volume of tissue irradiated) while increasing image quality by limiting scatter.

**Dose-Reduction Techniques.** The radiologist or cardiologist can reduce exposure during cine procedures by:

- Shortening the time of the cine or digital run
- Using fluoroscopy, when possible, to locate the catheter

When fluoroscopy is used, intermittent pulsed exposures to verify the location and movement of the catheter between exposures can also limit total fluoroscopy time. Some equipment features such as the last-frame-hold feature, in which the most recent fluoroscopic image remains in view as a guide to the radiologist when the x-ray beam is off, also promote lower patient dose by decreasing the total fluoroscopic beam-on time.

**Patient Dose Determined by Procedure.** The typical dose delivered to the patient depends on the procedure. In selective coronary arteriography, most of the radiation exposure is from cine. In other procedures, although the dose rate is lower, the dose from fluoroscopy may exceed the dose from cine if the total fluoroscopy time is substantially longer. This is often the case in percutaneous transluminal angioplasty.

## RADIATION SAFETY OF DIGITAL FLUOROSCOPIC EQUIPMENT, DEVICES, AND ACCESSORIES

### Digital Fluoroscopy

**Use of Pulsed Progressive Systems for Dose Reduction.** Various methods are used to obtain digital images in some fluoroscopic equipment. The electrical signal from the video camera attached to the output phosphor may be digitized. Alternatively, the TV camera may be replaced by a digital device such as a CCD camera or other digital detector. However the digital image is acquired, the use of digital technology offers the possibility of some methods of dose reduction. One such method makes use of the fact that a brief high-intensity pulse of radiation may create an entire image on the output phosphor. The lines composing the image are progressively scanned (i.e., the image on the camera, namely the TV lines, is scanned or painted in a natural sequence, from left to right followed by right to left and so on from top to bottom) to provide the picture that appears on a monitor during a brief time period (one sixtieth of a second). The x-ray beam is turned off while the image is being scanned, thereby decreasing patient dose, and then pulsed back on for the next image. These systems are known as "pulsed progressive" systems and are commonly used to lower patient dose.

**Use of Last-Image-Hold Feature for Dose Reduction.** Another dose-reduction technique that is particularly effective in DF systems is last image hold. In a digital system, this image could be composed of several frames of information that have been added together to reduce the effect of quantum noise that would be particularly apparent in a single frame.

## RADIATION SAFETY FOR HIGH-LEVEL-CONTROL INTERVENTIONAL PROCEDURES

### High-Level-Control Interventional Procedures

**Justification for Use of High-Level-Control Interventional Procedures.** Interventional procedures are invasive procedures performed by a physician with the aid of fluoroscopic imaging. The interventional physician, usually a radiologist or cardiologist, inserts catheters into vessels or directly into patient tissues for the purpose of:

- Drainage
- Biopsy
- Alteration of vascular occlusions or malformations

For these procedures, **high-level-control fluoroscopy (HLCF)** is often employed. HLCF is an operating mode for state-of-the-art fluoroscopic equipment in which exposure rates are substantially higher than those normally allowed in routine procedures. The higher exposure rate allows visualization of smaller and lower contrast objects that do not usually appear during standard fluoroscopy. HLCF therefore is used for interventional procedures in which visualization of fine catheters or not easily seen structures is crucial. An audible signal constantly reminds personnel that the HLC mode is engaged.

**Public Health Advisory about the Dangers of Overexposure of Patients and Exposure Rate Limits.** Some fluoroscopically guided therapeutic interventional procedures have the potential for substantial patient exposure. On September 30, 1974, the Food and Drug Administration (FDA) issued a public health advisory to alert health care workers to the dangers of overexposure of patients through the use of high-level fluoroscopy. The FDA x-ray equipment standards, issued in 1994, limited the tabletop exposure rate of fluoroscopic equipment for routine procedures to 100 $mGy_a$/min (10 R/min) unless an HLC mode was present, in which case routine fluoroscopy was limited to 50 $mGy_a$/min (5 R/min) when the system was not in HLC mode and unlimited when it was in HLC mode.[15] The authors of the standards believed that the high-level capability was necessary for certain vital situations involving therapeutic interventional procedures in which the potential risks to the patient of increased radiation exposure would be subordinate to a successful medical outcome of an intervention. Although the HLC mode allowed unlimited exposure, it required continuous, positive-pressure manual operation (e.g., continuously depressing a foot switch) and a continuous audible signal to remind personnel that the high-level fluoroscopic mode was in use. In this mode, patient exposure rates have been estimated to range from 200 to 1200 mGy$_a$/min (20 to 120 R/min). When the rule was issued, total patient exposure was limited by the heat-loading capabilities of the x-ray tube. The thinking was that the tube would reach its heat limit before any detectable deterministic radiation injury could occur. By the early 1990s, advances in x-ray tube technology and the development of vascular interventional procedures that require long fluoroscopy times (Box 11-4) had created a situation in which serious skin reactions had been reported in some patients. Radiogenic skin

injuries such as erythema (diffuse reddening) or desquamation (sloughing off of skin cells) are deterministic effects in which the severity of the disorder increases with radiation dose. As the data in Table 11-2 show, a half hour of total beam-on time at one location on a patient's skin is sufficient to produce erythema. The effect does not appear for approximately 10 days. Because manifestations of skin injury are delayed, a radiologist would not usually be the first person to observe the onset of the symptoms. Therefore, patient monitoring, radiation dosimetry, and accurate record keeping are important for the future medical management of adverse reactions. The FDA has recommended that a notation be placed in the patient's record if a skin dose in the range of 1 to 2 Gy$_t$ is received. The location of the area of the patient's skin that received the absorbed dose should also be noted using:

- A diagram
- Annotated photograph
- Narrative description

Since 2000, however, alarmed state regulatory agencies have imposed a restriction on high-level radiation exposure rates; with the image intensifier at a distance of 30 cm (12 inches) above the tabletop, the maximum continuous fluoroscopic entrance exposure rate permitted is 200 mGy$_a$/min (20 R/min).

**Use of Fluoroscopic Equipment by Nonradiologist Physicians.** Fluoroscopic devices are capable of subjecting the patient, the equipment operator, and other personnel near the fluoroscopic equipment to substantial doses of ionizing radiation. These devices include:

- C-arm fluoroscopes
- Fluoroscopes on stationary equipment with HLC mode used for interventional procedures
- Biplane interventional fluoroscopic systems

Because of the possibility of very high radiation doses from procedures using these machines, ongoing education and training in the safe use of fluoroscopic equipment are mandatory for nonradiologist physicians and equipment operators.

---

| BOX 11-4 | Procedures Involving Extended Fluoroscopic Time |
|---|---|

Percutaneous transluminal angioplasty
Radiofrequency cardiac catheter ablation
Vascular embolization
Stent and filter placement
Thrombolytic and fibrinolytic procedures
Percutaneous transhepatic cholangiography
Endoscopic retrograde cholangiopancreatography
Transjugular intrahepatic portosystemic shunt
Percutaneous nephrostomy
Biliary drainage
Urinary or biliary stone removal

From the U.S. Food and Drug Administration (FDA): *Public health advisory: avoidance of serious x-ray-induced skin injuries to patients during fluoroscopically guided procedures,* Rockville, Md, September 30, 1994, FDA.

| TABLE 11-2 | Radiation-Induced Skin Injuries | | | |
|---|---|---|---|---|
| | | **Hours of Fluoroscopic "On Time" to Reach Threshold\*** | | |
| **Effect** | **Typical Threshold Absorbed Dose $(Gy_t)^†$** | **Usual Fluoroscopic Dose Rate of 0.02 $Gy_a$/min** | **High-Level Dose Rate of 0.2 $Gy_a$/min** | **Time to Onset of Effect‡** |
| Early transient erythema | 2 | 1.7 | 0.17 | Hours |
| Temporary epilation | 3 | 2.5 | 0.25 | 3 wk |
| Main erythema | 6 | 5.0 | 0.50 | 10 days |
| Permanent epilation | 7 | 5.8 | 0.58 | 3 wk |
| Dry desquamation | 10 | 8.3 | 0.83 | 4 wk |
| Dermal atrophy | 11 | 9.2 | 0.92 | 0.14 wk |
| Telangiectasis | 12 | 10.0 | 1.00 | 0.52 wk |
| Moist desquamation | 15 | 12.5 | 1.25 | 4 wk |
| Late erythema | 15 | 12.5 | 1.25 | 6-10 wk |
| Dermal necrosis | 18 | 15.0 | 1.50 | 0.10 wk |
| Secondary ulceration | 20 | 16.7 | 1.67 | 0.6 wk |

Modified from Wagner LK, Eifel PJ, Geise RA: Potential biological effects following high x-ray dose interventional procedures, *J Vasc Interv Radiol* 5:71, 1994.
\*Time required to deliver the typical threshold dose at the specified dose rate.
†The unit for absorbed dose is the gray $(Gy_t)$ in the International System of Units.
‡Time after single irradiation to observation of effect.

Some of the causes of high radiation exposures to personnel during interventional procedures include:

- Operation of the fluoroscopic tube for longer periods of time in continuous mode in place of pulsed mode
- Failure to use the protective curtain or floating shields on the stationary fluoroscopic equipment's image intensifier as a means of protection
- Extensive use of cine as a recording medium

Monitoring and documenting procedural fluoroscopic time are essential. The responsibility for this documentation generally belongs to the radiographer assisting with the procedure. In addition, if a physician loses track of how long a procedure is taking, and how much radiation is being delivered to a localized area of the patient's body, it becomes the radiographer's ethical responsibility to call this to the physician's attention in the interest of the safety of all concerned. In the event of a critical situation in which there is excessive fluoroscopic operation time,

the radiographer is responsible for notifying an appropriate supervisor, who should then follow the imaging facility's established protocol.

The National Cancer Institute and the Society of Interventional Radiology have conjointly designed some guidelines to assist physicians in developing strategies that will enable them to fulfill their interventional clinical objectives while controlling patient radiation dose and minimizing exposure to occupationally exposed personnel and any other assisting personnel. These strategies are listed in Box 11-5.

## SUMMARY

- A diagnostic-type protective tube housing protects the patient and imaging personnel from off-focus, or leakage, radiation by restricting the emission of x-rays to the area of the useful, or primary, beam.
- Leakage radiation from the tube housing measured at 1 m from the x-ray source must not exceed 1 $Gy_a$/hr (100 mR/hr) when the tube is operated at its highest

| BOX 11-5 | Strategies to Manage Radiation Dose to Patients, Operators, and Staff during Interventional Fluoroscopy |
|---|---|

| Immediate | Long-Term |
|---|---|
| **Optimize Dose to Patient** | |
| Use proper radiologic technique:<br>• Maximize distance between x-ray tube and patient<br>• Minimize distance between patient and image receptor<br>• Limit use of electronic magnification<br>Control fluoroscopic time:<br>• Limit use to necessary evaluation of moving structures<br>• Employ last-image-hold function to review findings<br>Control images:<br>• Limit acquisition to essential diagnostic and documentation purposes<br>Reduce dose:<br>• Reduce field size (collimate) and minimize field overlap<br>• Use pulsed fluoroscopy and low frame rate | Include medical physicist in decisions:<br>• Machine selection and maintenance<br>Incorporate dose-reduction technologies and dose-measurement devices in equipment<br>Establish a facility quality improvement program that includes an appropriate x-ray equipment quality assurance program, overseen by a medical physicist, which includes equipment evaluation/inspection at appropriate intervals |
| **Minimize Dose to Operators and Staff** | |
| Keep hands out of the beam<br>Use movable shields<br>Maintain awareness of body position relative to the x-ray beam:<br>• Horizontal x-ray beam: operator and staff should stand on the side of the image receptor<br>• Vertical x-ray beam: the image receptor should be above the table<br>Wear adequate protection:<br>• Protective well-fitted lead apron<br>• Leaded glasses | Improve ergonomics of operations and staff:<br>• Train operators and staff in ergonomically good positioning for use of fluoroscopy equipment; periodically assess their practice<br>• Identify and provide the ergonomically best personal protective gear for operators and staff<br>• Urge manufacturers to develop ergonomically improved personal protective gear<br>• Recommend research to improve ergonomics for personal protective gear |

From the National Cancer Institute, Division of Cancer Epidemiology and Genetics, Radiation Epidemiology Branch: *Interventional fluoroscopy: reducing radiation risks for patients and staff,* NIH Publication No. 05-5286, Rockville, Md, 2005, National Institutes of Health.

voltage at the highest current that allows continuous operation.

- The control panel, or console, must be located behind a suitable protective barrier that has a radiation-absorbent window that permits observation of the patient during any procedure.
  - This panel must indicate the conditions of exposure and provide a positive indication when the x-ray tube is energized.[1]
- The radiographic examination tabletop must be of uniform thickness, and for undertable tubes as used in fluoroscopy, the patient support surface also should be as radiolucent as possible so that it will absorb only a minimal amount of radiation, thereby reducing the patient's radiation dose.
  - The tabletop is frequently made of a carbon fiber material.
- Radiographic equipment must have a source-to–image receptor distance (SID) indicator.
- X-ray beam limitation devices must be used to confine the useful beam before it enters the anatomic area of clinical interest.
  - The light-localizing variable-aperture rectangular collimator, aperture diaphragms, cones, and extension cylinders are the beam limitation devices used.

- The patient's skin surface should always be at least 15 cm below the collimator to minimize exposure to the epidermis.
- Good coincidence between the x-ray beam and the light-localizing beam of the collimator is necessary; both alignment and width dimensions of the two beams must correspond to within 2% of the SID.
- According to most state regulatory standards currently in effect, 2% of the SID is required with positive beam limitation (PBL) devices. Some states may require 3% of the SID with PBL devices.
- Exposure to the patient's skin may be reduced through proper filtration of the radiographic beam.
  - Inherent filtration amounting to 0.5 mm aluminum equivalent is required.
  - Together, the inherent filtration and added filtration comprise the total filtration. Stationary x-ray units operating at above 70 kVp are required to have a total filtration of 2.5 mm aluminum equivalent.
  - The half-value layer (HVL) of the beam is measured to determine whether an x-ray beam is adequately filtered.
- Compensating filters are used in radiography to provide uniform imaging of body parts when considerable variation in thickness or tissue composition exists.
- Diagnostic x-ray units must have exposure reproducibility, or the ability to duplicate certain radiographic exposures for any given combination of kVp, mA, and time.
- Exposure linearity is essential. When a change is made from one mA to a neighboring mA station, the most linearity can vary is 10%.
- When screen-film image receptors are used, intensifying screens used in conjunction with matching radiographic film are predominantly rare-earth screens. Carbon fiber is frequently used as a front material in a radiographic cassette.
- Radiographic grids increase patient dose in radiography. Their use for examination of thicker body parts is a fair compromise because they remove scattered radiation emanating from the patient that would otherwise degrade the recorded image.
  - Because of increased sensitivity of photostimulable phosphor to scatter radiation before and after exposure to a radiographic beam, a grid may be used more frequently during computed radiography (CR) imaging. The use of a grid does increase patient dose but significantly improves radiographic contrast and visibility of detail.
- To limit the effects of inverse square falloff of radiation intensity with distance during a mobile radiographic examination, an x-ray source–to–skin distance (SSD) of at least 30 cm (12 inches) must be used.
- With digital radiography, the latent image formed by x-ray photons on a radiation detector is actually an electronic latent image. It is called a *digital image* because it is produced by computer representation of anatomic information. The image receptor is divided into small detector elements that make up the two-dimensional picture elements, or pixels, of the digital image. The pixels collectively produce a two-dimensional display of the information contained in a particular x-ray projection.
- Radiographers must select correct technical exposure factors the first time to avoid overexposing patients when digital images are obtained.
- Computed radiography results when the invisible, or latent, image generated in conventional radiography is produced in a digital format using computer technology.
- The digital image can be displayed on a monitor for viewing, and it can be printed on a laser film when hard copy is needed.
- Fluoroscopic procedures produce the greatest patient radiation exposure rate in diagnostic radiology.
  - Minimize patient exposure time whenever possible.
  - Limit the size of the fluoroscopic field to include only the area of anatomy that is of clinical interest.

- Employ the practice of intermittent, or pulsed, fluoroscopy to reduce the overall length of exposure.
- Select the correct technical exposure factors to help minimize the amount of radiation received by a patient.
- Ensure that the SSD is no less than 38 cm (15 inches) for stationary (fixed) fluoroscopes and no less than 30 cm (12 inches) for mobile fluoroscopes.
- During C-arm fluoroscopic procedures, the patient–image intensifier distance should be as short as possible.
- Cinefluorography can result in the highest patient doses of all diagnostic procedures.
  - Reduce patient dose by using intermittent activation of the fluoroscope to locate the catheter, limiting the time of the cine or digital run, and using the last-image-hold feature to view the most recent image.
- During digital fluoroscopy the use of pulsed progressive systems lowers patient dose.
  - Use of the last-image-hold feature is another dose-reduction technique.
- High-level-control fluoroscopy (HLCF) is used for interventional procedures.
  - The operating mode uses exposure rates that are substantially higher than those allowed for routine fluoroscopic procedures.
  - If skin dose is received in the range of 1 to 2 $Gy_t$ the U.S. Food and Drug Administration (FDA) requires that a notation be placed in the patient's record.
  - The radiographer generally has the responsibility for monitoring and documenting procedural fluoroscopic time when fluoroscopic equipment is used by nonradiologist physicians.

## REFERENCES

1. Bushong SC: *Radiologic science for technologists: physics, biology and protection*, ed 9, St. Louis, 2008, Mosby.
2. Bushong SC: *Radiologic science for technologists: physics, biology and protection*, ed 10, St. Louis, 2014, Mosby.
3. Carlton RR, Adler AM: *Principles of radiographic imaging: an art and a science*, ed 5, Albany, NY, 2013, Delmar Cengage Learning, p 432.
4. Frank ED, Long BW, Smith BJ: *Merrill's atlas of radiographic positioning and procedures*, ed 12, vol 1, St. Louis, 2012, Mosby.
5. Kebart RC, James CD: Benefits of increasing focal film distance. *Radiol Technol* 62:434, 1991.
6. Edwards C, Statkiewicz-Sherer MA, Ritenour ER: *Radiation protection for dental radiographers*, Denver, 1984, Multi-Media.
7. National Council on Radiation Protection and Measurements (NCRP): *Medical x-ray, electron beam and gamma ray protection for energies up to 50 MeV: equipment design, performance, and use*, Report No. 102, Bethesda, Md, 1989, NCRP.
8. Eastman Kadak Company, Kodak Hyper Speed G Medical Triple Film, Rochester, NY. Available at: http://www.ti-ba.com/up-content/uploads/2010/11/KODAK_Hyper_Speed_G_Medical_Film_conversion_and optimization_Guid-e.pdf. Accessed June 26, 2013.
9. Bushong SC: *Radiologic science for technologists: physics, biology and protection*, ed 8, St. Louis, 2004, Mosby.
10. Roberts TD: The effect of computers in imaging and radiation safety. Available at: http://e-edcredits.com/xraycredits/article.asp?testID=17. Accessed June 7, 2013.
11. Johnston JN, Fauber TL: *Essentials of radiographic physics and imaging*, St. Louis, 2012, Mosby.
12. Seeram E: Digital image processing. *Radiol Technol* 75:6, 2004.
13. Cullinan AM, Cullinan JE: *Producing quality radiographs*, ed 2, Philadelphia, 1994, Lippincott.
14. Carlton RR, Adler AM: *Principles of radiographic imaging: an art and a science*, ed 5, Albany, NY, 2013, Delmar Cengage Learning, p 352.
15. Office of the Federal Register: *Federal Register* August 15, 1972 (37 FR 16461), Washington, DC, 1972, U.S. Government Printing Office.

## GENERAL DISCUSSION QUESTIONS

1. What are the x-ray tube housing construction requirements when a tube is operated at its highest voltage at the highest current that allows continuous operation?
2. What must the control panel, or console, indicate?
3. How do light-localizing variable-aperture rectangular collimators, aperture diaphragms, and cones and cylinders reduce the amount of scattered radiation being

produced during a radiographic examination?

4. How does filtration of the radiographic beam reduce exposure to the patient's skin and superficial tissues?

5. When should the half-value layer of a diagnostic x-ray tube be measured?

6. What filters are recommended for use with a molybdenum anode when a mammographic examination is performed on a patient with larger or dense breasts?

7. What is exposure linearity?

8. Why does the use of carbon fiber in a radiographic film cassette lower patient dose?

9. Why is the use of a radiographic grid a fair compromise if its use increases patient dose?

10. What can a radiographer do to avoid overexposing the patient when a computed radiographic system is used?

11. What effect does the use of intermittent, or pulsed, fluoroscopy have on patient dose?

12. Why is there concern over the use of mobile C-arm fluoroscopes during surgical, vascular, interventional, and other potentially lengthy procedures?

13. What dose-reduction techniques can radiologists or cardiologists implement to reduce exposure during cinefluorographic procedures?

14. What strategies can physicians use during interventional fluoroscopic procedures to control patient radiation dose and minimize exposure of occupationally exposed personnel and any other assisting personnel?

15. During digital fluoroscopy, how does the use of a pulsed progressive system lower patient dose?

## REVIEW QUESTIONS

1. The radiographic beam should be collimated so that it is which of the following?
   A. Slightly larger than the image receptor
   B. No larger than the image receptor
   C. Twice as large as the image receptor
   D. Four times as large as the image receptor

2. Both alignment and length and width dimensions of the radiographic and light beams must correspond to within:
   A. 1% of the SID.
   B. 2% of the SID.
   C. 5% of the SID.
   D. 10% of the SID.

3. What is the function of a filter in diagnostic radiology?
   A. To permit only alpha rays to reach the patient's skin
   B. To permit only beta particles to interact with the atoms of the patient's body
   C. To decrease the x-radiation dose to the patient's skin and superficial tissue
   D. To remove gamma radiation from the useful beam

4. HVL may be defined as the thickness of a designated absorber required to do which of the following?
   A. Increase the intensity of the primary beam by 50% of its initial value
   B. Increase the intensity of the primary beam by 25% of its initial value
   C. Decrease the intensity of the primary beam by 50% of its initial value
   D. Decrease the intensity of the primary beam by 25% of its initial value

5. When compared with conventional screen-film systems, the photostimulable phosphor in the computed radiography imaging plate is much more sensitive to scatter radiation before and after it is sensitized through exposure to a radiographic beam. Because of this increased sensitivity, which of the following is true?
   1. Five millimeters of added aluminum equivalent filtration must always be used during routine CR imaging.
   2. A radiographic grid may be used more frequently during CR imaging.
   3. Any source-to–image receptor distance can be used during CR imaging without adjustment in technical exposure factors.
   A. 1 only
   B. 2 only
   C. 3 only
   D. 1, 2, and 3
6. To minimize skin exposure to electrons produced by photon interaction with the collimator, how far below the collimator should the patient's skin surface be?
   A. At least 1 cm below
   B. At least 5 cm below
   C. At least 10 cm below
   D. At least 15 cm below
7. Which of the following aluminum equivalents for total permanent filtration meets the minimum requirement for mobile diagnostic and fluoroscopic equipment?
   A. 0.5 mm aluminum equivalent
   B. 1.0 mm aluminum equivalent
   C. 2.0 mm aluminum equivalent
   D. 2.5 mm aluminum equivalent
8. The trough, or bilateral wedge, filter, which is used in some dedicated chest radiographic units, is an example of which of the following?
   A. Compensating filter
   B. Filter used in all digital imaging systems
   C. Filter used in all dedicated mammographic units
   D. Filter used in all computed tomography systems
9. To *decrease* patient exposure during fluoroscopic procedures, the fluoroscopist can:
   1. Limit the size of the fluoroscopic field to include only the area of anatomy that is of clinical interest.
   2. Employ the practice of intermittent, or pulsed, fluoroscopy to reduce the overall length of exposure.
   3. Choose to use a conventional fluoroscope instead of an image intensification fluoroscope.
   A. 1 and 2 only
   B. 1 and 3 only
   C. 2 and 3 only
   D. 1, 2, and 3
10. A diagnostic-type protective tube housing must be constructed so that leakage radiation measured at a distance of 1 m from the x-ray source does *not* exceed _____ when the tube is operated at its highest voltage at the highest current that allows continuous operation.
    A. 5 $Gy_a$/hr
    B. 3 $Gy_a$/hr
    C. 1 $Gy_a$/hr
    D. 0.1 $Gy_a$/hr

# Management of Patient Radiation Dose during Diagnostic X-Ray Procedures

## OBJECTIVES

*After completing this chapter, the reader will be able to perform the following:*

- Explain the meaning of a holistic approach to patient care, and recognize the need for effective communication between imaging department personnel and the patient.
- Explain how voluntary motion can be eliminated or at least minimized and how involuntary motion can be compensated for during a diagnostic radiographic procedure.
- Explain the need for protective shielding during diagnostic imaging procedures, state the reason for using gonadal shielding or other specific area shielding, and compare the various types of shields available for use.
- Discuss the need to use the appropriate radiographic technical exposure factors for all radiologic procedures, and explain how these factors may be adjusted to reduce patient dose.
- Explain how a radiographer can achieve a balance in technical radiographic exposure factors to ensure the presence of adequate information in the recorded image and also minimize patient dose.
- Explain how adequate immobilization and correct image processing techniques reduce radiographic exposure for the patient.

- Compare the use of an air gap technique for certain examinations such as a cross-table lateral projection of the cervical spine with the use of a midratio grid (8:1).
- State the reason for reducing the number of repeat images, and describe the benefits of repeat analysis programs.
- List six nonessential radiologic examinations, and explain the reason why each is considered unnecessary.
- List four ways to indicate the amount of radiation received by a patient from diagnostic imaging procedures, and explain each.
- Discuss the concept of fluoroscopically guided positioning and explain why this is an unacceptable practice.
- Explain the concept of genetically significant dose (GSD).
- Discuss the protocol to be followed when irradiation of an unknown pregnancy occurs, and explain how the absorbed dose to the patient's embryo-fetus is determined.
- Discuss the value of mammography for the detection of breast cancer, state the maximum dose to the glandular tissue of a 4.5-cm compressed breast using a screen-film system, identify the value of digital mammography for

Copyright © 2014, Elsevier Inc.

imaging of patients with dense breasts, and describe how to achieve dose reduction.
- Compare the patient dose received from a succession of adjacent computed tomography (CT) scans with the patient dose received from a conventional series of diagnostic images of the adult cranium.
- State the goal of CT imaging from a radiation protection point of view.
- Discuss the Alliance for Radiation Safety in Pediatric Radiology and the Image Gently Campaign.

- Explain the reason children require special radiation protection when they undergo conventional diagnostic imaging procedures.
- Explain the difference between the Image Gently Campaign and the Image Wisely Campaign.
- Describe special precautions employed in radiography to protect the pregnant or potentially pregnant patient during an x-ray examination.

## CHAPTER OUTLINE

Protecting the Pregnant or
Potentially Pregnant Patient
   Position of the American
   College of Radiology on
   Abdominal Radiologic

Examinations of Female
Patients
Elective Examinations
Irradiation of an Unknown
Pregnancy

Irradiating a Known
Pregnant Patient
**Summary**

## KEY TERMS

air gap technique
Alliance for Radiation Safety
  in Pediatric Imaging
bone marrow dose
computed tomography (CT)
effective comunication
entrance skin exposure (ESE)

fluoroscopically guided
  positioning (FGP)
genetically significant dose
  (GSD)
gonadal dose
Image Gently Campaign

Image Wisely Campaign
repeat image
scattered radiation
skin dose
thermoluminescent dosimeters
  (TLDs)

During a diagnostic x-ray procedure, a holistic approach to patient care is essential. This means treating the whole person rather than just the area of concern. Holistic patient care must begin with effective communication between the radiographer and the patient. **Effective communication** is "an interaction that produces a satisfying result through an exchange of information."[1] This type of dialogue alleviates the patient's uneasiness and increases the likelihood for cooperation and successful completion of the procedure. To take care of all patients appropriately, the radiographer should develop easily understandable communication skills.

Radiographers must limit the patient's exposure to ionizing radiation by:

- Employing appropriate radiation reduction techniques
- Using protective devices that minimize radiation exposure

Patient exposure can be substantially reduced by:

- Use of proper body or part immobilization
- Motion reduction techniques
- Appropriate beam limitation devices
- Adequate filtration of the x-ray beam

- Use of gonadal or other specific area shielding
- Selection of suitable technical exposure factors used in conjunction with either high-speed screen-film combinations or computer-generated digital images
- Use of correct radiographic film processing techniques or appropriate digital image processing
- Elimination of repeat radiographic exposures

Chapter 11 describes and discusses imaging equipment, devices, and accessories that imaging professionals can use to reduce patient radiation exposure during diagnostic x-ray procedures. This chapter provides an overview of other methods and techniques that radiographers can also use to minimize the patient's exposure to radiation during radiologic examinations.

## EFFECTIVE COMMUNICATION

### Verbal Messages and Body Language

When verbal messages and unconscious actions or body language, or nonverbal messages, are understood as intended, communication between the radiographer and the patient is effective. Good communication:

- Encourages reduction in anxiety and emotional stress
- Enhances the professional image of the radiographer as a person who cares about the patient's well-being
- Increases the chance for successful completion of the x-ray examination

Everyone within the imaging department should always behave as a compassionate professional. Words and actions must demonstrate understanding and respect for human dignity and individuality.

## Importance of Clear, Concise Instructions

Patient protection during a diagnostic x-ray procedure should begin with clear, concise instructions (Fig. 12-1). When patients understand the procedure and their responsibilities, they can more fully cooperate. When health care professionals do not thoroughly explain procedures, patients fear the unknown and become anxious, especially during lengthy examinations. To alleviate the problem, the radiographer must take adequate time to explain the procedure in simple terms that the patient can understand. Patients should also be given the opportunity to ask questions. The radiographer must listen attentively to

these questions and answer them truthfully in an appropriate tone of voice and in accordance with ethical guidelines. This creates a sense of trust between the patient and the radiographer and encourages further communication.

## Appropriate Communication for Procedures That Will Cause Pain or Discomfort

If the radiographic procedure (e.g., angiocatheterization or another study requiring an injection of a contrast medium, such as an intravenous urogram) will cause pain, discomfort, or any strange sensations, the patient must be informed before the procedure begins (Fig. 12-2). However, to prevent the patient from imagining more pain

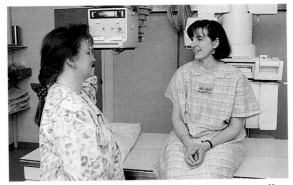

FIGURE 12-1  Clear, concise instructions promote effective communication between the radiographer and the patient.

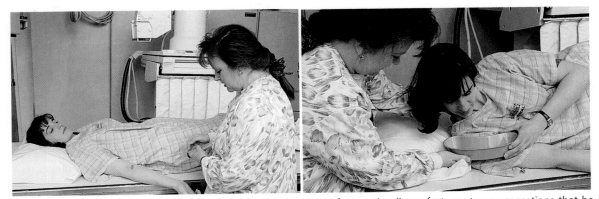

FIGURE 12-2  Before the procedure begins, inform the patient of any pain, discomfort, or strange sensations that he or she will experience during the procedure.

or discomfort than the procedure will actually cause, the radiographer should try not to overemphasize this aspect of the examination.

## Repeat Radiographic Exposures That Result from Poor Communication

Repeat radiographic exposures can sometimes be attributed to poor communication between the radiographer and the patient. Inadequate or misinterpreted instructions may prevent the patient from being able to cooperate. For example, during an interventional radiographic examination that creates some uncomfortable warmth, patients could move abruptly because they are surprised or want to inform the technologist or physician that something seems to be wrong. Such physical movement usually results in a repeat exposure. Effective communication between radiographer and patient will prevent this problem from occurring.

## IMMOBILIZATION

### Need for Patient Immobilization

If a patient moves during a radiographic exposure, the radiographic image will be blurred. Because blurred images have little or no diagnostic value, a repeat examination is necessary, even though it results in additional radiation exposure for the patient. Proper body or part immobilization and the use of motion reduction techniques can eliminate or at least minimize patient motion.

### Types of Patient Motion

Two types of patient motion exist:

- Voluntary
- Involuntary

Motion controlled by will is classified as *voluntary motion.* Lack of such control may be attributed to:

- The patient's age
- Breathing patterns or problems

- General anxiety
- Physical or mental discomfort
- Excitability
- Fear of the examination
- Fear of unfavorable prognosis
- Mental instability

To eliminate voluntary patient movement during radiography, the radiographer must gain the cooperation of the patient or adequately immobilize that individual during the radiographic exposure (Fig. 12-3). Various suitable restraining devices are available to immobilize either the whole body or the individual body part to be radiographed. These radiographic aids should be used whenever necessary.

*Involuntary motion,* caused by muscle groups such as those associated with the digestive organs or the heart, cannot be willfully controlled. Other

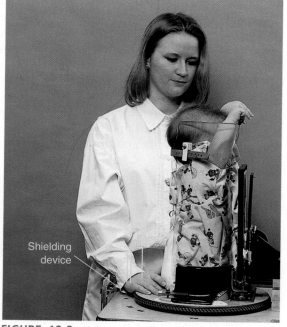

**FIGURE 12-3** Adequate immobilization during radiographic examinations eliminates or at least minimizes voluntary motion. This restraint has a shield *(left)* that may be adjusted to protect the child's reproductive organs from radiation exposure.

clinical manifestations also cause involuntary motion. These include:

- Chills
- Tremors such as those experienced by patients with Parkinson's disease
- Muscle spasms
- Pain
- Active withdrawal

Shortening the length of exposure time with an appropriate increase in milliamperes (mA) to maintain sufficient milliampere-seconds (mAs) for useful radiographic density or brightness and using very-high-speed imaging receptors can compensate for this type of motion.

## PROTECTIVE SHIELDING

### Need for Protective Shielding

The potential for radiation exposure to the radio-sensitive body organs or tissues of a patient requires the use of intelligent patient positioning and/or personal shielding (i.e., a device made of lead or lead-impregnated materials that will adequately attenuate ionizing radiation) to reduce or eliminate a radiation dose that would otherwise result in biologic damage. Areas of the body that should be shielded from the useful beam whenever possible are the:

- Lens of the eye
- Breasts
- Reproductive organs

### Gonadal Shielding

**Use of Gonadal Shielding Devices.** Gonadal shielding devices are used on patients during diagnostic x-ray procedures to protect the reproductive organs from exposure to the useful beam when these organs are in or within approximately 5 cm of a properly collimated beam. Gonadal shielding is used unless it will compromise the diagnostic value of the examination. It should be a secondary protective measure, not a substitute for an adequately collimated beam. Adequate collimation of the radiographic beam, to include

only the anatomy of interest (Fig. 12-4), must always be the first step in gonadal protection.

**Dose Reduction from the Use of Gonadal Shielding for Female and Male Patients.** As a consequence of their anatomic location, the female reproductive organs receive about three times more exposure during a given radiographic procedure involving the pelvic region than do the male reproductive organs. However, gonadal exposure for both male and female patients can be greatly reduced through the application of appropriate shielding. For female patients, the use of a flat contact shield placed over the reproductive organs reduces exposure by approximately 50% (Fig. 12-5, *A*). Primary beam exposure for male patients may be reduced as much as 90% to 95% when the gonads are also covered with a contact shield (Fig. 12-5, *B*). Gonadal shielding should always be used whenever it will not obscure necessary clinical information. Every imaging department should establish a written shielding protocol for each of its radiologic procedures. This reduces the cumulative population gonad dose.

**Placement of Gonadal Shielding Devices.** When a gonadal shield is used during a radiographic exposure, it must be correctly placed directly over the patient's reproductive organs to provide protection, as shown in Figure 12-5. External anatomic landmarks on the patient can be used to guide placement of a testicular or ovarian shield. For example, when a male patient is in the supine position, the symphysis pubis can be used to guide shield placement over the testes. For protection of the ovaries of a female patient, the shield should be placed approximately 2.5 cm (1 inch) medial to each palpable anterior superior iliac spine. If gonadal shields are not placed correctly, the reproductive organs will not be properly protected, and necessary anatomic information in the image could be obscured.

**Types of Gonadal Shielding Devices.** The following four basic types of gonadal shielding devices are used:

- Flat contact shields
- Shadow shields

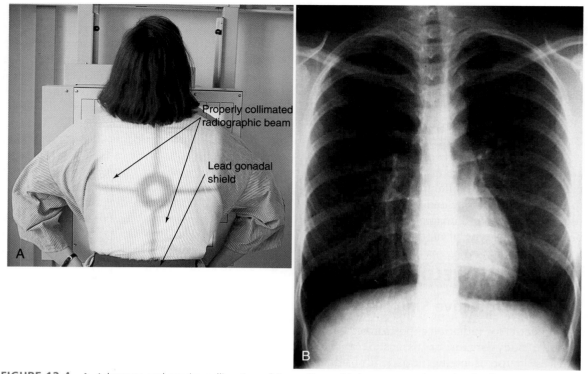

**FIGURE 12-4** **A,** Adequate and precise collimation of the radiographic beam must always be the first step in gonadal protection. **B,** When the gonads are not in the area of clinical interest, precise collimation of the radiographic beam reduces gonadal exposure.

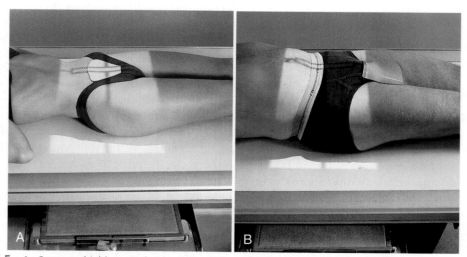

**FIGURE 12-5** **A,** Contact shield correctly placed over the reproductive organs of a female patient. **B,** Contact shield correctly placed over the reproductive organs of a male patient.

- Shaped contact shields
- Clear lead shields

*Flat Contact Shields.* Flat contact shields are made of lead strips or lead-impregnated materials 1 mm thick. These shields can be placed directly over the patient's reproductive organs (Fig. 12-6). These shields are most effective when they are used as protective devices for patients having anteroposterior (AP) or posteroanterior (PA) radiographs while in a recumbent position. Flat contact shields are not suited for nonrecumbent positions or projections other than AP or PA. If the flat contact shield is used during a typical fluoroscopic examination, it must be placed under the patient to be effective because the x-ray tube is located under the radiographic table. However, some fluoroscopic tubes are located above the patient and are referred to as "remote" rooms because personnel set up the patient for the examination and then leave the room before activating the x-ray tube. In these rooms, the shield should be placed over the patient.

*Shadow Shields.* Shadow shields are made of a radiopaque material (Fig. 12-7, *A*). Suspended from above the radiographic beam-defining system,

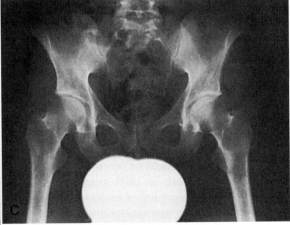

**FIGURE 12-6**  An uncontoured, flat contact shield of lead-impregnated material may be placed over the patient's gonads to provide protection from x-radiation during a radiographic procedure.

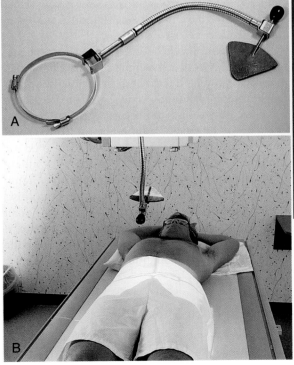

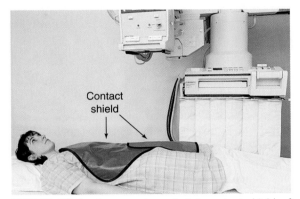

**FIGURE 12-7**  **A,** Shadow shield components. **B,** A shadow shield suspended above the radiographic beam-defining system casts a shadow over the protected body area, the gonads. **C,** The radiographic image demonstrates effective gonadal shielding resulting from the use of a shadow shield.

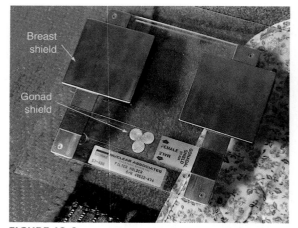

**FIGURE 12-8** Lead filter with a breast and gonad shielding device. This shield functions as a shadow shield.

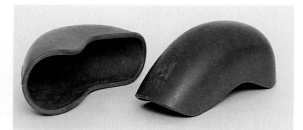

**FIGURE 12-9** Shaped contact shields (cuplike in shape) may be held in place with a suitable carrier.

these shields hang over the area of clinical interest to cast a shadow in the primary beam over the patient's reproductive organs (Fig. 12-7, *B* and *C*). The clear lead filter illustrated in Figure 12-8 functions as a shadow shield and is used to shield breasts and gonads. The beam-defining light casts the shadow of the shield over the anatomy. The beam-defining light must be accurately positioned to ensure correct placement of the shadow shield. When the shield is correctly positioned, it provides protection from the radiographic beam as efficiently as does the contact shield. The shadow shield is not suitable for use during fluoroscopy because no localizing light field exists and the field of view is usually moved about during a study. However, the shadow shield can be used effectively to provide gonadal protection in a sterile field or when incapacitated patients are examined. Shadow shields have the advantage of reducing patient embarrassment by generally eliminating the need for the radiographer to palpate the patient's anatomy in the area of the reproductive organs before placing the shield in the appropriate position.

***Shaped Contact Shields.*** Shaped contact shields, containing 1 mm of lead, are contoured to enclose the male reproductive organs. Disposable or washable athletic supporters or jockey-style briefs function as carriers for these shields. The carriers each contain a pouch into which the

shield is placed (Fig. 12-9). The cuplike shape of the shield permits it to be placed comfortably over the scrotum and penis whether the patient is in a recumbent or a nonrecumbent position. To ensure privacy and reduce embarrassment, the patient can don the garment containing the shield in the confines of the dressing room.

Because the carrier securely holds the shaped contact shield in place, AP, oblique, and lateral projections may be obtained with maximal gonadal protection. This shield is also suitable for use during nonposterior fluoroscopic examinations. Shaped contact shields are not recommended for PA projections because the shield covers only the anterior and lateral surfaces of the reproductive organs.

***Clear Lead Shields.*** Some of the basic gonadal shielding devices such as the previously described shaped contact shield and first-generation, or earliest type of, shadow shield are being replaced by clear lead gonad and breast shielding (see Fig. 12-8). These shields are made of transparent lead-acrylic material impregnated with approximately 30% lead by weight. Examples of gonad and breast shielding are provided in Figure 12-10, which demonstrates a full spinal scoliosis examination. Along with the clear lead gonad and breast shields, a lightweight, fully transparent clear lead filter is incorporated to provide uniform density throughout the spinal canal (see Fig. 12-10).

## Specific Area Shielding

**Need for Specific Area Shielding.** Radiosensitive organs and tissues, other than the

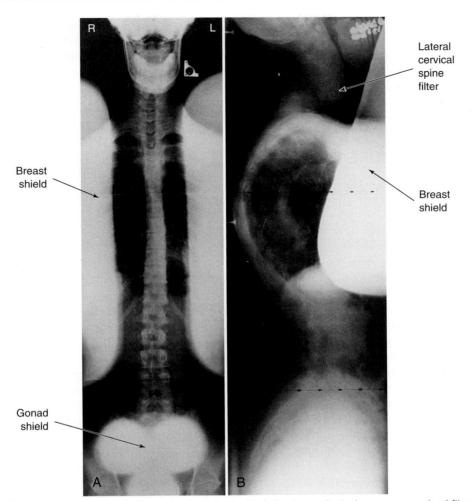

**FIGURE 12-10    A,** Anteroposterior radiograph of a patient with full-spine scoliosis demonstrates a lead filter with breast and gonad shields. **B,** Lateral radiograph of patient with full-spine scoliosis, with a lateral cervical filter and breast shield.

reproductive organs, may also be selectively shielded from the primary beam during a diagnostic radiographic examination. Shields for the lens of the eye are always of the contact type and are positioned directly on the patient.[2] They can reduce or entirely eliminate exposure to that highly sensitive area.

Areas of breast tissue may be shielded by using a clear lead shadow shield (see Fig. 12-8). This shielding is of vital importance in providing protection during juvenile scoliosis examinations. Radiation dose to the breast of a young patient may be further reduced by performing the scoliosis examination with the radiographic beam entering the posterior surface of the patient's body instead of the anterior surface. The use of the PA projection results in a much lower radiation dose to the anterior body surface, thereby significantly reducing the dose to the patient's breasts.

**Benefit of Specific Area Shielding.**  In summary, effective shielding programs can be established in any health care facility by providing the appropriate shields. Patients with the potential to reproduce should be gonadally shielded during x-ray procedures whenever the diagnostic value of the examination is not compromised. This action minimizes the number of potentially deleterious x-ray–induced mutations expressed in future generations. Specific area shielding for selected body areas other than the gonads significantly reduces radiation exposure to those areas and should also be used whenever possible.

## TECHNICAL EXPOSURE FACTORS

### Selection of Appropriate Technical Exposure Factors

The selection of appropriate technical exposure factors for each x-ray examination is essential to ensure a diagnostic image with minimal patient dose. For both digital and nondigital imaging, a high-quality image has sufficient density or brightness to display anatomic structures, an appropriate level of subject contrast to differentiate among the anatomic structures, the maximum amount of spatial resolution,* and a minimal amount of distortion. In addition, with respect to digital imaging, limiting the amount of quantum noise or mottle,† caused when too few x-rays reach the image receptor, is a concern.[3]

The appropriate technical factors are determined by considerations such as those listed in Box 12-1.

### Use of Standardized Technique Charts

When automatic exposure control (AEC) is not used, to ensure uniform selection of technical x-ray exposure factors, efficient imaging departments use standardized technique charts for each x-ray unit. A digital image receptor is capable of responding to a large variance in x-ray intensities exiting the patient. As a result, the digital image receptor is said to have a wide dynamic range.

---

*Spatial resolution is basically the recorded detail in the radiographic image.
†Quantum noise or mottle is a blotchy radiographic image that results when an insufficient quantity of x-ray photons reaches the image receptor.

| BOX 12-1 | Technical Exposure Factor Considerations |
|---|---|

1. Mass per unit volume of tissue of the area of clinical interest
2. Effective atomic numbers and electron densities of the tissues involved
3. Screen-film combination or other type of image receptor
4. Source-to–image receptor distance (SID)
5. Type and quantity of filtration employed
6. Type of x-ray generator used (single phase, three phase, or high frequency)
7. Balance of radiographic density or brightness and contrast required

Furthermore, computer processing produces acceptable images even when significant overexposure has occurred. Because of this, the standardization of technique charts has become even more important. Radiology departments cannot rely on vendors and other agencies to set technical standards. Establishing their own protocols helps radiology departments ensure consistency in the diagnostic quality of digital examinations and minimizes the potential for exposure technique selection errors.[3]

The radiographer is responsible for consulting the technique chart before making each radiographic exposure, to ensure a diagnostic image with minimal patient dose. Neglecting to use standardized technique charts necessitates estimating the technical exposure factors, which may result in:

- Poor-quality images
- Repeat examinations
- Additional and unnecessary exposure of the patient

Standardizing exposure techniques, however, does not mean that radiographers use the same protocol for all patients in all situations. Exposure techniques must be adjusted for a patient's specific condition and history. Appropriate and consistent use of exposure technique charts, adequate peak kilovoltage (kVp), and a well-calibrated AEC are essential to producing quality

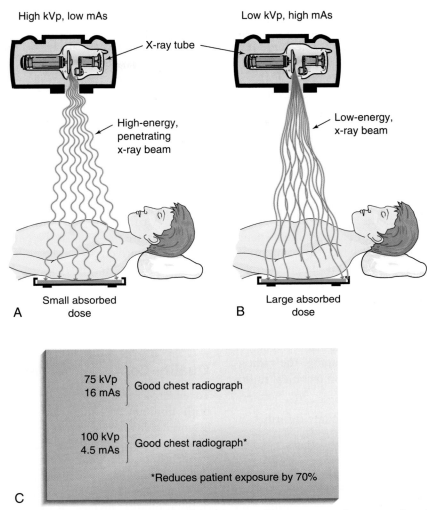

High kVp, low mAs

Low kVp, high mAs

X-ray tube

High-energy, penetrating x-ray beam

Low-energy, x-ray beam

**A**  Small absorbed dose

**B**  Large absorbed dose

75 kVp
16 mAs  }  Good chest radiograph

100 kVp
4.5 mAs  }  Good chest radiograph*

*Reduces patient exposure by 70%

**C**

**FIGURE 12-11**  The use of higher kilovoltage (kVp) and lower milliamperage and exposure time in seconds (mAs) reduces patient dose. **A,** The use of high kVp and low mAs results in a high-energy, penetrating x-ray beam and a small patient absorbed dose. **B,** The use of low kVp and high mAs results in a low-energy x-ray beam, the majority of which the patient will easily absorb. **C,** Example of a higher-kVp, lower-mAs technique resulting in a 70% reduction in patient exposure without significantly compromising radiographic quality.

diagnostic images consistently while minimizing patient radiation exposure.[3]

## Use of High-kVp and Low-mAs Exposure Factors to Reduce Dose to the Patient

Technical exposure factors that minimize the radiation dose to the patient should be selected whenever possible. The use of higher kVp and lower milliamperage and exposure time in seconds (mAs)* reduces patient dose (Fig. 12-11, *A* and *B*). For digital radiography (DR), kVp and mAs should be selected in the same manner as for

---

*Milliampere-seconds (mAs) are the product of x-ray electron tube current and the amount of time in seconds that the x-ray beam is on.

screen-film imaging. In screen-film imaging, as kVp increases and mAs decreases, radiographic contrast is reduced. Consequently, the amount of diagnostically useful information in the recorded image is less.

However, this is not the case in digital imaging, in which the amount of exposure (mAs) to the digital image receptor does not directly affect the amount of density or brightness produced, because of computer processing. Adequate penetration of the anatomic part (kVp dependent) is needed to create the differences in x-ray intensities exiting the part relative to that from adjacent structures to produce the desired level of contrast. As long as the part is adequately penetrated, changing kVp will have less of an effect on the contrast of the digital image. Consequently, the use of higher kVp than with screen-film, along with an appropriate decrease in mAs, is an advocated practice. Increasing kVp by 15% with a corresponding decrease in mAs reduces patient radiation exposure. Whether using screen-film or digital imaging, the radiographer must achieve a balance in technical radiographic exposure factors to:

- Ensure the presence of adequate information in the recorded image
- Minimize patient dose

To achieve this balance, the radiographer should always select the highest practical kVp within the optimal range for the position and part, coupled with the lowest mAs that will yield sufficient information for each radiographic examination (Fig. 12-11, C).

## PROCESSING OF THE RADIOGRAPHIC IMAGE

### Need for Correct Radiographic Image Processing

When screen-film image receptor systems are used, correct radiographic film processing enhances image quality by making invisible diagnostic information visible on the finished radiograph.

Correct processing also promotes archival quality of the film whereby it will not deteriorate over time but will remain in its original condition. Poorly processed radiographs offer inadequate diagnostic information, leading to:

- Repeat examinations
- Unnecessary patient exposure

When digital images are acquired, correct image postprocessing is also essential to produce a high-quality diagnostic image. For this, any artifacts produced by the image receptor, software, or patient-related problems must be controlled. Artifacts are unwanted densities in the image that are not part of the patient's anatomy and may negatively affect the ability of a radiologist to interpret the image correctly. Failure to eliminate these defects or at least to reduce them significantly can result in an unacceptable digital image and can therefore necessitate a repeat examination, thus increasing patient dose.

## Quality Control Program

To ensure standardization in the processing of both film and digital images, it is absolutely essential that every imaging department establish a *quality control program* that includes regular monitoring and maintenance of all processing and imaging display equipment in the facility. Such a program ensures the production of optimal-quality images. Radiographers are the operators of complex imaging equipment and therefore are the individuals who may first recognize equipment malfunction. Problems that occur in digital imaging (computed radiography [CR] and DR) tend to be systematic, which can affect the quality of every image and the degree of radiation exposure of every patient until the problems are identified and corrected. Acceptance testing, regular calibration, and proactive and consistent quality control can prevent these systematic errors.[3] Excellent reviews have been written on this subject. These reviews include step-by-step procedures for performance, monitoring, and continuing quality control.[2-7]

## AIR GAP TECHNIQUE

### Reduction of Scattered Radiation

The **air gap technique** is an alternative procedure to the use of a radiographic grid for reducing **scattered radiation** during certain examinations (e.g., cross-table lateral projection of the cervical spine, areas of chest radiography, and selected special procedures such as cerebral angiography in which some degree of magnification is acceptable). This technique removes scatter radiation by using an increased object-to–image receptor distance (OID). The removal of scatter radiation improves radiographic image contrast. If magnification is not desired, a complementary increase in source-to–image receptor distance (SID) may be made.

To perform an air gap technique, the image receptor is placed 10 to 15 cm (4 to 6 inches) from the patient, and the x-ray tube is placed approximately 300 to 366 cm (10 to 12 feet) away from the image receptor. The scattered

x-rays from the patient are disseminated in many directions at acute angles to the primary beam when the radiographic exposure is made. Because of the increased distance between the anatomic structures being imaged and the image receptor, a higher percentage of the scattered x-rays produced is then less likely to strike the image receptor (Fig. 12-12). This air gap method results in an adequate grid-type scatter cleanup effect. In general, the use of an air gap technique requires the selection of technical exposure factors that are comparable to those used with an 8:1 ratio grid. Therefore, when patient dose is compared with a nongrid technique, it is higher, but when compared with the patient dose resulting from the use of a midratio grid (8:1), the dose from an air gap technique is about the same.

### High–Peak Kilovoltage Radiography

In high-kVp radiography that employs kVp settings of 90 or above, air gap techniques are for the most part not as effective. Still, some facilities

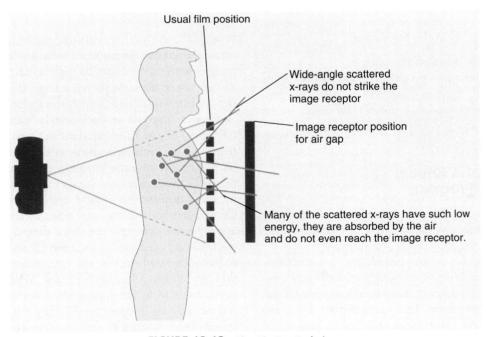

FIGURE 12-12 **The Air Gap Technique.**

that perform chest radiography by using kVp of 120 to 140 do successfully use air gap techniques. In general, when x-rays are scattered through greater angles, such as occurs for radiographs produced at less than 90 kVp, air gap techniques are more useful.

## REPEAT IMAGES

### Consequence of Repeat Images

A **repeat image** is any image that must be performed more than once because of human or mechanical error during the production of the initial image. This additional imaging unfortunately increases patient dose. If the patient's gonads were included in the imaged area, then the gonads would have received a double dose. This is of course true for any other sensitive included areas. Repeat images must be minimized. Occasionally, an additional image is permissible, when it is recommended by the radiologist for the purpose of obtaining additional diagnostic information. However, repeat exposures resulting from carelessness or poor judgment on the part of the radiographer must be eliminated. The radiographer must, from the beginning:

- Correctly position the patient
- Select the appropriate technical radiographic exposure factors that will ensure the production of optimal images for each initial examination

### Benefit of a Repeat Analysis Program

Health care facilities can benefit significantly by implementing and maintaining a *repeat analysis program*. By determining the number of repeats and the reasons for producing unacceptable radiographic images, existing problems and conditions in an imaging department are identified. Many categories may be established for discarded images. These categories are listed in Box 12-2.

The benefits of an aggressive repeat analysis program in an imaging department are listed in

---

| BOX 12-2 | Categories for Discarded Images |
|---|---|

1. Images too dark or too light because of inappropriate selection of technical exposure factors
2. Incorrect patient positioning
3. Incorrect centering of the radiographic beam
4. Patient motion during the radiographic exposure
5. Improper collimation of the radiographic beam
6. Presence of external foreign bodies
7. Processing artifacts

---

| BOX 12-3 | Benefits of a Repeat Analysis Program |
|---|---|

1. The program increases awareness among staff and student radiographers of the need to produce optimal-quality recorded images.
2. Radiographers generally become more careful in producing their radiographic images because they are aware that the images are being reviewed.
3. When the repeat analysis program identifies problems or concerns, in-service education programs covering these specific topics may be designed for imaging personnel.

---

Box 12-3. A quality control radiographer, or other designated person, reviews discarded film images with co-workers to determine the causes of various repeats. At the very least, this practice should lead to an improvement in technical skills.

Repeat analysis is particularly important in CR and DR. In these modalities, repeat images for improper technique, however, are not usually necessary. Because the images are digital, overexposed or underexposed images can be adjusted by the computer to appear technically normal. Consequently, it is important for the delivery of appropriate patient exposures that a qualified medical physicist measures these values, by using techniques employed at the site, to ensure that they are within acceptable ranges. When repeats occur with film, the film itself is set aside, and repeat analysis is done periodically with the collected films. With CR or DR, it is necessary to develop a policy whereby retaken image files can be recovered for analysis because this would not happen automatically. Analysis of the department's repeats rate:

- Provides valuable information for process improvement
- Helps minimize patient exposure
- Improves the overall performance of the department[3]

# UNNECESSARY RADIOLOGIC PROCEDURES

## Benefit versus Risk

As discussed in Chapter 1, the responsibility for ordering a radiologic examination lies with the referring physician. In making this decision, the physician must determine whether the benefit to the patient, in terms of medical information gained, sufficiently justifies subjecting the patient to the risk of the absorbed radiation resulting from the procedure.

## Nonessential Radiologic Examinations

Some radiographic examinations are performed in the absence of definite medical indications. This practice unnecessarily exposes the patient to radiation because there is virtually no benefit to the patient in terms of useful information gained from the procedure. Examples of nonessential radiologic examinations are described in Box 12-4.

# AMOUNT OF RADIATION RECEIVED BY PATIENTS UNDERGOING DIAGNOSTIC IMAGING PROCEDURES

## Concern about Risk of Exposure from Diagnostic Imaging Procedures

Because increased numbers of people in the United States are undergoing diagnostic imaging

---

**BOX 12-4 | Unnecessary Radiologic Procedures**

1. A chest x-ray examination on scheduled admission to the hospital. This examination should not be performed without clinical indications of chest disease or another important concern that justifies exposing the patient to ionizing radiation. This includes presurgical patients. A panel of physicians appointed by the Food and Drug Administration (FDA)[8] concluded that a chest x-ray examination is not necessary for every presurgical patient. Patients admitted for treatment of pulmonary problems or diseases, however, may benefit from a preadmission chest x-ray examination.
2. A chest x-ray examination as part of a preemployment physical. Very little information about previous illness or injury can be gained through this examination, and it is unlikely to be useful to the employer.
3. Lumbar spine examinations as part of a preemployment physical. As with the preemployment chest x-ray examination, this examination provides very little information about previous illness or injury that would be useful to an employer.
4. Chest x-ray examination or other unjustified x-ray examinations as part of a routine health checkup. Radiologic procedures should not be performed unless

a patient exhibits symptoms that merit radiologic investigation.

5. Chest x-ray examination for mass screening for tuberculosis (TB). Such examinations are of little value for most people. Testing for TB may be done with more efficient procedures. However, Bushong indicated that some x-ray screening is still acceptable. This applies to high-risk groups such as members of the medical and paramedical community, people working in fields such as education and food preparation, and selected groups of workers such as miners and workers dealing with material such as asbestos, beryllium, glass, and silica.[2]
6. Whole-body multislice spiral computed tomography (CT) screening. Patients may elect to undergo this type of CT procedure for screening purposes without an order from a referring physician. They may simply locate a facility that offers this service to the general public. At the time of this writing, the disease detection rate simply does not justify the relatively high radiation dose received by the patient from this procedure. Until there is evidence of a significant disease detection rate, this whole-body multislice spiral CT screening procedure should not be done.[2]

procedures each year, concern about the risk of radiation exposure from these procedures is growing. Imaging personnel must reduce the risk to patients whenever possible by employing methods that produce high-quality images with lower radiation exposure.

## Ways to Specify the Amount of Radiation Received by a Patient from a Diagnostic Imaging Procedure

In general, the amount of radiation received by a patient from diagnostic imaging procedures may be specified in three ways:

1. Entrance skin exposure (ESE) (includes skin and glandular)
2. Bone marrow dose
3. Gonadal dose

Although each type of specification has significance in estimating the risk to the patient, ESE is the most frequently reported because it is the simplest to determine.

### Entrance Skin Exposure

***Conversion of Entrance Skin Exposure to Patient Skin Dose.*** Entrance skin exposure (ESE) may be converted to patient skin dose by using well-documented multiplicative factors. As discussed later, ESE measurements are relatively easy to obtain. When actual patient measurements are not available, reasonably accurate estimates can still be made, which is why ESE is so widely used in assessing the amount of radiation received by a patient.

***Measuring Skin Dose Directly.*** Thermoluminescent dosimeters (TLDs) are the sensing devices most often used to measure skin dose directly. (The characteristics, components, and function of the TLD are described in Chapter 5). A small, relatively thin pack of TLDs is secured to the patient's skin in the middle of the clinical area of interest and exposed during a radiographic procedure. Because lithium fluoride (LiF), the sensing material in the TLD, responds in a manner similar to human tissue when exposed to ionizing radiation, an accurate determination of

surface dose can be made. (See Tables 2-4 and 2-5 for a list of permissible skin entrance exposures for various radiographic examinations). In fluoroscopy, the amount of radiation that a patient receives is usually estimated by measuring the radiation exposure rate at the tabletop and multiplying this by the fluoroscopy time.

**Skin Dose.** Skin dose in general represents the absorbed dose to the most superficial layers of the skin. This region is called the *epidermis*. It is composed of five layers:

1. Horny, or outer, layer
2. Translucent, or clear, layer
3. Granular layer
4. Prickle cell layer
5. Germinal, or basal, cell layer

The thickness of the epidermis varies from one anatomic area to another. It is greater in areas such as the palms of the hands and soles of the feet. The primary function of the epidermis is to protect underlying tissues and structures.

### Gonadal Dose

***Difference in Gonadal Dose Received by Human Male and Female Patients.*** Because genetic effects may result from exposure to ionizing radiation, protection of the reproductive organs is of particular concern in diagnostic radiology. (See Table 2-4 for a list of typical gonadal doses from various radiographic examinations). For several examinations identified in Table 2-4, differences in dose received exist between human male and female patients. Protection of the ovaries by overlying tissue accounts for these differences. In diagnostic radiology, the relatively low **gonadal dose** for a single human is considered insignificant. However, when the low gonadal dose is applied to the entire population, the dose becomes far more significant.

***Genetically Significant Dose.*** The concept of **genetically significant dose** (GSD) is used to assess the impact of gonadal dose. *GSD is the equivalent dose (EqD) to the reproductive organs that, if received by every human, would be expected to bring about an identical gross genetic injury to the total population, as does the sum of the actual doses received by exposed individual* *members of the population.* In other words, if a maximum of 500 people inhabited the earth and each person were to receive an EqD of 0.005 Sv (0.5 rem) of gonadal radiation, the gross genetic effect would be identical to the effect that would occur if 50 individual inhabitants each were to receive 0.05 Sv (5 rem) of gonadal radiation and the other 450 inhabitants were not to receive an EqD. In simple terms, the GSD concept suggests that the consequences of substantial absorbed doses of gonadal radiation become significantly less when averaged over an entire population rather than applied to just a few of its members.

***Genetically Significant Dose Considerations.***
The GSD takes into consideration that some people receive radiation to their reproductive organs during a given year, whereas others do not. In addition, it accounts for the fact that radiation exposure in members of the population who cannot bear children (e.g., those who are beyond reproductive years) has no genetic impact. Hence the GSD is the average annual gonadal EqD to members of the population who are of childbearing age. It includes the number of children who may be expected to be conceived by members of the exposed population in a given year. According to the U.S. Public Health Service, the estimated GSD for the population of the United States is approximately 0.20 millisievert (mSv) (20 millirem).

**Bone Marrow Dose.** In humans, bone marrow is of great importance because it contains large numbers of stem, or precursor, blood cells that could be depleted or destroyed by substantial exposure to ionizing radiation. The **bone marrow dose** is a dose of radiation delivered to that organ. Because radiation dose to bone marrow may be responsible for radiation-induced leukemia, the dose to this organ becomes very significant.[2] Bone marrow dose may also be referred to as the *mean marrow dose,* which is defined as "the average radiation dose to the entire active bone marrow."[2] For example, if in the course of performing a specific radiographic procedure, 25% of the active bone marrow were in the useful beam and received an average absorbed dose of 0.8 mGy$_t$ (80 mrad), the mean marrow dose would be 0.2 mGy$_t$ (20 mrad). The radiation dose absorbed by an organ such as bone marrow cannot be measured accurately by a direct method; it can only be estimated. In diagnostic radiology, the bone marrow dose provides an estimate of patient absorbed dose even though hematologic effects are generally negligible for doses associated with this modality.

Table 2-4 provides typical bone marrow doses for various radiographic examinations performed on human adults. The levels indicated in Table 2-4 are usually less for children because the active bone marrow is more evenly spread out, and significantly lower technical radiographic exposure factors are used. Although each dose listed in Table 2-4 results from fragmentary exposure of the human body, it is averaged over the whole body.

## Fluoroscopically Guided Positioning

**Fluoroscopically guided positioning** (FGP) is the practice of using fluoroscopy to determine the exact location of the central ray before taking a radiographic exposure.[9] Some Radiologic Technologists (RTs) believe that the use of FGP results in less dose to the patient than does a repeat radiograph. However, the American Society of Radiologic Technologists (ASRT) adopted the following positioning statement:

> *"The ASRT recognizes that the routine use of fluoroscopy to ensure proper positioning for radiography prior to making an exposure is an unethical practice that increases patient dose unnecessarily and should never be used in place of appropriate skills required of the competent Radiologic Technologist."*[10]

Even though the ASRT does not condone FGP, some imaging facilities continue to allow RTs to use fluoroscopy as a positioning aid because they believe that it:

- Is faster than having a repeat exposure
- Reduces the number of repeat exposures
- Provides less radiation exposure to the patient

The Standard of Ethics as published by the American Registry of Radiologic Technologists (ARRT) serves as a guide for practicing technologists in maintaining a high level of ethical conduct and in providing for the protection, safety, and comfort of patients.[11]

Blind positioning, or positioning using the radiographer's skill and anatomic landmarks, without a repeat exposure, provides the patient with the lowest dose. However, some technologists argue that the chance of repeating the image is reduced when using FGP. This argument does not hold true according to the current repeat rates of 7% to 8%.[12] For example, if a technologist has a repeat rate of 10%, it would not be ethical to overexpose 90% of the patients in an attempt to lower the repeat rate. The repeat rate depends on the:

- Technologist's skills in the operation of the fluoroscopic equipment
- Communication between the technologist and the patient
- Patient's cooperation
- Patient's condition

Therefore, the risk of a repeat during an FGP examination is still present, and ultimately, it is the technologist's professional responsibility to reduce the amount of radiation exposure to all patients, not just those who may need to have a repeat examination.

Studies indicate that patient ESE increases with the use of FGP when a repeat exposure is needed.[13] Blind positioning provides the lowest patient ESE.

The current scientific consensus is that all dose levels of ionizing radiation have some detrimental effect. At the same time, however, procedures in radiology, such as fluoroscopy and other imaging modalities, are very capable of providing vital information to physicians for diagnosis or treatment of disease. Exposure of patients to medical x-rays is commanding increasing attention in our society for two reasons:

1. The frequency of x-ray examinations, among all age groups, is growing annually. This increase indicates that physicians are relying more and more on radiographic examinations to assist them in patient care and diagnosis.
2. Concern among public health officials is increasing regarding the risk associated with medical x-ray exposure, especially the possibility of late effects.[2]

Therefore, every effort should be made by the radiographer to practice ALARA. A review of the literature concluded the following:

- No diagnostic procedure using ionizing radiation should be conducted unless its benefits outweigh its risks.
- Exposures should be kept ALARA, with the procedure optimized to reduce radiation hazards.
- The ESE dose (ESE as given in SI units) levels set in regulations must not be exceeded.
- To maintain ALARA and follow the ASRT position statement and the ARRT code of ethics, technologists must not use FGP positioning of patients.

## THE PREGNANT PATIENT

## Determining the Possibility of Pregnancy

Whenever a female patient of childbearing age is to undergo an x-ray examination, it is essential that the radiographer carefully question the patient regarding any possibility of pregnancy. Part of this questioning involves asking the patient for the date of her last menstrual period (LMP). If the patient is to receive substantial pelvic irradiation, and there is some doubt about her pregnancy status, then, provided there are no overriding medical concerns, it is strongly recommended that the result of a pregnancy test be obtained before the pelvis is irradiated. For all female patients of childbearing age, using a gonadal shield when the uterus and ovaries are within the field of view is advisable, as long as the presence of the shield would not disrupt the interpretation of the image. A shield is also recommended if the ovaries and uterus are less than 5 cm from any edge of the field.

## Irradiation during an Unknown Pregnancy

Even with all these precautionary steps, it is likely that a radiographer will encounter many occasions when a patient who was absolutely certain that she could not be pregnant later found that she was so at the time of her x-ray examination. This discovery usually is communicated to the imaging department by the patient's obstetrician and is accompanied by a request for the amount of radiation dose that the patient's embryo-fetus received from the x-ray study. The following discussion attempts to illustrate in a simplified manner how the radiography team can appropriately respond to such queries, by presenting several case examples.

The first step in the process is to list the particulars of the x-ray examination in as much detail as possible. A useful form can be developed to assist in this process (Fig. 12-13). The information that is needed to develop this form is listed in Box 12-5.

Facility: _____

Imaging Department

**REQUEST FOR PATIENT RADIATION DOSE**
**PATIENT X-RAY EXAM RECORD**

Patient's name: _____  X-ray study #: _____
Date of birth: _____  Exam date: _____
Date of last menstrual period: _____
Referring physician: _____
Physician requesting radiation dose: _____
Radiologist: _____  Radiographer: _____
Examination: _____  X-ray room unit: _____

RADIOGRAPHIC

| Projection | Patient thickness | Film | kVp | mAs | SID | Number of images | Gonadal shield |
|---|---|---|---|---|---|---|---|
| | | | | | | | |

FLUOROSCOPIC

| Anatomic location | kVp (mean) | mA (mean) | Fluoro time | Exam description |
|---|---|---|---|---|
| | | | | |

SPOT FILMS

| Anatomic location | kVp | mA | Time (msec) | Number of spots | Special details |
|---|---|---|---|---|---|
| | | | | | |

**FIGURE 12-13**  **Request for Patient Radiation Dose Form.**

| BOX 12-5 | Information Needed to Develop the Request for Patient Radiation Dose Form |
|---|---|

1. The x-ray unit or units used for the study
2. The projections taken
3. The number of images associated with each projection
4. Each projection's technical exposure factors (kVp, mAs, image receptor size)
5. The source-to–image receptor distance (SID) for each projection
6. The patient's anteroposterior (AP) or lateral dimensions at the site of each projection
7. For fluoroscopic irradiation, the approximate kVp, mA, and especially the duration
8. For spot films, the number taken, the kVp and mA selected, and the approximate exposure time

## Procedure to Follow and Responsibility for Absorbed Equivalent Dose Determination to the Patient's Embryo-Fetus

When these details have been collected and listed on an appropriate summary form, they must be conveyed to the radiation safety officer or to the medical physicist providing x-ray quality assurance services. It is then that person's task to determine the absorbed EqD to the patient's embryo-fetus. The calculation process incorporates actual measurements of radiation output on the involved x-ray unit or units with the examination data list supplied by the radiographer. It also uses published absorbed dose data tables. What eventually is obtained and presented by the medical physicist, radiologist, or radiation safety officer to the patient's physician is a calculated estimate of the approximate EqD to the embryo-fetus as a result of the x-ray examination.

## Sample Cases to Estimate Approximate Equivalent Dose to the Embryo-Fetus

Several typical cases (somewhat simplified) are presented to illustrate one of the methods that

may be used to obtain this calculated estimate. It is not the purpose here to provide an advanced presentation but rather to offer a basic method that makes use of fundamental principles and demonstrates the importance of the radiographer's input in the process. The most significant principle is the correction to the measured radiation output at a given kVp as a result of the patient's thickness and the distance from the image receptor to the tabletop. The radiation output can now be specified in milligray in air per milliampere-second ($mGy_a/mAs$). The product of radiation output at the patient's radiation entrance surface and the milliampere-seconds used for the x-ray projection considered yields the $ESE_d$ for that view—the quantity that we seek to obtain for each x-ray exposure given to the patient. The most common measurement of milligray in air per milliampere-second is at a distance of 100 cm from the x-ray tube target. For a patient with thickness $T$ in centimeters and a typical distance of 8 cm from the image receptor to the tabletop, the radiation output at the patient's entrance surface as a function of selected milliampere-seconds is determined as shown in Figure 12-14, which illustrates all the geometric quantities of interest.

The x-ray tube output is usually determined in units of milligray per milliampere-seconds at 100 cm (40 inch) SID. In order to determine what the radiation exposure to the patient is at the patient's entrance, or skin surface, it is necessary to know the milligray per milliampere-seconds at that location. Because the skin surface is closer to the x-ray tube target, then the milligray per milliampere-seconds value will be greater than it is at 100 cm. How much greater is determined from the inverse square law and given in Equation 12-1:

**Equation 12-1**

$$(mGy_a/mAs) \text{ at skin surface} = (mGy_a/mAs) \text{ at } 100\,cm \times (100/[92-T])^2$$

As an example, assume the following values:

$$(mGy_a/mAs) \text{ at } 100\,cm = 0.06$$
$$T = 25\,cm$$

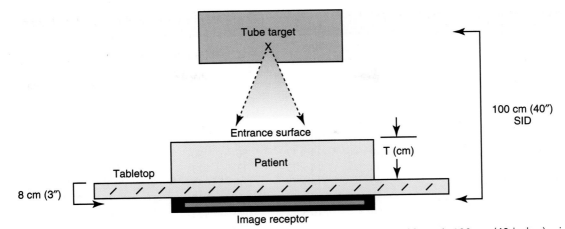

**FIGURE 12-14**   As the diagram shows, the distance from the tube target to the tabletop is 100 cm (40 inches) minus 8 cm (3 inches). The distance from the tube target to the top of the patient in inches is therefore equal to (100 − 8) − T (40 inches − 3 inches) − (T/2.54), where the patient's thickness, T, is specified in centimeters. *SID*, Source-to–image receptor distance.

Then:

$$(mGy_a/mAs \text{ at skin surface} = 0.06 \times (100/[92-25])^2$$
$$= 0.06 \times (100/67)^2$$
$$= 0.06 \times 2.23$$
$$= 0.13\,mGy/mAs$$

The patient's $ESE_d$ for an x-ray exposure is then given in Equation 12-2:

**Equation 12-2**

$$ESE_d = (mGy_a/mAs) \text{ at skin surface} \times mAs \text{ used}$$

Example:

$$mAs \text{ used} = 30$$
$$(mGy_a/mAs)_s = 0.13$$
$$ESE_d = 0.13 \times 30$$
$$= 3.9\,mGy$$

After the $ESE_d$ has been found for each x-ray exposure, it is necessary to obtain conversion factors that will yield a value for the uterine absorbed dose attributable to each exposure. In 1977 the National Council on Radiation Protection and Measurements (NCRP) published Report No. 54, *Medical Radiation Exposure of Pregnant and Potentially Pregnant Women.* Table 4 in this report has been a very useful resource for helping establish the uterine absorbed dose. Although other useful and more recent data tables exist, this table has been reproduced here as Table 12-1 to illustrate a simple method for fetal dose estimation. To use the table, it is necessary to know for each x-ray view the $ESE_d$, the anatomic location, the beam quality (half-value layer [HVL]), and the image receptor size.

## Sample Cases to Obtain an Approximate Estimate of the Fetal Equivalent Dose

Now some typical x-ray examinations are considered, and an approximate estimate of the fetal EqD resulting from each study is obtained. Examples are presented in Case A and Case B.

## OTHER DIAGNOSTIC EXAMINATIONS AND IMAGING MODALITIES

### Patient Dose in Mammography

Mammography is used to detect breast cancer that is not palpable by physical examination (Fig. 12-15). Experts agree that yearly mammographic screening of women 50 years of age and older leads to earlier detection of breast cancer. Earlier treatment saves lives and reduces suffering. The value of mammography in younger women is

| TABLE 12-1 | Embryo (Uterine) Doses for Selected X-Ray Projections (mcGy/R)*† | | | | | | | | |
|---|---|---|---|---|---|---|---|---|---|
| Anatomy or Study | Projection | SID (Inches) | Image Receptor Size (inches)‡ | Beam Quality (HVL mm aluminum) | | | | | |
| | | | | 1.5 | 2.0 | 2.5 | 3.0 | 3.5 | 4.0 |
| Pelvis, lumbopelvic | AP | 40 | 17 × 14 | 142 | 212 | 283 | 353 | 421 | 486 |
| | LAT | 40 | 14 × 17 | 13 | 25 | 39 | 56 | 75 | 97 |
| Abdominal§ | AP | 40 | 14 × 17 | 133 | 199 | 265 | 330 | 392 | 451 |
| | PA | 40 | 14 × 17 | 56 | 90 | 130 | 174 | 222 | 273 |
| | LAT | 40 | 14 × 17 | 13 | 23 | 37 | 53 | 71 | 91 |
| Lumbar spine | AP | 40 | 14 × 17 | 128 | 189 | 250 | 309 | 366 | 419 |
| | LAT | 40 | 14 × 17 | 9 | 17 | 27 | 39 | 53 | 69 |
| Hip | AP (1) | 40 | 10 × 12 | 105 | 153 | 200 | 244 | 285 | 324 |
| | AP (2) | 40 | 17 × 14 | 136 | 203 | 269 | 333 | 395 | 454 |
| Full spine (chiropractic) | AP | 40 | 14 × 36 | 154 | 231 | 308 | 384 | 457 | 527 |
| Urethrogram | AP | 40 | 10 × 12 | 135 | 200 | 265 | 327 | 386 | 441 |
| Upper GI | AP | 40 | 14 × 17 | 9.5 | 16 | 25 | 34 | 45 | 56 |
| Femur (one side) | AP | 40 | 7 × 17 | 1.6 | 3.0 | 4.8 | 6.9 | 9.4 | 12 |
| Cholecystography | PA | 40 | 10 × 12 | 0.7 | 1.5 | 2.6 | 4.1 | 6.0 | 8.3 |
| Chest | AP | 72 | 14 × 17 | 0.3 | 0.7 | 1.3 | 2.0 | 3.1 | 4.3 |
| | PA | 72 | 14 × 17 | 0.3 | 0.6 | 1.2 | 2.0 | 3.0 | 4.5 |
| | LAT | 72 | 14 × 17 | 0.1 | 0.3 | 0.5 | 0.8 | 1.2 | 1.8 |
| Ribs, barium swallow | AP | 40 | 14 × 17 | 0.1 | 0.3 | 0.5 | 0.9 | 1.4 | 2.0 |
| | PA | 40 | 14 × 17 | 0.1 | 0.3 | 0.5 | 0.9 | 1.5 | 2.2 |
| | LAT | 40 | 14 × 17 | 0.03 | 0.08 | 0.2 | 0.3 | 0.4 | 0.6 |
| Thoracic spine | AP | 40 | 14 × 17 | 0.2 | 0.4 | 0.8 | 1.4 | 4.1 | 3.0 |
| | LAT | 40 | 14 × 17 | 0.04 | 0.1 | 0.2 | 0.4 | 0.5 | 0.8 |
| Skull, cervical spine, scapula, shoulder, humerus | — | 40 | — | <0.01 | <0.01 | <0.01 | <0.01 | <0.01 | <0.01 |

Data modified from National Council on Radiation Protection and Measurements (NCRP): *Medical radiation exposure of pregnant and potentially pregnant women,* Report No. 54, Washington, DC, 1977, NCRP.

*AP,* Anteroposterior; *GI,* gastrointestinal; *HVL,* half-value layer; *LAT,* lateral; *PA,* posteroanterior; *SID,* source-to–image receptor distance.

*Average dose to the uterus millicentigray per 1 roentgen entrance skin exposure (free-in-air) ($ESE_d$). The latter value is essentially equal in these energy ranges to 10 mGy $ESE_d$ or 1 cGy $ESE_d$.

†Adapted from NCRP report No. 54 Rosenstein (1976).

‡Field size is collimated to the image receptor.

§Includes retrograde pyelogram; kidney, ureter, and bladder (KUB); barium enema, lumbosacral spine, intravenous pyelogram (IVP); renal arteriogram.

| CASE A | **OBSTRUCTION SERIES** |
|---|---|

X-ray projection details:

(Although an 180-cm (72 inches) source-to–image receptor distance (SID) would normally be used for a postero-anterior (PA) upright chest projection, for purposes of simplifying the calculation we will keep the SID = 100 cm (40 inches) the same for all x-ray projections in this series.)
  PA chest radiograph
(1) 80 kVp, 10 mAs, 100 cm SID, 35 × 43-cm cassette, 25-cm patient thickness
  Erect anteroposterior (AP) abdomen
(1) 75 kVp, 32 mAs, 100 cm SID, 35 × 43-cm cassette, 20-cm patient thickness
  Supine abdomen
(1) 70 kVp, 50 mAs, 100 cm SID, 35 × 43-cm cassette, 20-cm patient thickness

The first step is to obtain the value of $mGy_a/mAs$ for each projection. To determine this value, a reference value $(mGy_a/mAs)_{100\text{-}cm}$ is needed for the x-ray unit involved and the kVp used. To comply with state rules and regulations, a medical physicist measures these values yearly for each x-ray tube. If the measured reference $mGy_a/mAs$ values for the three projections are 0.01, 0.04, and 0.04, respectively, then substituting these numbers into Equation 12-1 along with the corresponding SIDs and patient thicknesses yields: $(mGy_a/mAs)_s$ PA chest = 0.02 $(mGy_a/mAs)_s$, erect AP abdomen = 0.08, and supine abdomen = 0.08, respectively. From Equation 12-2 the entrance skin exposure dose $(ESE_d)$ value is then given by:

$ESE_d$ PA chest: $0.02 \times 10 = 0.2\,mGy = (0.02\,cGy)$

$ESE_d$ erect AP abdomen: $0.08 \times 32 = 2.6\,mGy\ (0.26\,cGy)$

$ESE_d$ supine abdomen: $0.08 \times 50 = 4\,mGy\ (0.4\,cGy)$

For the chest field, the half-value layer (HVL) is approximately 3 mm aluminum (Al), whereas for the abdominal fields, 2.5 and 2.0 mm Al, respectively, are used. Then from Table 12-1 the embryo/uterine dose conversion factors are 2 mcGy/cGy of $ESE_d$, 265 mcGy/cGy of $ESE_d$, and 199 mcGy/cGy of $ESE_d$. Multiplying these values by the $ESE_d$ for each view gives a fetal dose estimate (FDE) for each, namely:

PA chest FDE $= 0.02 \times 2 = 0.04\,mcGy\ (.04\ millirads)$

Erect AP abdomen FDE$=0.26 \times 265 = 69\,mcGy\ (69\ millirads)$

Supine abdomen FDE$=0.4 \times 199 = 79.6\,mcGy\ (79.6\ millirads)$

The total FDE is therefore $0.04 + 69 + 79.6 = 149\,mcGy$. For diagnostic x-rays, 1 mcGy is the same as an equivalent dose (EqD) of 10 microsieverts (1 millirem), and consequently the calculated approximate EqD to the patient's embryo-fetus from her obstruction series is 149 mcGy or 1.49 mSv.

For reference purposes, this value of EqD to the embryo-fetus is substantially less than the 5 mSv (500 mrem) recommended by the National Council on Radiation Protection and Measurements as a maximum EqD to the embryo-fetus during the 9-month gestation period.

---

somewhat controversial. The controversy has little to do with radiation risk (induction of breast cancer by radiation). Although it is still mentioned occasionally in the popular press, cancer researchers generally agree that radiation risk resulting from the small doses associated with mammography is negligible in all women.[14-16] Federal regulations for U.S. Food and Drug Administration (FDA) certification of screening mammography facilities state that the mean dose to the glandular tissue of a 4.5-cm compressed breast using a screen-film mammography system should not exceed 3 $mGy_t$ per view.[17] Studies have shown that well-calibrated mammographic systems are capable of providing excellent imaging performance with an average glandular

dose of not more than 2 $mGy_t$.[18] The age recommendation for screening is controversial because mammography is less accurate in the detection of breast cancer in younger women and is likely to result in many false-positive readings, leading to unnecessary biopsies in that population. The increased density of the breast of younger women tends to reduce radiographic contrast, and therefore conventional screen-film mammography is frequently less sensitive in the average younger woman than in the average older woman. Digital mammography units, which can enhance contrast with image gray-level manipulation, offer substantial improvement for patients with dense breasts. Earlier detection of more aggressive cancers will save lives in general. Consequently,

## CASE B    MODIFIED UPPER GASTROINTESTINAL EXAMINATION

X-ray projection details:
Fluoroscopy: 115 kVp, 4.5 mA (mean values), 3.5 minutes
Spot films (4): 110 kVp, 200 mA, 20 msec (mean values)

### Calculation Details

Suppose that from measured data on the involved fluoroscopic unit, the entrance exposure rate dose to the patient is about 12.5 mGy per milliampere minute. Therefore, the entrance skin exposure dose ($ESE_d$) for the delivered fluoroscopic radiation is obtained from the product:

$$12.5\,mGy/mA\text{-}min \times 4.5\,mA \times 3.5\,min = 197\,mGy\ (19.7\,cGy)$$

From measured spot film radiation output, for the technique factors used in this study, let the x-ray output at the patient's entrance surface be 0.5 mGy/mAs.* Therefore, the total $ESE_d$ for the four spot films is given by:

$$4 \times 0.5\,mGy/mAs \times 200\,mA \times 0.020\,sec = 8\,mGy = (0.8\,cGy)$$

Using half-value layer (HVL) values of 4.0 and 3.5 mm aluminum (Al), respectively, the uterine dose rates obtained from Table 12-1 are as follows:

Averaged fluoroscopic irradiation: 56 mcGy/cGy entrance = 56 mrem/cGy
Spot films: 45 mcGy/cGy entrance = 45 mrem/cGy

The estimated approximate equivalent dose (EqD) to the embryo-fetus from this modified upper gastrointestinal (UGI) study is then:

$$56 \times 19.7 + 45 \times 0.8 = 1139\,mrem = 1.14\,rem = 11.4\,mSv$$

For this modified UGI study on a heavy patient, we have obtained a fetal EqD estimate that is more than twice the National Council on Radiation Protection and Measurements recommended maximum fetal EqD of 5 mSv (0.5 rem). This result, however, is far below the range between 100 and 200 mSv (10 and 20 rem) at which therapeutic abortion has historically been considered. If the embryo-fetus were in its most sensitive stage (i.e., early first trimester), then possibly some genetic studies could be undertaken. Otherwise, in most situations, increased follow-up would be the course of action.

*For the spot films the entrance surface of the patient is only about 46 cm (18 inches) from the x-ray tube target, and that is why the value of mGy/mAs can be so high.

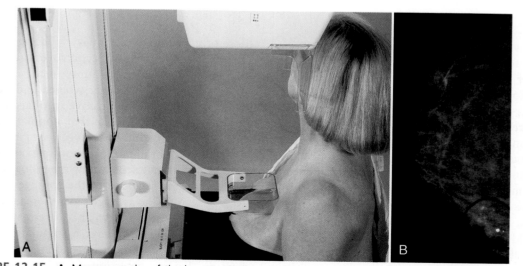

**FIGURE 12-15**  **A,** Mammography of the breast using the craniocaudal projection. **B,** Mammography can be used to detect breast cancer.

the efficacy of screening mammography in women less than 50 years old is a subject that has generated a great deal of interest.

**Mammography Screening.** We support the recommendations of the American College of Radiology (ACR), the American Cancer Society, and the American Medical Association. These groups advocate annual mammography screening or mammography screening at least every other year for women age 40 to 49 years. Before the onset of menopause, a baseline mammogram is also highly recommended for comparison with mammograms taken at a later age. The interested reader should contact these organizations for their latest policy statements on this subject.

**Dose Reduction in Mammography.** Dose reduction in mammography can be achieved by limiting the number of projections taken. Axillary projections should be done only on request of the radiologist. If mammography is performed as a routine screening procedure, it is prudent to perform only craniocaudal and mediolateral projections of each breast with adequate compression to demonstrate breast tissue uniformly from the nipple to the most posterior portion.

**Digital Mammography.** A description of DR is provided in Chapter 11. In the latest (and most expensive) systems that are used for breast imaging, digital mammography has replaced film-based mammography to provide optimal-quality images.

## Patient Dose in Computed Tomography

**Radiation Exposure.** Computed tomography (CT) is defined as "the process of creating a cross-sectional tomographic plane of any part of the body."[19] This computer-reconstructed image of a patient is created by an "x-ray tube and detector assembly rotating 360 degrees about a specified area of the body."[19] CT was previously referred to as *computed axial tomography (CAT)* because the first generation of scanners produced only axial images. The term *computed tomography* is now more appropriate because "images can now be created in multiple planes."[19]

Although a discussion of CT equipment, function, and procedure is not within the scope of this text, patient dose resulting from exposure to ionizing radiation is relevant because CT is a frequently employed diagnostic x-ray imaging modality that is considered to be a relatively high radiation exposure examination. Currently, this is of even more concern because of the increasing use of multislice spiral (helical) CT scanners employing small slice thickness. With higher radiation exposure to the patient, there is an increased associated cancer risk. For this reason, physicians ordering such procedures must weigh the benefits of the procedure for the patient in terms of medical information gained and determine whether these benefits outweigh the risk.

**Concerns Related to Patient Dose: Skin Dose and Dose Distribution.** Two concerns relate to patient dose in CT scanning. One concern is the skin dose, and the other is the dose distribution during the scanning procedure. The dose at the edge of a beam does not decrease to zero immediately; some extra radiation is delivered at the edge of the slice. Because of this, the skin dose for a succession of adjacent scans is greater than the skin dose from a single scan. The neighboring slices contribute some dose from both sides. When a patient undergoes an ordinary but complicated non-CT x-ray examination, many images involving different projections are obtained. If the doses from this extensive radiographic series are added together, the sum could be comparable to the dose from a CT examination.

Still another consideration exists. CT examinations generally expose a smaller mass of tissue than that exposed during an ordinary x-ray series. This is because the CT x-ray beam is more tightly collimated than the conventional radiographic beam. The entrance exposure from a CT examination also may be compared with the entrance exposure received during a routine fluoroscopic examination. In this instance, the entrance exposure received during a CT examination is generally considerably less than that received during a routine fluoroscopic procedure.

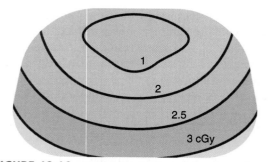

**FIGURE 12-16** Typical distribution of the doses deposited in a single-slice computed tomography examination. For multiple contiguous slices, the doses may be twice these values.

The dose distribution resulting from a CT scan is not the same as the dose distribution occurring in routine radiologic procedures (Fig. 12-16). In radiography or fluoroscopy, skin dose at the entrance surface of the patient is much higher than at the exit surface. In abdominal imaging, for example, the entrance skin dose is approximately 100 times the exit dose. For CT, because the tube rotates around the patient, the dose is much more uniform throughout the patient. Because CT scanners use an x-ray beam that is tightly collimated, the amount of scatter radiation generated is lower than the scatter produced by the less tightly collimated radiographic beam. Also because of this, the mass of human tissue exposed to radiation falls off rapidly outside the plane of interest during the production of any given scan. Although in a single-slice scanner only one cross-sectional tomographic plane (slice) is exposed and imaged at a time (note: in current scanners, multiple slices [e.g., 4, 16, 64, even as many as 128] can be acquired simultaneously), some overlap of the margins of the x-ray beam occurs when each single tomographic section is made. When a series of adjacent slices is obtained, some radiation scatters from the slice being made into the adjacent slices (interslice scatter). Both these factors contribute to dose increase and are the reasons that a succession of adjacent tomographic sections (slices) imparts a higher absorbed dose than would a single tomographic section.

**Approximate Doses for Head and Body Computed Tomography Imaging.** Depending on the type of CT imaging system and the examination technique, Bushong identified typical average CT dose ranges of 30 to 50 mGy during head imaging and 20 to 40 mGy during body imaging.[2] Actual doses delivered during any CT scanning procedure depend on the type of scanner being used and especially the radiation technical exposure factors selected. The tight collimation of the CT beam makes possible its accurate placement relative to the area of anatomy to be studied, which permits CT technologists to avoid exposing selected radiosensitive organs (e.g., the eyes).

**Direct Patient Shielding.** Direct patient shielding is not typically used in CT. Because of the rotational nature of the exposure, a shield is no more effective than the collimators that already exist on the device. Because the beam is so tightly collimated to the slice thickness, exposure to the anatomy outside the field of view is usually caused only by internal scatter. Generally in CT, anatomy does not appear in the primary x-ray beam unless it is part of the intended field of view.

**Spiral, or Helical, Computed Tomography.** Spiral CT presents a greater challenge for assessing patient dose than does conventional CT. It is defined as a "data acquisition method that combines a continuous gantry rotation with a continuous table movement to form a spiral path of scan data."[19] It is also called *helical CT*.

When the spiral scan pitch ratio (also just known as *pitch*), which is the relationship between the movement or advance of the patient couch (also known as table increment I) and the x-ray beam collimator dimension (Z; pitch = I/Z) is approximately 1, the spiral CT patient dose is comparable to that produced by conventional or axial CT. However, when the pitch ratio is higher (e.g., 2:1), patient dose is reduced in comparison with conventional CT because less of the patient is exposed during the scan. The reverse also is true; patient dose increases at a lower pitch.

**Other Factors That Influence Patient Dose.** Patient dose also may be influenced by other factors. Changes in noise level (the random variation in pixel brightness seen when an image is made of too few photons—that is, if the mA setting is too low in a CT scan), pixel (individual picture element) size, and slice thickness all affect patient dose. The use of smaller pixel sizes for better resolution, the selection of thinner slices, and the increase of tube mA all increase the patient's absorbed dose. These relationships are summarized as follows.

$$D = K\left(\frac{SNR^2}{e^3h}\right)$$

where SNR is the signal-to-noise ratio (i.e., the comparison of the average CT number in a region with the statistical variation of CT number in that region), e is the size of the smallest resolvable object, and h is the slice thickness. K is simply a constant of proportionality that depends on the special properties or characteristics of each scanner. The value of this constant is determined by measurement. The SNR is an indicator of the "smoothness" of the image and is related to the ability to detect low-contrast objects (e.g., a liver tumor within liver tissues). The equation shows that the dose is proportional to the square of the SNR, and therefore an attempt to increase the SNR (by increasing the tube mA) results in a noticeably higher patient dose. The dose also increases if CT technologists attempt to resolve smaller objects by setting thinner slice widths without sacrificing any SNR.

**Computed Tomography Dose Parameters.** In order to approximate the effective radiation dose to a patient who has undergone a CT study, the values of two CT-specific dose markers or quantities need to be determined for each scan series. The following discussion introduces and briefly defines all the relevant parameters, describes how their values can be obtained, and shows their relationships to one another. The relevant dose parameters are as follows:

- CT dose index (CTDI)
- $CTDI_W$
- $CTDI_{VOL}$
- Dose length product (DLP)

The last two items are the required dose markers. Their values directly depend on the details of the performed CT scan and are displayed by the scanner's software for each completed patient scan. There is a direct progressive relationship among all four of the listed parameters, as demonstrated in the following paragraphs.

The CTDI is determined by an ionization measurement using a 1-cm diameter and 10-cm (100 mm) long cylindric pencil-like ionization chamber that has been inserted into a shaped cavity within a cylindric acrylic phantom. The phantom, which can be similar in diameter to either a human head or a human abdomen, is then generally single-slice scanned with technique factors (kVp, mAs, and slice thickness) that are equivalent to those used for a patient study. The irradiated pencil chamber is attached to an electrometer whose ionization charge reading when multiplied by several correction factors will then be given in milligray (mGy) units. Dividing this number by the scan direction collimation* will make this ionization measurement representative of the localized dose from a multiple slice examination.

$CTDI_W$ is simply a weighted average of two measured CTDI values, one that is obtained with the pencil chamber placed in the central cavity of the acrylic phantom and the other derived from the average of four peripheral (only 1-cm-deep) cavity measurements that are located at the 3, 6, 9, and 12 o'clock positions.

$$CTDI_W = \tfrac{1}{3}(CTDI_{center}) + \tfrac{2}{3}(CTDI_{periph})$$

$CTDI_{VOL}$ is the average absorbed dose within the scanned volume. Its value is directly related to $CTDI_W$ by the following expression:

$$CTDI_{VOL} = CTDI_W / PITCH$$

---

*Scan direction collimation is equal to the product of the number of data channels used during one axial acquisition (N) and the nominal slice width of one axial image (T). For example, in a single-slice scanner for a 10-mm slice thickness selection, N = 1 and T = 10, so NT = 10. In a multislice CT scanner with selected scan thickness parameters 5 mm, 4i ("4i" means four 5-mm slices acquired simultaneously), then N = 4, T = 5, and NT = 20.

For nonhelical or axial scans such as those normally used in adult head scan sequences, the pitch (P) equals 1, and therefore $CTDI_{VOL} = CTDI_W$; but for typical helical scans, P is usually greater than 1 (e.g., 1.375 is quite common), so the magnitude of $CTDI_{VOL}$ will be less than that of $CTDI_W$.

The previous discussion demonstrates how a medical physicist can obtain a value for $CTDI_{VOL}$ by measurement. However, at the conclusion of each patient CT scan sequence, the built-in computer software accesses a database that supplies a numeric value of the $CTDI_{VOL}$ for that scan sequence. Also supplied is the value of a quantity called the *dose length product* (DLP).

DLP represents the product of the $CTDI_{VOL}$ and the irradiated scan length. It is expressed in milligray-centimeters (mGy-cm). DLP characterizes the volumetric extent along the patient's body that has been irradiated with an average absorbed dose. As such it has significance for estimating future cancer risk as a result of radiation doses unavoidably delivered to sensitive organs from CT examinations. Mathematically, $DLP = CTDI_{VOL} \times$ scan length. Scan length, which may be considered as approximately the superior-inferior extent of the patient's irradiation, can be derived from the product of slice width times number of slices times pitch. Thus a helical scan that is composed of 60 5-mm slices with a pitch of 1.5 has an approximate scan length of $60 \times 0.5 \times 1.5 = 45$ cm. If instead this were an axial scan, then the scan length would be just $60 \times 0.5 = 30$ cm.

**Effective Computed Tomography Dose.** What follows uses a table of scan region–specific conversion factors (Table 12-2), generated by the European Union,[20] that when combined with the dose information supplied by the CT software for each delivered scan sequence will yield an effective dose (EfD) value for that CT scan. The simple expression to be used for calculation of EfD is given by the following equation:

$$EfD = DLP \times EfDLP$$

where EfDLP is the normalized EfD associated with a specific scan region of the body. EfDLP is expressed in millisieverts per milligray-centimeter ($mSv/mGy^{-1}$-$cm^{-1}$) and represents a conversion factor from a patient's CT scan DLP to the EfD received by the patient as a result of that scan. Experimentally determined numeric values for these factors are given in Table 12-2.

Using the values in Table 12-2 and the information displayed on the dose page printout for a patient's CT scan, the EfD to the patient from that scan can be calculated. Several examples of using such data from actual patient CT scans are demonstrated in Cases 1 to 3. For greater ease

| TABLE 12-2 | Scan Region–Specific Conversion Factors |
|---|---|
| **Body Region Scanned** | **Normalized Effective Dose (EfDLP)** |
| Head | 0.0023 |
| Neck | 0.0054 |
| Chest | 0.017 |
| Abdomen | 0.015 |
| Pelvis | 0.019 |

---

**CASE 1  HEAD SCAN (AXIAL)**

Scan data*: $CTDI_{VOL}$ = 60.8 mGy, DLP = 373 mGy-cm (portion of scan series at 140 kVp)

$CTDI_{VOL}$ = 49.1 mGy, DLP = 351 mGy-cm (portion of scan series at 120 kVp)

From Table 12-2, EfDLP = 0.0023.

Therefore, the EfD to this patient is given by the following equation:

$$(373 + 351) \times 0.0023 = 1.67 \text{ mSv } (0.167 \text{ rem})$$

*See text for abbreviations.

---

**CASE 2  CHEST SCAN (HELICAL)**

Scan data*: $CTDI_{VOL}$ = 8.5 mGy, DLP = 323 mGy-cm

From Table 12-2, EfDLP = 0.017.

Therefore, the EfD to this patient is given by the following equation:

$$323 \times 0.017 = 5.49 \text{ mSv } (0.549 \text{ rem})$$

*See text for abbreviations.

| CASE 3 | ABDOMINAL SCAN (HELICAL) |
| --- | --- |

Scan data*: $CTDI_{VOL}$ = 17.5 mGy, DLP = 839 mGy-cm
   From Table 12-2, EfDLP = 0.015.
      Therefore, the EfD to this patient is given by the following equation:

$$839 \times 0.015 = 12.6 \, mSv \, (1.26 \, rem)$$

*See text for abbreviations.

of reading, some references to traditional units are included throughout the remainder of this chapter.

**Risk of Future Cancer.** According to the results of BEIR V (Biological Effects of Ionizing Radiation Committee V), published in 1989, the risk of cancer death associated with exposure to ionizing radiation is 0.08% per 10 mSv (1 rem) EfD for doses received rapidly, such as would be delivered by an x-ray–producing machine. This value represents an average estimate for both men and women for all ages and all types of cancers. Because of certain assumptions about the relationship between low radiation doses and cancer induction, uncertainties are associated with this BEIR V risk value. Consequently, other scientific groups have come up with different results. On close inspection, however, all these results are reasonably close. Therefore, if the BEIR V risk estimate value is applied to the three CT scan cases discussed in the previous paragraph, we can obtain a risk estimate of cancer death associated with the doses from those scans. Before we do this, it should be realized that in the United States the death rate from cancer is approximately 20%. Consequently, if we consider groups of 100,000 U.S. citizens, then on average approximately 20,000 of each group will die of cancer. Let us then see what the effect on such a group could be as a result of the EfD received from the CT scan cases.

- Case 1: EfD = 0.167 rem. Risk estimate = 0.0008 × 0.167 = 0.000134
  - In a population of 100,000 people, the extra cancer deaths that could occur from exposure of the population to such CT examinations would be 100,000 × 0.000134 = 13, or 20,013 deaths from cancer could be expected to occur instead of 20,000.
- Case 2: EfD = 0.549 rem. Risk estimate = 0.0008 × 0.549 = 0.000439
  - In a population of 100,000 people, the extra cancer deaths that could occur from exposure of the population to such CT examinations would be 100,000 × 0.000439 = 44, or 20,044 deaths from cancer could be expected to occur instead of 20,000 deaths.
- Case 3: EfD = 1.26 rem. Risk estimate = 0.0008 × 1.26 = 0.00101
  - In a population of 100,000 people, the extra cancer deaths that could occur from exposure of the population to such CT examinations would be 100,000 × 0.00101 = 101, or 20,101 deaths from cancer could be expected to occur instead of 20,000 deaths.

**Goal of Computed Tomography Imaging from a Radiation Protection Point of View.** In summary, from a radiation protection point of view, the goal of CT imaging should be to obtain the best possible image while delivering an acceptable level of ionizing radiation to the patient (optimize the dose to the patient). In the absence of specially designed scan protocols, the fulfillment of this responsibility lies with the technologist performing the examination.

**Alliance for Radiation Safety in Pediatric Imaging.** The **Alliance for Radiation Safety in Pediatric Imaging** was founded in 2007. It is a partnership of medical societies whose overall common purpose is to reduce the dose for pediatric patients. Its first goal is to raise awareness among nonradiology users of CT. If a child is placed in a CT scanner and adult protocols are used, the child will receive a higher dose than an adult, but the image will appear to be of acceptable quality—it will not appear overexposed, as a film would. Radiologists have been aware of this for some time, and many practices have altered their protocols for pediatric patients.

However, as of 2007, many referring physicians and nonradiology owners of CT scanners were not aware of the problem. Since 2007, the Alliance for Radiation Safety in Pediatric Imaging has continued in their pursuit to raise awareness of the need for dose reduction for pediatric patients among nonradiology users of CT. A recent study was performed to determine the general prevalence of the use of CT in the pediatric emergency department from 2003 to 2010. While an increase in the prevalence of the use of CT was demonstrated during that period of time, it was also demonstrated "in areas where alternative non-radiation-based modalities were options, there were decreased trends in CT use and increased use of alternative non-radiation-based modalities."[21]

**Increased Radiation Sensitivity of Children.** Although reducing dose is important for all patients, some information clearly indicates that children are significantly more radiation sensitive than adults and that exposure early in life, at levels found in CT and even lower, leads to a measurable increase in cancer incidence as the subjects age into their 50s and 60s. A study from the Radiation Effects Research Foundation published in March 2008, in which a particular number of subjects were followed, showed that exposure in utero (n = 2452, where n is the number of subjects followed from childhood exposure from the atomic bombs of Hiroshima and Nagasaki) and as a child (≤6 years old, n = 15,288) was associated with a significantly increased risk of fatal cancer in adulthood.[22] Even older children were affected. A study of patients with scoliosis (in which the mean age at exposure was 10.6 years, the mean dose received was 0.11 Gy, and the number of subjects exposed was 4822) who were followed up into adulthood found 70 cases among the exposed individuals when 35 cases were expected from comparison with a control group.[23] The National Academy of Science's most recent report on the Biological Effects of Ionizing Radiation summarized the available data as follows[24]: The same radiation in the first year of life for boys produces three to four times the cancer risk as exposure between the ages of 20 and 50 years. For girls, the difference is six to eight times. For children in general, the risk is approximately three times.

**Image Gently Campaign.** On January 22, 2008 the Alliance kicked off the **Image Gently Campaign.** The campaign includes dissemination of information on pediatric CT dose reduction among the various medical specialties that refer patients for CT examinations or even operate their own CT scanners. It also included the establishment of the Image Gently website. The website (www.imagegently.org) delivers the message that CT saves children's lives, but that patient dose should be lowered by "child sizing" the kV and mA settings, by scanning only the indicated area (e.g., if ultrasound demonstrates a possible dermoid in the upper abdomen and a follow-up CT is ordered, there is rarely a need to scan the entire abdomen and pelvis), and by removing multiphase scans from the pediatric protocol (e.g., precontrast, postcontrast, and delayed CT scans rarely add additional information in children yet can double or triple the dose). The website also contains a downloadable worksheet that allows a medical physicist to determine the technique factors that will ensure that the pediatric dose on different manufacturer's scanners is no higher than the adult dose. Input for the worksheet is a series of measurements made on the CT scanner by a medical physicist. With use of these techniques, the pediatric dose may be reduced by as much as 50% with no reduction in image quality. Even greater dose reductions are possible if the viewer is willing to tolerate an increase in noise in the image. A high-contrast imaging situation such as bone imaging or verification of tube placement may be successfully interpreted in the presence of increased noise.

The Alliance consists of more than 24 medical societies, including the ASRT and the American Association of Physicists in Medicine. Therefore, it represents more than 600,000 physicians, medical physicists, and technologists. The Alliance has held summit meetings with all the major vendors of CT equipment and has lobbied for features that encourage the use of dose-reduction techniques, more training of the vendor's application specialists in dose-reduction techniques, and display of patient dose for patients of all sizes.

**Image Wisely Campaign.** The American College of Radiology (ACR) and the Radiological Society of North America (RSNA) formed the Joint Task Force on Adult Radiation Protection to address concerns about the increase of public exposure to ionizing radiation from medical imaging. The Joint Task Force collaborated with the American Association of Physicists in Medicine (AAPM) and the ASRT to create the **Image Wisely Campaign** with the objective of lowering the amount of radiation used in medically necessary imaging studies and eliminating unnecessary procedures. In December of 2012, Minnesota became the first state in the United States of America to endorse the Image Wisely and Image Gently campaigns.

Image Wisely offers resources and information to radiologists, medical physicists, other imaging practitioners, and patients.[25]

## PEDIATRIC CONSIDERATIONS DURING CONVENTIONAL X-RAY IMAGING

### Vulnerability of Children to Radiation Exposure

With regard to the potential for biologic damage from exposure to ionizing radiation, children are much more vulnerable to both the late somatic effects and genetic effects of radiation than are adults. Hence children require special consideration when they undergo diagnostic x-ray studies. Appropriate radiation protection methods must be used for each procedure. Some of these methods are described in the following sections. Because children have a greater life expectancy, they may easily survive long enough to develop leukemia induced by radiation or develop a radiogenic malignancy such as lung or thyroid cancer. In fact, according to studies published by Beebe and others in 1978, the risk of a radiation-induced leukemia in children after a substantial dose of ionizing radiation is approximately two times that of adults.[26] For low doses such as those generally encountered in ordinary diagnostic radiology, data are still inconclusive (see Chapter 9). With this consideration in mind, radiographers must take every precaution to minimize exposure in all pediatric patients.

### Children Require Smaller Radiation Doses than Do Adults

In general, smaller doses of ionizing radiation are sufficient to obtain useful images in pediatric imaging procedures than are necessary for adult imaging procedures. For example, an entrance exposure below 5 mcGy results from an AP projection of an infant's chest,[27] whereas the same projection or a PA projection of an adult's chest yields an entrance exposure ranging from 10 to 25 mcGy (see Table 2-5).

### Patient Motion and Motion Reduction Methods

Patient motion is frequently a problem in diagnostic pediatric radiography. Because of the limited ability of children to understand the radiologic procedure and, in most cases, their limited ability to cooperate, children are less likely to remain still during a radiographic or fluoroscopic exposure. To solve or at least minimize this problem, the radiographer must employ very short exposure times by selecting a high-mA station and also using effective immobilization techniques. For some examinations, such as chest radiography, special pediatric immobilization devices are available to hold the pediatric patient securely and safely in the required position, thus providing adequate immobilization (see Fig. 12-3). The use of such techniques, along with the use of appropriate radiographic or fluoroscopic technical exposure factors and correct image processing methods, greatly reduces or eliminates the need for repeat examinations that will increase patient dose.

## Gaining Cooperation during the Procedure

The presence of technologists who have experience working with children is helpful. Rooms specially earmarked for pediatric studies also are beneficial. Such rooms contain not only the appropriate restraint devices but also suitable entertainment and distracting devices such as cartoon posters and puppets. The examination progresses most efficiently with the best hope for patient cooperation when the child feels less intimidated.

## Gonadal Shielding and Gonadal Dose

The radiographer should be familiar with particular difficulties related to gonadal shielding in pediatric studies. First, if the gonadal tissue is more than 2 cm from the edge of the field of view (assuming good collimation), the use of a gonadal shield does not significantly affect the gonadal dose because in that case the dose is caused mainly by internal scatter. In small girls, the variation in anatomic location of the ovaries requires shielding of the iliac wings as well as the sacral area when shielding is needed.[27] Effective shielding may not be possible for some studies because it obscures the anatomic area of interest.

## Collimation

Collimation is especially important in pediatric studies. The automatic collimation system reduces the radiation field size to the dimensions of the image receptor, but because many pediatric patients are significantly smaller than the image receptor, further manual adjustment of collimation is sometimes necessary. As in any other radiographic study, reducing the field size to the anatomic features of interest not only reduces patient exposure but also increases recorded image quality by decreasing scatter. Projection orientation also is important. Female patients who may be imaged in either PA or AP projection

will receive significantly lower doses to the breast tissues in a PA projection.[28]

## Patient Protection for Adults and Children: Similarities and Necessary Changes

Essentially, the same patient protection methods used to reduce the radiation exposure in adults may be employed to reduce the radiation exposure in pediatric patients. In general, the techniques discussed in this chapter may be applied to meet the needs of infants or children. It should also be strongly noted that CT technical exposure factors normally used for adults are not appropriate for young children. The scan kVp can be lowered as well as the mAs per obtained slice. Unfortunately, many facilities have in the past routinely used the same factors for both adults and small children and continue to do so today. There is an unwillingness to develop new scanning protocols because of the conflicting demands of multiple pediatric protocols. Mindful of the overall enhanced vulnerability of children to ionizing radiation, it is imperative that facilities and imaging personnel make every conscious effort to develop and use protocols that are in the best interest of the children entrusted to their care.

# PROTECTING THE PREGNANT OR POTENTIALLY PREGNANT PATIENT

## Position of the American College of Radiology on Abdominal Radiologic Examinations of Female Patients

Because much evidence suggests that the developing embryo-fetus is very radiation sensitive, special care is taken in radiography to prevent unnecessary exposure of the abdominal area of pregnant women. Unfortunately, many women are not aware that they are pregnant during the earliest stage of pregnancy, and this means that exposure of the abdominal area of potentially pregnant (i.e., fertile) women is a concern. The official position of the ACR, the major professional organization of radiologists in the United States, is as follows: "Abdominal radiological exams that have been requested after full consideration of the clinical status of a patient, including the possibility of pregnancy, need not be postponed or selectively scheduled."[29]

## Elective Examinations

When the referring physician does not consider radiologic procedures urgent, they may be regarded as elective examinations and can be booked at an appropriate time to meet patients' needs and safety requirements. In NCRP Report No. 102, a recommendation was made to facilitate scheduling of elective examinations.[30,31] This recommendation states that elective abdominal examinations of women of childbearing years should be performed during the first few days after the onset of menses to minimize the possible irradiation of an embryo (Box 12-6).

## Irradiation of an Unknown Pregnancy

In the event that a pregnant patient is inadvertently irradiated, a radiologic physicist should perform the calculations necessary to determine fetal exposure. This may include taking measurements using phantoms to simulate the patient and using ion chambers to record exposure. The following question sometimes arises: Should a therapeutic abortion be performed to prevent the birth of an infant because of radiation exposure during pregnancy? Studies of groups such as the atomic bomb survivors of Hiroshima have shown that damage to the newborn is unlikely for doses below 0.2 Gy. Because most medical procedures result in fetal exposures of less than 0.01 Gy, the risk of abnormality is small. The position of the NCRP is stated in Box 12-7.[30]

## Irradiating a Known Pregnant Patient

If the physician believes it is in the best interest of a pregnant or potentially pregnant patient to undergo a radiologic examination, the examination should be performed without delay. Under such circumstances, special efforts should be

| BOX 12-6 | **Recommendation from National Council of Radiation Protection and Measurements to Facilitate Scheduling of Elective Procedures** |
| --- | --- |

Ideally, an elective abdominal examination of a woman of childbearing age should be performed during the first few days after the onset of menses to minimize the possibility of irradiating an embryo. In practice, the timeliness of medical needs should be the primary consideration in deciding the timing of the examination.

From National Council of Radiation Protection and Measurements (NCRP): *Medical x-ray, electron beam, and gamma-ray protection up to 50 MeV (equipment, design, performance, and use)*, Report No. 102, Bethesda, Md, 1989, NCRP.

| BOX 12-7 | **Position of the National Council of Radiation Protection and Measurements Concerning Risk and Fetal Exposure with Regard to Termination of Pregnancy** |
| --- | --- |

This risk is considered to be negligible at a fetal absorbed dose of 5 cGy or less when compared with other risks during pregnancy. The chance of malformations is significantly increased above control levels only at doses beyond 15 cGy. Therefore, the exposure of the fetus to radiation arising from diagnostic procedures would rarely be cause, by itself, for terminating a pregnancy. If there are reasons other than possible radiation effects to consider a therapeutic abortion, the attending physician should discuss those reasons with the patient so that it is clear that the radiation exposure is not being used as an excuse for terminating the pregnancy.

Adapted from National Council on Radiation Protection and Measurements (NCRP): *Radiation protection in pediatric radiology*, Report No. 68, Washington, DC, 1977, NCRP.

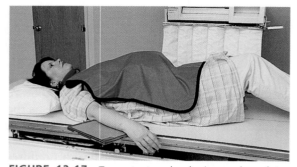

**FIGURE 12-17** To protect a developing embryo-fetus from unnecessary radiation exposure, place a lead apron over the female patient's lower abdomen and pelvic regions when these sites do not have to be included in the area to be irradiated.

made to minimize the dose of radiation the patient receives to her lower abdomen and pelvic regions. This can be accomplished by restrictively selecting technical exposure factors that, while still appropriate for the examination, will produce the smallest exposure needed for a diagnostically useful image and by precisely collimating the radiographic beam to include only the anatomic area of interest. When the patient's lower abdomen and pelvic regions do not have to be included in the area to be irradiated, they should be protected with a lead apron or other suitable protective contact shield so that a developing embryo-fetus does not receive unnecessary radiation exposure (Fig. 12-17).

## SUMMARY

- Effective communication with the patient is the first step in holistic patient care.
  - Imaging procedures should be explained in simple terms.
  - Patients must have an opportunity to ask questions and receive truthful answers within ethical limits.
- Adequate immobilization of the patient is necessary to eliminate voluntary motion.
  - Restraining devices are available to immobilize either the whole body or the individual body part to be radiographed.

- Involuntary motion can be compensated for by shortening exposure time with an appropriate increase in mA and by using very-high-speed image receptors.
- Protective shielding may be used to reduce or eliminate radiation exposure of radiosensitive body organs and tissues.
  - The reproductive organs should be protected from exposure to the useful beam when they are in or within approximately 5 cm of a properly collimated beam, unless this would compromise the diagnostic value of the study.
  - Correctly placed, appropriate gonadal shielding can greatly reduce the exposure received by patients of both sexes (50% reduction for female patients, 90% to 95% reduction for male patients).
- The clear lead shadow shield and a postero-anterior (PA) projection can significantly reduce the dose to the breast of a young patient undergoing a scoliosis examination.
- Appropriate technical exposure factors for each examination must be selected.
  - Techniques chosen should ensure a diagnostic image of optimal quality with minimal patient dose.
  - Standardized technique charts should be available for each x-ray unit to help provide a uniform selection of technical exposure factors. High kVp and lower mAs should be chosen whenever possible to reduce the amount of radiation received by the patient yet maintain acceptable radiographic contrast to ensure the presence of adequate information in the recorded image.
- Correct image processing techniques reduce radiographic exposure for patients by decreasing the need for repeat examinations that result from poorly processed images.
  - Imaging departments should establish a quality control program to ensure standardization in film-processing techniques and processing of digital images.
- An air gap technique can be used as an alternative to the use of a grid.

- Repeat radiographic exposures must be minimized to prevent the patient's skin and gonads from receiving a double dose of radiation.
- Radiographic examinations should be performed only when patients will benefit from useful information gained from the procedure. Nonessential radiologic examinations should not be performed.
- The amount of radiation received by a patient from diagnostic imaging procedures may be specified as entrance skin exposure (ESE) (including skin and glandular), gonadal dose, or bone marrow dose.
  - ESE is the easiest to obtain and most widely used.
  - The estimated genetically significant dose (GSD) for the population of the United States is approximately 0.20 mSv (20 millirem).
- Fluoroscopically guided positioning is an unethical and unacceptable practice that leads to increased patient radiation dose.
- A radiographer should carefully question female patients of childbearing age regarding any possibility of pregnancy before they undergo an x-ray examination.
  - If irradiation of an unknown pregnancy occurs, a calculated estimate of the approximate equivalent dose to the embryo-fetus as a result of the examination should be obtained.
- Nonpalpable breast cancer may be detected through mammography.
  - Federal regulations state that the mean dose to the glandular tissue of a 4.5-cm compressed breast using a screen-film mammography system should not exceed 3 $mGy_t$ per view.
  - Digital mammography units with the ability to enhance contrast with image gray-level manipulation offer improvement for patients with dense breasts.
- Computed tomography (CT) scanning is considered a relatively high-radiation exposure diagnostic procedure because of increasing use of multislice spiral (helical) CT scanners employing small slice thickness.
- Skin dose and dose distribution are two concerns.
- In spiral CT, patient dose is comparable to that of conventional CT when the pitch ratio is approximately 1; patient dose is reduced when pitch is higher and increased when pitch is lower.
- From a radiation protection point of view, the goal of CT imaging should be to obtain the best possible image while delivering an acceptable level of ionizing radiation to the patient.
- The goal of the Alliance for Radiation Safety in Pediatric Imaging is to increase awareness of the need to reduce patient dose for pediatric patients, especially in CT imaging.
- The Image Gently Campaign advocates lowering patient dose by "child sizing" the kV and mA, scanning only the indicated area, and removing multiphase scans from pediatric protocols.
- The objective of the Image Wisely Campaign is to lower the amount of radiation used in medically necessary imaging studies and to eliminate unnecessary procedures.
- Children are much more vulnerable than adults to both the late somatic and genetic effects of ionizing radiation.
  - Use a PA projection to protect the breasts of female patients.
  - In small girls, shielding of the ovaries requires shielding of the iliac wings as well as the sacral area when shielding is needed.
  - Adequate collimation of the radiographic beam to include only the area of clinical interest is essential, and effective immobilization techniques should be used when necessary. The use of a high-mA station and a short exposure time also helps to minimize patient motion.
- A developing embryo-fetus is especially sensitive to exposure from ionizing radiation
  - Use the smallest technical exposure factors that will generate a diagnostically useful radiographic image, carefully collimate

the beam to include only the anatomic area of interest, and cover the lower abdomen and pelvic regions with a suitable contact shield if they do not need to be included in the examination.

- Abdominal radiologic examinations that have been requested after full consideration of the clinical status of a patient, including the possibility of pregnancy, need not be postponed or selectively scheduled.[29]

- Elective abdominal examinations of women of childbearing years should be performed during the first few days after the onset of menses to minimize the possible irradiation of an embryo.

- A radiologic physicist should determine fetal dose if a pregnant patient is inadvertently irradiated.

## REFERENCES

1. Torres LS: *Basic medical techniques and patient care for radiologic technologists*, ed 5, Philadelphia, 1997, Lippincott Williams & Wilkins.
2. Bushong SC: *Radiologic science for technologists: physics, biology and protection*, ed 10, St. Louis, 2013, Mosby.
3. Herrman TL, Fauber TL, Gill J, et al: *White paper: best practices in digital radiography, 2012. American Society of Radiologic Technologists.* Available at: http://www.asrt.org/docs/whitepapers/asrt12_bstpracdigradwhp_final.pdf. Accessed April 12, 2013.
4. Gray J, et al: *Quality control in diagnostic imaging*, Baltimore, 1983, University Park Press.
5. Hendee WR, et al: *Radiologic physics equipment and quality control*, Chicago, 1977, Year Book.
6. McKinney W: *Radiographic processing and quality control*, Philadelphia, 1988, Lippincott.
7. Carter CE, Veale BL: *Digital radiography and PACS*, St. Louis, 2008, Mosby.
8. U.S. Food and Drug Administration (FDA): *Presurgical chest x-ray screening examinations*, FDA Publication No. 86-8265, Washington, DC, 1986, U.S. Government Printing Office.
9. Haynes K, Curtis T: Fluoroscopic vs. blind positioning: comparing entrance skin exposure. *Radiol Technol* 81:1, 2009.
10. American Society of Radiologic Technologists: *ASRT organizational issues: fluoroscoping for positioning.* Available at: http://www.asrt.org/docs/governance/hodpositionstatements66FE1F374C63.pdf. Accessed February 18, 2013.
11. American Registry of Radiologic Technologists: *ARRT Standards of Ethics.* Available at: http://arrt.org/pdfs/Governing-Documents/Standards-of-Ethics.pdf. Accessed on February 18, 2013.
12. Adler A, et al: An analysis of radiographic repeat and reject rates. *Radiol Technol* 63:308, 1992.
13. Leeming BW, et al: A comparison of fluoroscopically controlled patient positioning and conventional positioning, including comparative dosimetry. *Radiology* 124:231, 1977.
14. Huda W, et al: Radiation doses due to breast imaging in Manitoba: 1978-1988. *Radiology* 177:813, 1990.
15. Ritenour ER, Hendee WR: Screening mammography: a risk vs risk decision. *Invest Radiol* 24:17, 1989.
16. Taubes G: The breast-screening brawl. *Science* 275:1056, 1997.
17. Office of the Federal Register: *Federal Register* 67FR (5446) subpart B, section 900.12, e5 (vi), Feb 6, 2002, Washington, DC, U.S. Government Printing Office.
18. Yaffe M, Mawdslwy GE: Equipment requirements and quality control for mammography, in specification, acceptance testing and quality control of diagnostic x-ray imaging equipment. In Siebert JA, Barnes GT, Gould RG, editors: *American Association of Physicists in Medicine medical physics monograph, No. 20,* College Park, Md, 1994, American Association of Physicists in Medicine.
19. Frank ED, et al: *Merrill's atlas of radiographic positioning and procedures*, ed 12, vol 3, St. Louis, 2012, Mosby.
20. European Union, EUR 16262 EN: *European guidelines on quality criteria for computed tomography, May, 1999.* http://w3.tue.nl/fileadmin/sbd/Documenten/Leergang/BSM/European_Guidelines_Quality_Criteria_Computed_Tomography_Eur_16252.pdf. Accessed July 2, 2013.
21. Menoch MJA, et al: *Trends in* computed tomography utilization in the pediatric emergency department, *Pediatrics,* 2012; 129; e690 originally, published on line February 13, 2012, DOI: 10.1542/peds.2011-2545. http://pediatrics.aappublications.org/content/129/3/e690.full.html. Accessed July 2, 2013.
22. Preston DL, et al: Solid cancer incidence in atomic bomb survivors exposed in utero or as young children. *J Natl Cancer Inst* 100:428, 2008.
23. Doody MM, Lonstein JE, Stovall M, et al: Breast cancer mortality after diagnostic radiography: findings from the U.S. Scoliosis Cohort Study. *Spine (Phila Pa, 1976)* 25:2052, 2000.
24. National Academy of Sciences Committee on Biological Effects of Ionizing Radiation: *Report VII: health risks from exposure to low levels of ionizing*

*radiation*, Washington, DC, 2005, National Academies Press.

25. Image Wisely: http://www.imagewisely.org/. Accessed February 18, 2013.

26. Beebe GW, et al: Studies of the mortality of A-bomb survivors. 6. Mortality and radiation dose, 1950-1974. *Radiat Res* 75:138, 1978.

27. National Council on Radiation Protection and Measurements (NCRP): *Radiation protection in pediatric radiology*, Report No. 68, Washington, DC, 1981, NCRP.

28. Bontrager KL: *Textbook of positioning and related anatomy*, ed 4, St. Louis, 1997, Mosby.

29. Reynold FB: Prepared remarks for the October 20, 1976, American College of Radiology press conference.

30. National Council on Radiation Protection and Measurements (NCRP): *Medical x-ray, electron beam and gamma-ray protection up to 50 MeV (equipment design, performance and use)*, Report No. 102, Bethesda, Md, 1989, NCRP.

31. National Council on Radiation Protection and Measurements (NCRP): *Medical exposure of pregnant and potentially pregnant women*, Report No. 54, Washington, DC, 1977, NCRP.

## GENERAL DISCUSSION QUESTIONS

1. How does the patient benefit from effective communication with the radiographer during an imaging procedure?

2. What can the radiographer do to eliminate the problem of voluntary patient motion, and how can involuntary motion be compensated for during radiography?

3. When should gonadal shielding not be used during a diagnostic imaging procedure?

4. Why should a radiographer use a standardized technique chart to select technical exposure factors before performing an imaging procedure?

5. Why are correct radiographic processing and establishment of a quality control program important for imaging departments that use screen-film image receptors or digital imaging display equipment?

6. How does an air gap technique reduce scattered radiation?

7. How can the dose to the breast of a young female patient be reduced when a radiographic examination for scoliosis is performed?

8. When is a radiographic examination considered nonessential? Give some examples.

9. Describe three ways in which the amount of radiation received by a patient from diagnostic imaging procedures may be specified.

10. What does the genetically significant dose take into consideration?

11. Why is it unacceptable to use fluoroscopically guided positioning?

12. How should irradiation of an unknown pregnancy be handled?

13. How can dose reduction in mammography be achieved?

14. What is the goal of CT imaging from a radiation protection point of view?

15. How do children compare with adults with regard to the potential for biologic damage from exposure to ionizing radiation?

16. What steps in CT imaging are being taken to reduce radiation exposure for children?

17. What is the position of the American College of Radiology (ACR) regarding abdominal radiologic examinations of pregnant or potentially pregnant patients?

18. What are the benefits of using a pediatric designed x-ray room for young children?

19. How is a thermoluminescent dosimeter (TLD) used to measure skin dose?

20. What is meant by *standardized exposure techniques*?

## REVIEW QUESTIONS

1. As a consequence of their anatomic location, the female reproductive organs receive about _____ exposure during a given radiographic procedure involving the pelvic region than do the male reproductive organs.
   A. Three times less
   B. Three times more
   C. Ten times less
   D. Ten times more

**2.** In fluoroscopy, how is the amount of radiation that a patient receives usually estimated?
   A. By having the patient wear an optically stimulated luminescence (OSL) dosimeter during the procedure
   B. By measuring the radiation exposure rate at tabletop and multiplying this by the milliamperage (mA) and kilovoltage (kVp) settings
   C. By measuring the radiation exposure rate at tabletop and multiplying this by the fluoroscopy time
   D. By placing an ionization-type survey meter next to the patient during the procedure to record the dose received

**3.** Direct patient shielding is not typically used in:
   A. CT.
   B. Conventional fluoroscopy.
   C. Digital fluoroscopy.
   D. Digital radiography.

**4.** In which of the following projections will a young female patient receive a significantly lower dose to her breast tissue during a chest x-ray study?
   A. AP
   B. AP lordotic
   C. PA
   D. Lateral

**5.** A woman who is 3 months pregnant has been in a motor vehicle accident. The emergency room physician suspects there is injury to her cervical spine and thus feels justified in ordering an x-ray examination to aid in determining the extent of the patient's injury. Because the patient is pregnant, the radiographer should:
   1. Select the smallest technical exposure factors that will produce a diagnostically useful image.
   2. Adequately and precisely collimate the radiographic beam to include only the anatomic area of interest.
   3. Shield the patient's lower abdomen and pelvic region with a suitable protective contact shield.

   A. 1 only
   B. 2 only
   C. 3 only
   D. 1, 2, and 3

**6.** Pediatric patients require special consideration and appropriate radiation protection procedures because they are more vulnerable to which of the following?
   A. Both the late somatic effects and genetic effects of radiation
   B. Only the late somatic effects of radiation
   C. Only the genetic effects of radiation
   D. Only the early somatic effects of radiation

**7.** The use of the PA projection during a juvenile scoliosis radiographic examination results in which of the following?
   A. Higher entrance exposure dose to the anterior body surface, thereby significantly increasing the dose to the breast
   B. Lower entrance exposure dose to the anterior body surface, thereby significantly reducing the dose to the breast
   C. Poorer-quality images that necessitate a repeat examination
   D. Images that do not adequately demonstrate spinal curvature

**8.** Federal regulations in the United States for Food and Drug Administration Certification of screening mammography facilities state that the mean dose to the glandular tissue of a 4.5-cm compressed breast using a screen-film mammography system should *not* exceed which of the following?
   A. 1 $mGy_t$ per view
   B. 3 $mGy_t$ per view
   C. 5 $mGy_t$ per view
   D. 7 $mGy_t$ per view

**9.** Which of the following examinations are considered to be unnecessary radiologic procedures?
   1. Chest x-ray study as part of a preemployment physical

2. Screening mammography
3. Whole-body multislice spiral CT
   screening
A. 1 and 2 only
B. 1 and 3 only
C. 2 and 3 only
D. 1, 2, and 3

**10.** If a maximum of 500 people were inhabiting the earth and each person were to receive an equivalent dose (EqD) of 0.005 Sv gonadal radiation, the gross genetic effect would be _____ the effect occurring if 50 individual inhabitants were each to receive 0.05 Sv of gonadal radiation and no equivalent dose were received by other inhabitants.
A. Greatly different from
B. Slightly different from
C. Almost the same as
D. Identical to

## CHAPTER 13

# Management of Imaging Personnel Radiation Dose during Diagnostic X-Ray Procedures

## OBJECTIVES

*After completing this chapter, the reader will be able to perform the following:*

- State the annual occupational effective dose limit for whole-body exposure of diagnostic imaging personnel during routine operations, and explain the significance of the ALARA (as low as reasonably achievable) concept for these individuals.
- Explain the reason that occupational exposure of diagnostic imaging personnel must be limited, and state the most important reason for allowing a larger equivalent dose for radiation workers than for the population as a whole.
- Identify the type of x-radiation that poses the greatest occupational hazard in diagnostic radiology, and explain the various ways this hazard can be significantly reduced.
- Explain how the various methods and techniques that reduce patient exposure during a diagnostic examination can also reduce exposure for the radiographer and any other personnel.
- Discuss the responsibilities of the employer for protecting declared pregnant diagnostic imaging personnel from radiation exposure.

- List and explain the three basic principles of radiation protection that can be used for personnel exposure reduction.
- State and explain the inverse square law, and solve mathematical problems applying this concept.
- Explain the purpose of a diagnostic-type protective tube housing, differentiate between a primary and a secondary protective barrier, and list examples of such barriers.
- Describe the construction of protective structural shielding, and list the factors that govern the selection of appropriate construction materials.
- List and describe the protective garments that may be worn to reduce whole-body or partial-body exposure, and discuss the circumstances in which such garments are worn.
- Explain the various methods and devices that may be used to reduce exposure for personnel during routine fluoroscopic examinations and during interventional procedures that use high-level-control fluoroscopy.
- Explain the various methods and devices that may be used to reduce the radiographer's exposure when performing a mobile radiographic examination.

Copyright © 2014, Elsevier Inc.

- Explain the variation in dose rate caused by scatter radiation near the entrance and exit surfaces of the patient during C-arm fluoroscopy, and discuss methods of dose reduction for C-arm operators.
- Describe methods used to provide patient restraint during a diagnostic x-ray procedure, and identify individuals who could use these methods.
- List the three categories of radiation sources that may be generated in an x-ray room; list

the considerations on which the design of radiation-absorbent barriers should be based; and explain the importance of each.
- Differentiate between a controlled area and an uncontrolled area.
- Discuss current approaches to shielding design.
- Discuss the requirements for posting caution signs for radioactive materials and radiation areas.

## CHAPTER OUTLINE

## KEY TERMS

Bucky slot shielding device
control-booth barrier
controlled area
cumulative effective dose
    (CumEfD) limit
diagnostic-type protective tube
    housing
distance

genetically significant dose
    (GSD)
inverse square law (ISL)
leakage radiation
occupancy factor (T)
occupational risk
primary protective barrier
primary radiation

scatter radiation
secondary protective barrier
shielding
time
uncontrolled area
use factor (U)
workload (W)

While fulfilling professional responsibilities associated with diagnostic imaging, radiographers may be exposed to secondary radiation (scatter or leakage). Some x-ray procedures increase the radiographer's risk of exposure (Box 13-1). When participating in any procedure that may result in occupational exposure, the radiographer must employ appropriate methods of protection against ionizing radiation. This chapter presents an overview of methods that can be used to reduce exposure for imaging professionals during diagnostic x-ray procedures.

## ANNUAL LIMIT FOR OCCUPATIONALLY EXPOSED PERSONNEL

### Effective Dose Limits

Federal government standards, following a recommendation of the National Council on Radiation

Protection and Measurements (NCRP) (discussed in Chapter 10), permit diagnostic imaging personnel to receive an "annual occupational effective dose (EfD) of 50 millisievert (mSv) (5 rem)"[1] for whole-body exposure during routine operations. However, in keeping with the as low as reasonably achievable (ALARA) policy, and diligent supervision of personnel cumulative radiation exposure records, no radiographer should ever occupationally approach this effective dose level. This effective dose does not include:

- Personal medical exposure
- Natural background exposure

To ensure that the lifetime risk of occupationally exposed personnel remains acceptable, an additional recommendation indicates that the *lifetime effective dose* in millisieverts should not exceed 10 times the person's age in years. Hence a **cumulative effective dose (CumEfD) limit** has been established for the whole body that limits a radiation worker's lifetime effective dose to his or her age in years times 10 mSv (years × 1 rem).

### Annual Occupational and Nonoccupational Effective Dose Limits

The annual occupational effective dose limit of 50 mSv is an upper boundary limit. It is greater than the annual effective dose limit allowed for

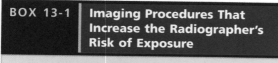

| BOX 13-1 | Imaging Procedures That Increase the Radiographer's Risk of Exposure |
|---|---|

- General fluoroscopy
- Interventional procedures that employ high-level-control fluoroscopy (HLCF)
- Mobile examinations
- General radiographic procedures
- C-arm fluoroscopy

individual members of the general population not occupationally exposed. That limit is:

- 1 mSv (0.1 rem) for continuous or frequent exposures from artificial sources other than medical irradiation and natural background radiation[1]
- 5 mSv (0.5 rem) for infrequent annual exposure[1]

The 1-mSv annual effective dose limit set for members of the general public is designed to limit that exposure "to reasonable levels of risk comparable with risks from other common sources—i.e., about $10^{-4}$ to $10^{-6}$ annually"[1] ($10^{-4}$ to $10^{-6}$ means an excess cancer risk of 1 chance in 10,000 to 1 chance in 1 million per year). The 5-mSv maximal annual effective dose limit recommendation "is made because annual exposures in excess of the 1-mSv recommendation, usually to a small group of people, need not be regarded as especially hazardous, provided it does not occur often to the same groups and that the average exposure to individuals in these groups does not exceed an average annual effective dose of about 1 mSv."[1] Both these limits "will keep the annual equivalent dose to those organs and tissues that are considered in the effective dose system below levels of concern for deterministic effects."[1]

## Allowance for a Larger Equivalent Dose for Radiation Workers

Valid reasons exist for allowance of a larger equivalent dose (EqD) (the product of the average absorbed dose [D] in a tissue or organ in the human body and its associated radiation weighting factor [$W_R$] chosen for the type and energy of the radiation in question [see Chapter 4 for additional information]) for radiation workers. Among the most important of these reasons is that the workforce in radiation-related jobs is small when compared with the population as a whole.

Thus, the amount of radiation received by this workforce can be larger than the amount received by the general public without alteration in the **genetically significant dose (GSD)**, the average annual gonadal EqD to members of the population who are of childbearing age (see Chapter 12). Although the radiographer and other diagnostic imaging personnel are allowed to absorb more radiation, the EqD received must be minimized whenever possible. This reduces the potential for:

- Somatic damage
- Genetic (hereditary) damage

## ALARA CONCEPT

In addition to the effective dose limiting system, another radiation protection principle exists—the ALARA concept. As defined in Chapter 10, this concept holds that actual effective and EqD values of the radiographer and other occupationally exposed persons, with consideration of economic and social factors, should be kept well below their allowable maximal limits. The best way for radiologists and radiographers to do this is to conscientiously employ all appropriate radiation-control procedures such as:

- Whenever applicable, applying the basic principles of time, distance, and shielding
- Always adequately collimating the radiographic beam (Fig. 13-1)

Because continual use of such radiation protection awareness procedures ensures a high degree of safety from most radiation exposures, radiography is not considered a hazardous profession. The **occupational risk** that nevertheless always resides in the background is the possibility, however slight, of developing a future radiogenic cancer or the induction of a genetic defect as a consequence of whatever cumulative radiation exposure is received. For monitored diagnostic imaging personnel it may be compared with the occupational risk for persons employed in other industries generally considered reasonably safe such as:

- Government
- Trade

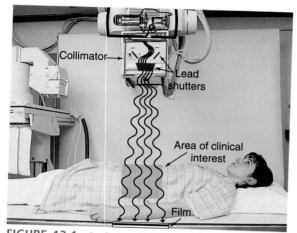

**FIGURE 13-1** Radiographic beam collimation (restricting the x-ray beam to the area of clinical interest) limits the production of scattered radiation. This radiation-control procedure helps keep the radiographer's occupational exposure as low as reasonably achievable (ALARA).

These jobs have a risk of fatal accidents generally estimated to be approximately $1 \times 10^{-4} \ y^{-1}$.[1] The annual risk for radiation workers who conscientiously apply their skills is unlikely to exceed this rate.

## DOSE-REDUCTION METHODS AND TECHNIQUES

### Avoiding Repeat Examinations

Methods and techniques that reduce patient exposure can also reduce exposure for the radiographer. For example, when using digital imaging systems or conventional screen-film portable (mobile) systems, minimizing repeat exposures will decrease the chance of additional occupational exposure. Other such considerations are identified in this chapter.

### The Patient as a Source of Scattered Radiation

During any diagnostic x-ray examination, the patient becomes a source of scattered radiation as a consequence of the Compton interaction process (see Chapter 3). At a 90-degree angle to the primary x-ray beam, at a distance of 1 m, the scattered x-ray intensity is generally approximately $\frac{1}{1000}$ of the intensity of the primary x-ray beam.

## Scattered Radiation—Occupational Hazard

Because scattered radiation poses the greatest occupational hazard in diagnostic radiology, the use of any device or appropriate technique that lessens the amount of scattered radiation significantly reduces occupational exposure of diagnostic imaging personnel. Beam limitation devices, such as automatic collimation or positive beam limitation (PBL), restrict the size of the radiographic beam so that its margins do not extend beyond the image receptor. This reduction in beam size decreases the number of x-ray photons available to undergo Compton scatter. Because scatter is reduced, the radiographer's occupational exposure is diminished.

## Filtration of the Diagnostic X-Ray Beam

When a radiographic beam is properly filtered, nonuseful low-energy photons are removed from the primary beam. Without proper filtration, a relatively high percentage of the normally excluded low-energy photons will interact with the tissues of the patient's body. Some of these photons undergo Compton scatter. The radiographer's EqD could therefore increase as a result of exposure to this excess scattered radiation. Most of these low-energy photons, however, are absorbed in the patient, thereby increasing the patient's absorbed dose and contributing nothing to the radiographic image. Thus filtration primarily benefits the patient.

## Protective Apparel

Protective lead aprons (Fig. 13-2, *A*) and shielded barriers (Fig. 13-2, *B*) function as gonadal shields for diagnostic imaging personnel. These devices protect personnel from secondary (scatter and leakage) radiation. Like protective gloves that are used to cover the hands of radiologists or

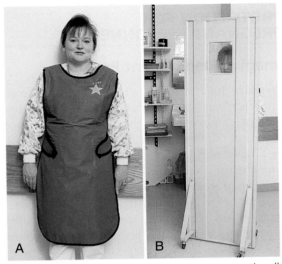

**FIGURE 13-2** **A,** A lead apron protects occupationally exposed personnel from scattered radiation. **B,** A lead mobile x-ray barrier of 0.5- or 1.0-mm lead equivalent provides protection from scattered radiation. It may be used during special procedures, in the operating room, and in cardiac units.

| TABLE 13-1 | Physical Attributes of Protective Lead Aprons | | | |
|---|---|---|---|---|
| **Percentage X-Ray Attenuation** | | | | |
| **Lead Equivalent Thickness (mm)** | **Weight (kg)** | **Kilovolts at Peak** | | |
| | | **50** | **75** | **100** |
| 0.25 | 1-5 | 97 | 66 | 51 |
| 0.50 | 3-7 | 99.9 | 88 | 75 |
| 1.00 | 5-12 | 99.9 | 99 | 94 |

At 100 kVp, x-ray attenuation for a 0.50-mm lead equivalent apron and a 1-mm lead equivalent apron is 75% and 94%, respectively.

Modified from Bushong SC: *Radiologic science for technologists: physics, biology and protection,* ed 10, St. Louis, 2013, Mosby.

radiographers when they must be in or near the primary x-ray beam, the garments are available in various thicknesses such as 0.25, 0.5, and 1 mm of lead equivalent.[2] Higher lead equivalents in protective apparel provide greater protection from radiation exposure. However, for practical use in the clinical setting, the weight of the garment must also be considered, along with the approximate length of time that it will be worn. An apron containing 1 mm lead equivalent may weigh as much as 12 kg.[2] Wearing this protective device for a lengthy procedure can result in considerable back strain for the wearer. Depending on the energy range of the radiation for a specific procedure, an apron containing the standard lead equivalent of 0.5 mm or an apron containing the minimum required lead equivalent of 0.25 mm may be sufficient for use. The standard 0.5-mm lead equivalent apron, traditionally worn during routine fluoroscopic procedures, weighs 3 to 7 kg, whereas the 0.25-mm minimum lead equivalent apron can weigh 1 to 5 kg.[2] Some physical attributes of protective lead aprons, including the percentage of x-ray attenuation at selective peak kilovoltages (kVps), are listed in Table 13-1.

In the event that any personnel could have the posterior surface of their body turned toward the x-ray source during a radiologic procedure, a wrap around-style apron would afford the best protection. However, this style of apron, encircling the body and covering it from the shoulders to the knees with a 1 mm lead equivalent, has a considerable amount of weight. When taking both the amount of protection provided by an apron and its weight into consideration, the 0.5-mm lead equivalent apron provides a relatively good compromise for use.

To preserve the integrity of all protective apparel, it must be stored correctly when not in use. Lead aprons should be hung on racks or draped over a bar designed for storage to prevent unnecessary damage. They should never be folded or crunched up in any fashion because this poor practice will lead to damage to the leaded material such as cracks or breaks, thus compromising the device's effectiveness for protection from radiation. To ensure the integrity of protective apparel, all aprons should be inspected on a yearly basis for cracks or other defects either by fluoroscopy or by radiographing each area of the apparel with a high-kVp technique.

## Technical Exposure Factors

Technical exposure factors can influence the quantity of scattered radiation produced and reaching imaging personnel. For lower kVps, more mA is needed to secure a high-quality image, and therefore there are greater numbers of low-energy photons present. These characteristics of the x-ray beam lend themselves to the production of increased large-angle scatter radiation. Conversely, higher-kVp techniques:

- Increase the mean energy of the photons comprising the radiographic beam
- Require lower photon beam intensity (i.e., lower mA)

As the average energy of the beam increases, the percentage of radiation that is forward-scattered increases. Therefore, less side-scattered radiation is available to strike imaging personnel, and their EqD is reduced.

## Use of High-Speed Image Receptor Systems

When high-speed image receptor systems are used, smaller radiographic exposure is required. Consequently, fewer x-ray photons are available to produce Compton scatter, and as a result personnel exposure is decreased.

## Repeats in Digital Imaging

Chapter 11 noted that because the image contrast and overall brightness in digital imaging can be manipulated after image acquisition, the need for almost all repeats as a result of improper technique selection has been eliminated. However, repeats necessitated by mispositioning can still occur, resulting in a repeat examination that will cause additional radiation exposure to both the patient and possibly the technologist. Care must be taken by the technologist to correctly position the patient and the equipment initially.

## Correct Processing of Radiographic Images

Correct processing of radiographic images also leads to a decrease in the number of repeat examinations required.

# PROTECTION FOR PREGNANT PERSONNEL

## Imaging Department Protocol

Pregnant staff members should be able to continue performing their duties without interruption of employment if they follow established radiation safety practices. Most health care facilities have policies for protecting pregnant personnel from radiation. Under these policies, an imaging professional who becomes pregnant first informs her supervisor. After this voluntary declaration has been made, the health care facility officially recognizes the pregnancy. The facility, through its radiation safety officer:

- Provides essential counseling
- Furnishes an appropriate additional radiation monitor or badge

This secondary dosimeter is to be attached at the waist level during all radiation procedures. When a protective lead apron is used, the dosimeter should be worn at waist level beneath the garment. The purpose of this additional monitor is to ensure that the monthly EqD to the embryo-fetus does not exceed 0.5 mSv (0.05 rem). This EqD limit excludes both:

- Medical radiation
- Natural background radiation

It is designed to significantly restrict the total lifetime risk of leukemia and other malignancies in persons exposed in utero.

## Acknowledgment of Counseling and Understanding of Radiation Safety Measures

After receiving radiation safety counseling, the pregnant radiologic technologist must read and sign a form acknowledging that she has received counseling and understands the practices to be followed to ensure the safety of the embryo-fetus. For monitoring of pregnant personnel, dosimeter companies provide a separate monthly report that tracks the exposure of the worker and the embryo-fetus. A copy of this report is sent to the health care facility's radiation safety officer.

## Protective Maternity Apparel

Protective maternity apparel, when needed, should be available for pregnant radiologists and radiographers. Specially designed maternity protective aprons consist of 0.5-mm lead equivalent over their entire length and width and also have an extra 1 mm lead equivalent protective panel that runs transversely across the width of the apron to provide added safety for the embryo-fetus.

Wraparound protective aprons of 0.5 mm lead equivalent can also be used during pregnancy. The overall physical size of the apron must be appropriate for the pregnant worker to ensure safety and provide reasonable comfort.

## Work Schedule Alteration

In accordance with ALARA guidelines, work schedules are designed to distribute radiation exposure risk evenly to all employees. If a declared pregnant radiographer is reassigned to a lower radiation exposure risk area (e.g., removed from interventional fluoroscopy and assigned to general radiography), then the remaining radiographers in the higher risk area who must fill in can be subject to increased risk. Therefore, the declared pregnant radiographer does not necessarily need to be reassigned to a lower radiation exposure position as a direct consequence of a declared pregnancy. However, it is imperative that, while remaining in her current position, the EqD to the embryo-fetus from occupational exposure of the mother not exceed the NCRP recommended monthly EqD limit of 0.5 mSv (0.05 rem) or a limit of 5.0 mSv (0.50 rem) during the entire pregnancy (see Chapter 10).

## BASIC PRINCIPLES OF RADIATION PROTECTION FOR PERSONNEL EXPOSURE REDUCTION

As stated in Chapter 1, the three basic principles of radiation protection are:

- Time
- Distance
- Shielding

Occupational radiation exposure of imaging personnel can be minimized by the use of these cardinal principles. Decreasing the length of time spent in a room where x-radiation is being produced, standing at the greatest distance possible from an energized x-ray beam, and interposing radiation-absorbent material between oneself and the source of radiation reduce occupational exposure.

## Time

The amount of radiation a worker receives is directly proportional to the length of **time** the individual is in the path of ionizing radiation. During fluoroscopy, reduced exposure time will decrease both:

- Patient exposure
- Personnel exposure

For this reason, most fluoroscopic x-ray units are equipped with 5-minute timers to alert the radiologist or other authorized equipment operator that a specific period of time has elapsed. To minimize radiation exposure, a radiographer therefore should be present in a fluoroscopy room only when needed to perform relevant patient care and to fulfill the respective duties associated with the procedure. Otherwise, the radiographer should remain behind a protective barrier.

## Distance

**Distance** is the most effective means of protection from ionizing radiation. Imaging personnel receive significantly less radiation exposure by standing farther away from a source of radiation because there is a significant decrease in the radiation level.

**Application of the Inverse Square Law.** The **inverse square law** (ISL) expresses the relationship between distance and intensity (quantity) of

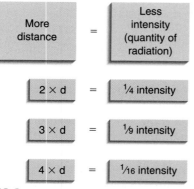

**FIGURE 13-3**  As the distance between the source of radiation and any given measurement point increases, radiation intensity (quantity) measured at that point decreases by the square of the relative change in distance between the new location and the old.

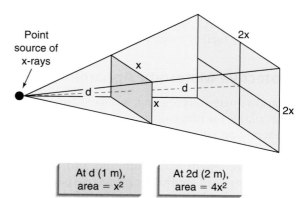

**FIGURE 13-4**  When the distance from a point source of radiation is doubled, the radiation at the new location spans an area four times larger than the original area. However, the intensity at the new distance is only one fourth of the original intensity.

radiation and governs the dose received. The law is stated as "The intensity of radiation is inversely proportional to the square of the distance from the source."

To be more precise, as the separation between the radiation source and a measurement point increases, the quantity of radiation measured at the more distant position decreases by the square of the ratio of the original distance from the source to the new distance from the source (Fig. 13-3). This decrease in radiation intensity physically occurs because the area, which the same flux of x-rays at the original location now covers at the new location, has increased by the square of the relative distance change. For example, when the distance from the x-ray target, a point source* of radiation, is doubled, the radiation at the new location spans an area four times

larger than the original area. However, because the same amount of radiation exists to cover this larger area, the intensity at the new distance consequently decreases by a factor of four (Fig. 13-4).

The ISL may be stated as a formula, shown in the equation in Box 13-2. A mathematical example is also provided. The ISL should be used, whenever possible, to reduce the radiographer's exposure from sources of x-radiation. (This law also may be applied to sources of gamma and neutron radiation.)

The ISL also implies that if a radiographer moves closer to a source of radiation, his or her radiation exposure dramatically increases. For example, if the radiographer stands 2 m away from an x-ray source instead of 6 m away, the radiographer's radiation exposure increases by a factor of $(6/2)^2 = 9$.

## Shielding

When it is not possible to use the principles of time and/or distance to minimize occupational radiation exposure, protective **shielding** of appropriate thickness may be used to provide protection from radiation. The most common materials used for structural protective barriers are:

---

*Point source: To be able to treat finite-sized radioactive sources as "point sources" correctly to facilitate the calculation of exposure rates at points of interest, it is necessary that the distance of such points from the radioactive source be at least equal to 10 times the largest dimension of the source. As an example of this concept, consider a spherical radioactive source whose diameter is 2.5 cm. Then the smallest distance away from this source at which it may be accurate enough to regard it mathematically as a "point source" will be 25 cm (10 inches).

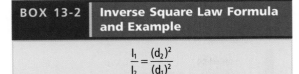

**BOX 13-2** | **Inverse Square Law Formula and Example**

$$\frac{I_1}{I_2} = \frac{(d_2)^2}{(d_1)^2}$$

where $I_1$ expresses the exposure (intensity) at the original distance, $I_2$ expresses the exposure (intensity) at the new distance, $d_1$ expresses the original distance from the source of radiation, and $d_2$ expresses the new distance from the source of radiation.

**Example:** If a radiographer stands 1 m away from an x-ray tube and is subject to an exposure rate dose* of 2 mGy$_a$ per hour, what will it be if the same radiographer moves to a position located 2 m from the x-ray tube?

Answer:

$$\frac{I_1}{I_2} = \frac{(d_2)^2}{(d_1)^2}$$

$$\frac{2}{I_2} = \frac{(2)^2}{(1)^2}$$

$$\frac{2}{I_2} = \frac{4}{1} \text{ (cross-multiply)}$$

$$4I_2 = 2$$

$$I_2 = 0.5 \, mGy_a/hr$$

*Exposure rate dose given in units of mGy$_a$ per hour is the same quantity as air kerma rate.

- Lead
- Concrete

Accessory protective devices are made of lead-impregnated vinyl. These accessory devices include:

- Aprons
- Gloves
- Thyroid shields
- Protective eyeglasses

This apparel provides protection from ionizing radiation when it is not possible to remain behind either a stationary or movable protective barrier. The effectiveness of shielding materials (i.e., their ability to attenuate radiation) depends on their atomic number, density, and thickness.

**Protective Structural Shielding.** Structural barriers such as walls and doors in an x-ray room have been designed to provide radiation shielding for both:

- Imaging department personnel
- The general public

This protection is necessary to ensure that occupational and nonoccupational annual effective dose limits are not exceeded. Lead sheets of appropriate thickness that are placed in the walls of the radiography or fluoroscopy room are generally used to provide proper shielding. A qualified medical physicist determines the exact protection requirements for a particular imaging facility. Radiographers should understand the concept of shielding but are not responsible for determining barrier thickness.

*Primary Protective Barrier.* The purpose of a **primary protective barrier** is to prevent direct, or unscattered, radiation from reaching personnel or members of the general public on the other side of the barrier. The primary beam is made up of the x-ray photons that follow straight-line paths through all sets of collimator shutters. Primary protective barriers are located perpendicular to the undeflected line of travel of the x-ray beam (Fig. 13-5).

If the peak energy of the beam is 130 kVp, the primary protective barrier in a typical installation:

- Consists of 1.6 mm (1/16 inch) lead
- Extends 2.1 m (7 feet) upward from the floor of the x-ray room, when the x-ray tube is 1.5 to 2.1 m (5 to 7 feet) from the wall in question

*Secondary Protective Barrier.* Secondary radiation consists of radiation that has been deflected from the primary beam. Leakage from the tube housing (photons that pass through the housing because the lead shielding around the tube for practical reasons cannot be made perfect) and scatter (primarily from the patient) make up the secondary radiation. A **secondary protective barrier** protects against leakage and scatter radiation. Any wall or barrier that is never struck by

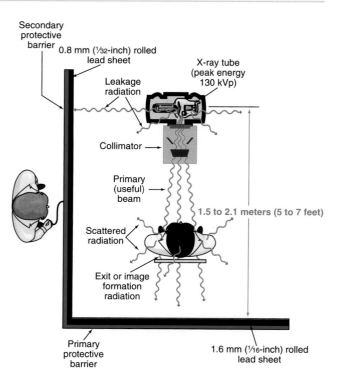

Secondary protective barrier
0.8 mm (1/32-inch) rolled lead sheet

X-ray tube (peak energy 130 kVp)

Leakage radiation

Collimator

Primary (useful) beam

1.5 to 2.1 meters (5 to 7 feet)

Scattered radiation

Exit or image formation radiation

Primary protective barrier

1.6 mm (1/16-inch) rolled lead sheet

**FIGURE 13-5** Protective barriers are lined with lead to protect personnel and the general public from radiation. The primary protective barrier is located perpendicular to the undeflected line of travel of the x-ray beam. The walls that are not in the direct line of travel of the primary beam are called *secondary protective barriers* because they are designed to shield against secondary (leakage and scattered) radiation.

the primary x-ray beam is classified as a secondary barrier (see Fig. 13-5). This does not mean that secondary radiation cannot hit primary barriers as well. A secondary barrier should overlap the primary protective barrier by approximately 1.27 cm (1/2 inch). In a typical installation, the secondary barrier consists of 0.8 mm (1/32 inch) lead.

*Control-Booth Barrier.* X-ray rooms housing permanent or nonportable radiographic equipment contain a **control-booth barrier** for the protection of the radiographer. This barrier must:

- Extend 2.1 m (7 feet) upward from the floor
- Be permanently secured to the floor

Diagnostic x-rays should scatter a minimum of two times before reaching any area behind this barrier. Because this booth is situated so that it intercepts leakage and scattered radiation only, it may be regarded as a secondary protective barrier. To ensure maximum protection during

radiographic exposures, personnel must remain completely behind the barrier. The radiographer may observe the patient through the lead glass window in the booth (Fig. 13-6). This window typically consists of 1.5 mm lead equivalent. With the appropriate lead equivalent in the barrier, exposure of the radiographer will not exceed a maximum allowance of 1 mSv (100 mrem) per week; in actual practice in a well-designed facility, exposure should not exceed 0.02 mSv (2 mrem) per week. For further protection, the exposure cord must be short enough that the exposure switch can be operated only when the radiographer is completely behind the control-booth barrier.

*Clear Lead-Acrylic Secondary Protective Barrier.* Clear lead-acrylic material impregnated with approximately 30% lead by weight may be fashioned into an effective secondary protective barrier, such as for the control booth (Fig. 13-7). This creates a modern appearance for the facility

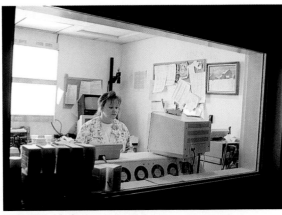

**FIGURE 13-6** While making a radiographic exposure with a stationary radiographic unit, the radiographer must remain completely within the control-booth barrier (behind the fixed protective barrier) for safety. The radiographer may observe the patient through the lead glass observation window in the control booth.

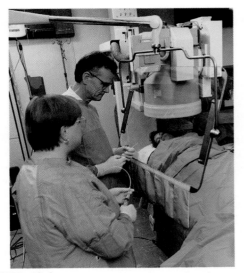

**FIGURE 13-8** A clear lead-acrylic overhead protective barrier used during special procedures and cardiac catheterization.

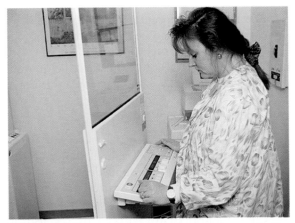

**FIGURE 13-7** A clear lead-acrylic secondary protective barrier impregnated with approximately 30% lead lends a modern appearance to the facility.

*Clear Lead-Acrylic Overhead Protective Barrier.* Clear lead-acrylic protective barriers also can be used as overhead x-ray barriers to provide an open view during special procedures and cardiac catheterization (Fig. 13-8). This shielding typically offers 0.5 mm lead equivalency protection.

**Accessory Protective Devices.** As mentioned previously, accessory protective shielding includes aprons, gloves, and thyroid shields made of lead-impregnated vinyl. These protective garments are available in a variety of:

- Shapes
- Sizes
- Thicknesses

As lead equivalent thickness increases, attenuation of the x-ray beam also increases when kVp remains the same. However, the physical burden from the protective apron grows as lead equivalent thickness increases. To reduce the possibility of back or neck problems, other materials may be used in the protective apron to lessen its weight. Some garments, for example, are impregnated with tin[2] or similar metals because the electron shell structures of these substances offer

and permits a panoramic view, allowing diagnostic imaging personnel to observe the patient more completely. Modular x-ray barriers:

- Are shatter resistant
- Can extend 2.1 m (7 feet) upward from the floor
- Are available in lead equivalency from 0.3 to 2 mm

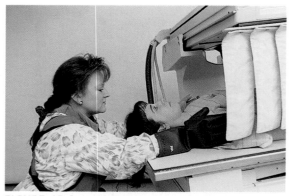

**FIGURE 13-9**    A lead apron, gloves, and thyroid shield protect the radiographer from scattered radiation.

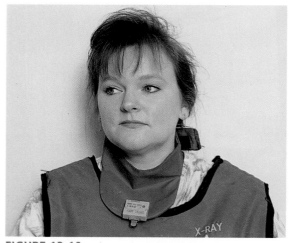

**FIGURE 13-10**    The neck and thyroid gland can be protected from radiation exposure through the use of a 0.5-mm lead equivalent protective shield.

advantages in terms of a more probable photoelectric interaction attenuation than does lead in the lower diagnostic x-ray energy range.

**Lead Aprons and Gloves.** If the radiographer's hands will be near the x-ray beam, protective lead aprons and leaded gloves should be used whenever the radiographer cannot remain behind a protective barrier during an exposure (Fig. 13-9). Historically from regulatory doctrine, if the peak energy of the x-ray beam was 100 kVp, then a protective apron must be equivalent to at least a 0.25-mm thickness of lead. An apron of 0.5 mm lead equivalent, however, affords much greater protection and is the most widely used and recommended thickness in diagnostic imaging and, in fact, is the minimum lead equivalent required for a protective garment worn by occupationally exposed individuals during fluoroscopic or interventional procedures. Thus regardless of this regulatory mention of 0.25-mm thicknesses of lead for some purposes, the need for 0.5 mm lead equivalent for fluoroscopy and interventional purposes and the recommendations from various authorities that 0.5 mm lead aprons are desirable for all purposes have induced most facilities to stock personal shielding devices of this nature only. This eliminates the possibility of personnel inadvertently selecting the wrong apron. Lead apron thicknesses of 0.25, 0.5, and 1.0 are all commercially available: 0.25 mm of lead is very appropriate for use in mammography; 1.0 mm, which offers the most protection,

is rarely used because of its weight. 0.5 mm has become the all-purpose apron of choice and in many cases should also be a wraparound style.

**Neck and Thyroid Shield.** A neck and thyroid shield (Fig. 13-10) can guard the thyroid area of occupationally exposed people during:

- General fluoroscopy
- X-ray special procedures

The neck and thyroid shield should be a minimum of 0.5 mm lead equivalent.

**Protective Eyeglasses.** Scatter radiation to the lens of the eyes of diagnostic imaging personnel can be substantially reduced by the use of protective eyeglasses (Fig. 13-11), with optically clear lenses that contain a minimal lead equivalent protection level of 0.35 mm. Side shields on the glasses are also available for procedures that require turning of the head. A wraparound frame containing optically clear lenses with 0.5 mm lead equivalent is also available.

## DIAGNOSTIC-TYPE PROTECTIVE TUBE HOUSING

Chapter 11 mentioned that a lead-lined metal **diagnostic-type protective tube housing** (see

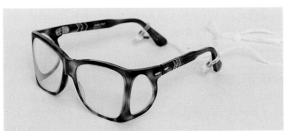

**FIGURE 13-11** Eyeglasses protect the lens of the eyes during general fluoroscopy and special procedures. (Shown are glasses with wraparound frames; other styles are also available.)

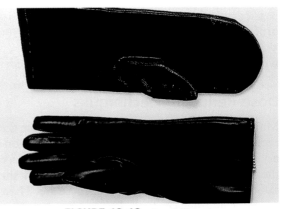

**FIGURE 13-12** Lead Gloves.

Fig. 11-1) is designed so that it protects both the radiographer and the patient from off-focus, or leakage, radiation by restricting the emission of x-rays to the area of the useful, or primary, beam.

Although the x-ray tube housing is also designed to protect the operator from the hazard of electric shock, the radiographer must be careful when handling this piece of equipment and its adjoining part, the collimator. While manipulating the tube housing for a radiographic examination, the radiographer should avoid handling or severely bending the high-tension cables that connect to the positive and negative terminals of the x-ray tube. No one should touch the tube housing or high-tension cables while a radiographic exposure is in progress.

## PROTECTION DURING FLUOROSCOPIC PROCEDURES

### Personnel Protection

To ensure protection from scattered radiation emanating from the patient during a fluoroscopic examination, the radiographer should:

- Stand as far away from the patient as is practical
- Move closer to the patient only when assistance is required

As mentioned earlier, a protective apron of at least 0.5 mm lead equivalent must be worn during all fluoroscopic procedures. Protective lead gloves of at least 0.25 mm lead equivalent

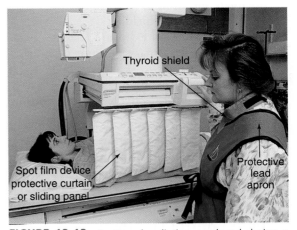

**FIGURE 13-13** Scattered radiation produced during a fluoroscopic examination can be absorbed by a spot film device protective curtain, or sliding panel, with a minimum of 0.25-mm lead equivalent placed between the fluoroscopist and the patient.

should be worn whenever the hands must be placed near the fluoroscopic field (Fig. 13-12). Imaging personnel assisting during a fluoroscopic examination also should wear thyroid shields of 0.5 mm lead equivalent, especially if they are standing in close proximity to the patient being examined (Fig. 13-13). If immediate presence assisting a radiologist during a fluoroscopic examination is not required near the x-ray table, the radiographer should either stand behind the radiologist, who is also wearing protective apparel, or stand behind the control-booth barrier until his or her services are required. To protect personnel who must move around the x-ray room during a fluoroscopic examination, a wraparound protective apron is recommended.

## Dose-Reduction Techniques

Many of the methods and devices that reduce the radiographer's exposure when operating stationary (fixed) radiographic equipment also reduce the dose received by the radiographer and the radiologist during a fluoroscopic procedure. These methods and devices include:

- Adequate beam collimation
- Adequate filtration
- Adequate gonadal shielding
- Control of technical exposure factors
- Use of high-speed image receptor systems
- Appropriate source-to-skin distance
- Use of a cumulative timing device
- Diagnostic-type protective x-ray tube housing

Some additional requirements are included in the federal government specifications for the use of fluoroscopic equipment to ensure adequate protection for both the radiographer and the radiologist.

## Remote Control Fluoroscopic Systems

In Chapter 11, possible arrangements of image-intensified fluoroscopic imaging systems are described. Of the fluoroscopic equipment arrangements discussed in Chapter 11, the remote control unit provides imaging personnel the best radiation protection opportunity. This system permits the radiologist and assisting radiographer to remain outside of the fluoroscopic room at a control console located behind a protective barrier until needed. This system improves imaging personnel safety because added distance and therefore the ISL are used as a means of increased protection. With remote equipment, the radiologist and assisting radiographer can view the patient directly through clear protective shielding and enter the x-ray room only when absolutely necessary to provide essential patient care or perform procedural functions.

## Spot Film Device Protective Curtain

A spot film device protective curtain, or sliding panel, with a minimum of 0.25 mm lead equivalent should normally be positioned between the fluoroscopist and the patient to intercept scattered radiation above the tabletop (see Fig. 13-13).

## Bucky Slot Shielding Device

A **Bucky slot shielding device** of at least 0.25 mm lead equivalent must automatically cover the Bucky slot opening in the side of the x-ray table during a standard fluoroscopic examination when the Bucky tray is positioned at the foot end of the table (Fig. 13-14). This shielding device

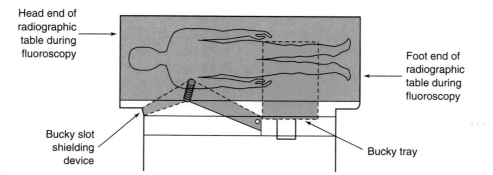

**FIGURE 13-14** To provide protection at the gonadal level for the fluoroscopist, the Bucky slot shielding device should be at least 0.25-mm lead equivalent.

protects the radiologist and radiographer at the gonadal level. Without this device and the spot film protective curtain in place, the exposure rate for the fluoroscopist would exceed 1 mGy$_a$/hr (100 mR/hr) at a distance of 0.6 m (2 feet) from the side of the x-ray table.

## Rotational Scheduling of Personnel

Diagnostic imaging personnel receive the highest occupational exposure during:

- Fluoroscopy
- Mobile radiography
- Special procedures
- Interventional surgery

Scheduling personnel to spend less time in these higher-radiation tasks can decrease this exposure. Radiographers may be assigned to clinical areas in a rotational pattern. This type of scheduling uses the cardinal principle of time as a means of additional radiation protection.

## PROTECTION DURING MOBILE RADIOGRAPHIC EXAMINATIONS

### Use of Protective Garments

Mobile radiographic equipment creates special radiation protection considerations for the radiographer. Suitable protective garments should be worn by the radiographer whenever structural protective shielding is unavailable. In fact some states (e.g., The state of Minnesota) require radiographers to wear lead aprons whenever they are performing mobile radiographic or fluoroscopic examinations.

A protective apron should be assigned to each mobile unit so that it is immediately available for the radiographer.

### Distance as a Means of Protection

Some mobile units are equipped with a remote control exposure device. This permits the radiographer to leave the immediate vicinity and uses distance as an effective means of protection from radiation. For most mobile units, which are not remote controlled, the cord leading to the exposure switch must be long enough to permit the radiographer to stand at least 2 m (approximately 6 feet) from the:

- Patient
- X-ray tube
- Useful beam

This permits the radiographer to take advantage of the ISL of exposure reduction with distance.

## Where the Radiographer Should Stand during a Mobile Radiographic Procedure

The radiographer should attempt to stand at a right angle (90 degrees) to the x-ray beam–scattering object (the patient) line; when the protection factors of distance and shielding have been accounted for, this is the place at which the least amount of scattered radiation is received (Fig. 13-15). However, because distance and shielding have much more influence on the reduction of exposure to the technologist, these factors should be addressed first.

## PROTECTION DURING C-ARM FLUOROSCOPY

### Personnel Exposure from Scattered Radiation

Safety procedures are particularly important when mobile fluoroscopy (C-arm) systems are used. Because patterns of exposure direction are less predictable and the equipment is frequently operated by physicians whose training and experience in radiation safety may not match those of an experienced radiologist, the radiographer should exercise special vigilance. For C-arm devices with similar fields of view, the dose rate for personnel located within a meter of the patient is comparable to that in routine

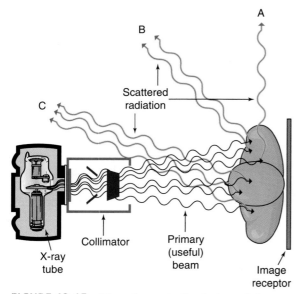

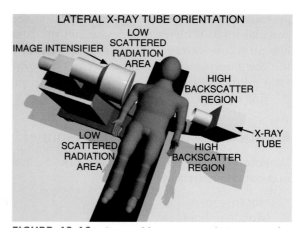

**FIGURE 13-16** Cross-table exposure during use of a C-arm fluoroscope. The exposure rate caused by scatter near the entrance surface of the patient (the x-ray tube side) exceeds the exposure rate caused by scatter near the exit surface of the patient (the image intensifier side). The location of lower potential scatter dose is on the side of the patient away from the x-ray tube (i.e., the image intensifier side).

**FIGURE 13-15** When the protective factors of distance and shielding have been accounted for, the radiographer will receive the least amount of scattered radiation by standing at a right angle (90 degrees) to the scattering object (the patient) (in position *A*). The most scattered radiation would be received at point *C* because of backscatter coming from the patient. (Intensity, or quantity, of x-ray exposure at any given point is indicated in this picture by the number of scattered x-rays reaching that point.)

## Need for Protective Apparel for All Personnel and Monitoring of Imaging Personnel

The C-arm fluoroscope can be manipulated into almost any position and remain in an energized state for long periods of time to accommodate, for example, an orthopedic surgeon performing an open reduction of a fractured hip in the operating room or a vascular surgeon performing an interventional procedure. When radiographers and other medical personnel participate in procedures that require this unit to be energized for long periods of time, they are subject to increased radiation exposure. In addition, the physical configuration of a C-arm fluoroscopic unit limits the methods that can be used to achieve protection from scattered radiation. For this reason, personnel who routinely operate a C-arm fluoroscope or those who are in the immediate area of the unit when it is energized must wear a lead apron instead of crowding behind a portable lead acrylic shield. This garment should be 0.5 mm lead equivalent to ensure adequate protection. A

fluoroscopy—approximately several milligray in air (mGy$_a$) per hour. Exposure of personnel is caused by scattered radiation from the patient. During operating room procedures in which cross-table exposures are used (Fig. 13-16), an understanding of the patterns of x-ray scatter is particularly useful. The exposure rate caused by scatter near the entrance surface of the patient (the x-ray tube side) exceeds the exposure rate caused by scatter near the exit surface of the patient (the image intensifier side). The difference in the amount of scatter, typically a factor of 2 or 3, is caused by the higher radiation intensity at the entrance surface of the patient. Thus the location of the lower potential scatter dose is on the side of the patient away from the x-ray tube (i.e., the image intensifier side). Obviously, the radiographer should never encounter the actual useful beam.

neck and thyroid shield of 0.5 mm lead equivalent should also be worn. Appropriate monitoring of imaging personnel (see Chapter 5) who are normally involved in C-arm fluoroscopic procedures is mandatory.

## Positioning of the C-Arm Fluoroscope

As discussed in Chapter 11, the positioning of a C-arm fluoroscope with the x-ray tube over the table and the image intensifier underneath the table results in higher exposure of the patient and increased scatter radiation. From the perspective of increased radiation safety, it is best to reverse the C-arm to place the x-ray tube under the table and the image intensifier over the table (see Fig. 11-26).

## Exposure Reduction for Personnel

At the start of each procedure, the equipment operator should set the unit's cumulative timer to zero so that it will be possible to be aware of the amount of beam-on time actually used.[3] When some type of image storage device (e.g., last image hold) is used in conjunction with the unit, beam-on time decreases and exposure reduction increases. If the image intensifier is positioned as close to the patient as possible, the required fluoroscopic x-ray beam intensity is minimized. This equipment-patient arrangement also permits the image intensifier to function more effectively as a scatter barrier between the patient and the person operating the C-arm fluoroscope. All these methods can lead to significant exposure reduction to both personnel and patient.

During a procedure involving the use of a C-arm fluoroscope, it is imperative that the patient's anatomic region of interest be oriented correctly with a minimal use of "positioning" fluoroscopy.[3] Furthermore, collimating the x-ray beam to the smallest area possible that includes the anatomic area of interest will decrease the amount of scattered radiation produced from the interaction of the x-ray beam with the patient, the actual scattering object.

Because distance from the source of radiation is the simplest method of protection for occupationally exposed personnel, C-arm operators should use it to their advantage whenever possible. Usually, this can be accomplished by using the foot pedal or the hand-held exposure switch with the cables extended away from the machine as far as possible when making x-ray exposures.

For better visualization of small body parts, C-arm fluoroscopes have the capability to magnify the image. However, the use of magnification usually requires mA, which produces additional radiation exposure. *Mag mode* should be used only on the request of the physician performing the procedure.[3]

## PROTECTION DURING HIGH-LEVEL-CONTROL INTERVENTIONAL PROCEDURES

### Increased Importance of Radiation Safety Techniques

All the standard precautions and procedures for the reduction of dose to personnel are applicable during interventional procedures. Here, these techniques take on an increased importance because of the extended length of some of these procedures (see Box 11-4), the large number of digital and cineradiographic images that may be taken, and, in certain studies, the frequent use of the high-level-control (boost) mode of operation. In boost mode, the exposure rate may significantly exceed the rate used in routine fluoroscopy (e.g., maximum allowed entrance exposure rate dose to a patient in regular fluoroscopy is 10 cGy/minute, whereas in high-level or boost mode this value can range upward to 20 to 40 cGy/minute).

### Knowledge of Dose-Reduction Techniques Required by the Radiographer

Although the duration of the procedure and the number of the exposures taken are under the control of the radiologist or other interventional physician, the radiographer should be knowledgeable in the application of dose-reduction techniques. The radiographer should verify that dose-reducing features are available and in good working order. These include the presence of:

- High-quality low-dose fluoroscopy mode
- Pulsed beam operation (e.g., using 7.5, 15, or 30 radiation pulses/second in place of continuous fluoroscopy radiation)
- Adequate collimation
- Correct beam filtration
- Removable grids
- Roadmapping*
- Time-interval differences[†]
- Last-image-hold mode

In last-image-hold mode, the image from the last exposure remains on the viewing monitor so the operator does not need to be exposed again simply to review the position of a catheter in relation to landmarks when no new information is needed. If possible, the beam entry side could be changed during the procedure to reduce the total dose to any one area of skin.

High-level control is to be used sparingly and only when increased visualization is necessary

---

*Roadmapping is a method of digital image subtraction in which the frame that contains the greatest amount of contrast material in vessels is identified and is then subtracted from all subsequent images. Live fluoroscopic images of the catheter moving through the vasculature can then be seen even after the vessels contain less contrast. By using this equipment feature, overlaying of two images can be accomplished (e.g., a stored image and a current image). Thus, there is a decrease of procedure time because fewer mask images are needed. This leads to some reduction in radiation dose. In addition, choosing the roadmapping feature in place of cineradiography can also result in a lower radiation dose.

[†]Time-interval difference is a method of digital image subtraction in which each image is subtracted from an image a few frames in advance. This technique reveals vessels containing contrast material and suppresses soft tissue in the images. It is less sensitive to patient motion than when the first image is subtracted from all successive images. This feature can result in a reduction of fluoroscopy "on-time" because there is a time interval between the images. Less beam-on time decreases radiation dose.

during a critical maneuver such as embolization or deployment of devices such as stents.[4] As noted in Chapter 1, many standard and C-arm interventional fluoroscopic systems now possess the technical capability for standardized dose structure reporting.[5] This is accomplished through printouts from these units that yield an actual exposure record for every examination. For older equipment that does not have printout capability, records should be kept so that the cumulative fluoroscopic exposure time may be determined.

## How the Radiologist or Other Interventional Physician Can Reduce Radiation Exposure

The radiologist or other interventional physician can reduce radiation exposure by the following means:

- Decreasing the duration of the procedure and thereby reducing fluoroscopic beam-on time
- Taking fewer digital and cineradiographic images
- Reducing the use of continuous in contrast to pulsed mode of operation
- Keeping the protective curtain, if present, on the image intensifier or scatter shield in place during a procedure
- Regularly using the last-image-hold feature to view the most recent fluoroscopic image

These practices will substantially decrease exposure not only to all participating personnel but to the patient as well.

## Extremity Monitoring

Because the hands and forearms of physicians performing interventional procedures can be subject to large radiation exposures if the safety protocol is not carefully followed—and sometimes this may not be possible—it is important that extremities be monitored. Physicians need to be aware of the recommended dose limits that have been established for extremities. The NCRP currently recommends an annual EqD limit to localized areas of the skin and hands of

500 mSv (50 rem) (see Table 10-3). To avoid even remotely approaching this quite large limit and consequently increasing the possibility of future adverse effects, protective gloves should be worn whenever feasible by any physician whose hands will, of necessity, often be close to the fluoroscopic beam.

## PATIENT RESTRAINT

Radiographers must never stand in the primary (useful) beam to restrain a patient during a radiographic exposure (Fig. 13-17, *A*). When patient restraint is necessary, mechanical restraining devices should be used to immobilize the patient,

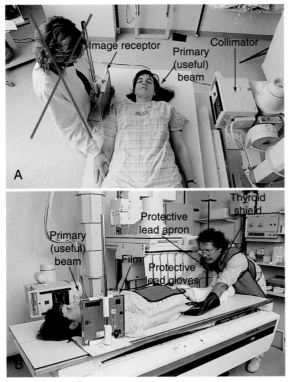

**FIGURE 13-17   A,** The radiographer should *never* stand in the primary (useful) beam to restrain the patient. **B,** A nonoccupationally exposed person restraining a patient during a radiographic exposure should wear a lead apron, gloves, and thyroid shield and stand outside the primary beam.

whenever possible. If mechanical means of restraint are not feasible, nonoccupationally exposed persons, wearing appropriate protective apparel, are to perform this function. These individuals should be positioned so that their lead-protected torsos are not struck by the primary, or direct, beam (Fig. 13-17, *B*). Holding patients may be necessary when they are unable to support themselves. For example, a weak elderly male patient may be unable to stand without assistance and raise his arms above his head for a lateral chest x-ray examination. In this situation, a nonoccupationally exposed person (relative or friend) can hold the patient in position during the exposure. A mechanical restraining device is often used to hold an infant in the upright position for chest radiographs. If such a device is not available, the child has to be physically held (usually by a parent) during the exposure. Pregnant women are never to be permitted to assist in holding a patient during an exposure.

## DOORS TO X-RAY ROOMS

Radiographic and fluoroscopic exposures should be made only when the doors are closed. This practice affords a substantial degree of protection for persons in areas adjacent to the room door because in most facilities room doors have attenuation for diagnostic energy x-rays equivalent to that provided by 0.8 mm (1/32 inch) of lead.

## DIAGNOSTIC X-RAY SUITE PROTECTION DESIGN

### Requirement for Radiation-Absorbent Barriers

To reduce the EfD to radiographers, nonoccupationally exposed personnel, and the general public to levels deemed statistically safe by both federal and international bodies, every room in which a diagnostic x-ray unit is housed must be equipped with radiation-absorbent barriers. The design of these barriers is based on considerations listed in Box 13-3.

| **BOX 13-3** | **Radiation-Absorbent Barrier Design Considerations** |
|---|---|

- The mean energy of the x-rays that will strike the barrier
- Whether the barrier is of a primary or a secondary nature
- The distance from the x-ray source to a position of occupancy 0.3 m from the barrier
- The workload of the unit
- The use factor of the unit
- The occupancy factor behind the barrier
- The intrinsic shielding (e.g., tube housing attenuation) of the x-ray unit
- Whether the area beyond the barrier is "controlled" or "uncontrolled"

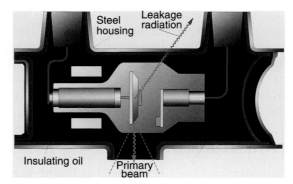

**FIGURE 13-18** Primary radiation emerges directly from the collimator and spreads throughout the room.

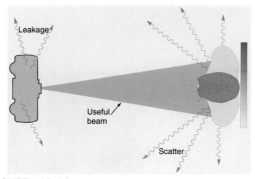

**FIGURE 13-19** Scatter radiation emerges from the patient and spreads in all directions.

## Reason for Overshielding

The shielding designer must take all the factors identified in Box 13-3 into account to meet necessary radiation protection standards. In addition, the designer should plan conservatively to satisfy future regulatory limits that may be more stringent. This and the ALARA principle are two reasons why many diagnostic x-ray facilities are overshielded. Spending extra money initially for additional shielding is far easier and much less expensive than adding it after the suite has been completed.

## Radiation Shielding Categories

Three categories of radiation sources can be generated in an x-ray room. They are classified as follows:

1. Primary radiation
2. Scatter radiation
3. Leakage radiation

The last two categories are collectively known as *secondary radiation.*

**Primary Radiation.** Primary radiation emerges directly from the x-ray tube collimator (Fig. 13-18) and moves without deflection toward a wall, door, viewing window, and so on. Because of this property, primary radiation also is known as *direct radiation.* Energy from direct radiation has not been degraded by scatter, and substantial

portions of the initial beam may not have been attenuated. Therefore, a wall in the path of direct radiation requires the most protective shielding to ensure the safety of personnel and the public. In a typical x-ray suite, the most important primary radiation barrier is that behind the wall Bucky unit.

**Scatter Radiation.** Scatter radiation results whenever a diagnostic x-ray beam passes through matter. Compton interactions between the x-ray photons and the electrons of the atoms within the attenuating object deflect x-ray photons from their initial trajectories. As a result, photons emerge from the object in all directions (Fig. 13-19). Scattered radiation is greatly reduced in intensity relative to the incident beam. It also is quite weakened in energy and consequently in penetrating power. The amount of shielding required to protect against scatter radiation is therefore almost always much less than that for primary radiation. In general, the patient is the major source of scatter radiation.

**Leakage Radiation.** Leakage radiation is radiation generated in the x-ray tube that does not exit from the collimator opening but rather penetrates the protective tube housing and, to some degree, the sides of the collimator (see Figs. 13-18 and 13-19). Leakage radiation is therefore always present in some amount. When shielding is planned for a secondary barrier, the potential contributions from leakage radiation must be added to those from the scatter radiation reaching that barrier.

## Calculation Considerations

**Workload.** Because a diagnostic x-ray unit does not produce radiation 24 hours per day, 7 days per week, a parameter that reflects the unit's radiation-on time has been used in the determination of barrier shielding requirements. The quantity is called its **workload (W)**. The workload is essentially the radiation output-weighted time that the unit is actually delivering radiation during the week. Workloads are specified either in units of milliampere-seconds (mAs) per week or milliampere-minutes (mA-min) per week. The following example illustrates this concept.

---

Example: A radiographic x-ray suite is in operation 5 days per week. The average number of patients per day is 20, and the average number of images per patient is 3. The average technical exposure factors are 90 kVp, 300 mA, and 0.1 sec. Find the weekly workload.

$$W = (300\,\text{mA} \times 0.1\,\text{sec}) \times (5\,\text{days/wk})$$
$$\times (20\,\text{patients/day}) \times (3\,\text{images/patient})$$
$$= 9000\,\text{mAs/wk}$$
$$= 150\,\text{mA-min/wk}$$

Note that the kVp is not used in the workload calculation. It is, however, an important parameter in the calculation of barrier-shielding thickness. (This is explicitly seen in an example illustrating the calculation of shielding for a wall in an x-ray suite.)

---

**Inverse Square Law.** Just as the perceived brightness of light source decreases with separation from its origin, the intensity of an x-ray beam is lessened as the distance from its source increases. The ISL, introduced earlier in this chapter, is the mathematical relation describing this property and is a fundamental component of radiation protection. As such, the ISL plays a major role in the design of radiation safety barriers. An example of its use for this purpose is shown here.

---

Example: At a distance of 1 m from an x-ray tube target, the dose rate measured by a radiation survey meter was 4.5 mGy per hour. What would that instrument read if it were moved back an extra 2 m? As already seen, the ISL is mathematically given by the following proportion:

$$\frac{I_1}{I_2} = \frac{(d_2)^2}{(d_1)^2}$$

If the given data are substituted into the relation and cross-multiplied, the following result is obtained:

$$3^2 \times I_2 = 4.5 \times 1^2$$
$$9\,I_2 = 4.5$$
$$I_2 = 0.5\,\text{mGy/hr}$$

This result demonstrates a substantial reduction in radiation intensity. Its direct consequence is a greatly reduced barrier shielding thickness requirement.

---

The ISL is actually built into the combined mathematical and empiric (i.e., experimentally derived) formulas that determine primary barrier thickness values and secondary barrier thickness values. Because these relations are constructed to give answer for broad-beam attenuation* rather than just for a very localized area, the ISL effect is slightly less than it would be for an idealized situation. A short discussion with an example

---

*As defined in NCRP Report 147 (see later), broad-beam attenuation refers to that occurring when the field area is large at the barrier and the point of measurement is near the barrier's exit surface.

illustrating the usage of this for a primary barrier is presented in the following pages. However, before this discussion, several other concepts of fundamental importance in the design of appropriate shielding have to be introduced.

**Use Factor.** If radiation, whether primary or secondary, is never directed at a particular wall or structure, then ordinary or existing construction is sufficient. Most structures in a diagnostic x-ray suite, however, are struck by radiation to some degree for some fraction of the weekly beam-on time. The **use factor** (U) is a quantity that was introduced to select this fractional contact time.

For primary radiation, the use factor represents the portion of beam-on time that the x-ray beam is directed at a primary barrier during the week. Consider a typical radiographic suite with a wall Bucky unit. If 50% of the x-ray examinations involve this device, the wall behind the Bucky unit has a U (*primary*) = ½.

Because scatter and leakage radiation emerge in all directions in the x-ray room, every wall, door, viewing window, and other surface will always be struck by some quantity of radiation. Therefore, U (*secondary*) = 1 for all radiation-accessible structures. Furthermore, if a particular wall is considered to be a primary barrier and its required shielding is designed on that basis, then in virtually all situations no supplementary shielding need be added for the secondary radiation that may also be striking this barrier.

Table 13-2 presents the most current recommended use factor values. The use factor also can be referred to as the *beam direction factor.*

**Occupancy Factor.** Radiation barriers are installed to protect personnel and the general public from radiation that otherwise would reach them uninhibited. If no one will ever be present beyond an existing wall in a particular area while the x-ray unit is being operated, the addition of supplementary shielding to that wall is unnecessary. This shielding design statement would be that *existing construction is sufficient.* An example of this is an outside wall facing a courtyard that "always" has zero occupancy. The opposite extreme is an area in which someone is

| TABLE 13-2 | Use Factors Recommended by the International Commission on Radiological Protection |
|---|---|
| **Use Factor** | **Primary Barrier** |
| Full use (U = 1) | Floors of radiation rooms except dental installations, doors, walls, and ceilings of radiation rooms exposed routinely to the primary beam |
| Partial use (U = ¼) | Doors and walls of radiation rooms not exposed routinely to the primary beam; also, floors of dental installations |
| Occasional use (U = 1/16) | Ceilings of radiation rooms not exposed routinely to the primary beam; because of the low use factor, shielding requirements for a ceiling usually determined by secondary rather than primary beam considerations |

From International Commission on Radiological Protection (ICRP): *Report of Committee III on protection against x-rays up to energies of 3 MeV and beta and gamma rays from sealed sources,* ICRP Publication No. 3, New York, 1960, Pergamon Press.

always present. When planning radiation protection shielding for a diagnostic x-ray suite, the designer must consider not only zero and full occupancy cases but also the more common partial occupancy situation. The **occupancy factor** (T) is used to modify the shielding requirement for a particular barrier by taking into account the fraction of the work week during which the space beyond the barrier is occupied. Table 13-3 lists the latest recommended values for T.

**Controlled and Uncontrolled Areas.** If a region adjacent to a wall of an x-ray room is used only by occupationally exposed personnel (e.g., radiographers), that location is designated as a **controlled area.** Conversely, a nearby hall or corridor that is frequented by the general public is classified as an **uncontrolled area.** For the latter, the weekly maximum permitted equivalent dose (MPED) is equal to 20 microsieverts (μSv) (2 mrem); for controlled areas, it is a much larger

| TABLE 13-3 | Suggested Occupancy Factors*† | |
|---|---|---|
| **Location** | | **Occupancy Factor (T)** |
| Administrative or clerical offices; laboratories, pharmacies, and other work areas fully occupied by an individual; receptionist areas, attended waiting rooms, children's indoor play areas, adjacent x-ray rooms, film reading areas, nurses' stations, x-ray control rooms | | 1 |
| Rooms used for patient examinations and treatments | | $\frac{1}{2}$ |
| Corridors, patient rooms, employee lounges, and staff rest rooms | | $\frac{1}{5}$ |
| Corridor doors‡ | | $\frac{1}{8}$ |
| Public toilets, unattended vending areas, storage rooms, outdoor areas with seating, unattended waiting rooms, patient holding areas | | $\frac{1}{20}$ |
| Outdoor areas with only transient pedestrians or vehicular traffic, unattended parking lots, vehicular drop-off areas (unattended), attics, stairways, unattended elevators, janitors' closets | | $\frac{1}{40}$ |

Adapted from National Council on Radiation Protection and Measurements (NCRP): *Structural shielding design for medical x-ray imaging facilities,* Report No. 147, Bethesda, Md, 2004, NCRP.

*For use as a guide in planning shielding where other occupancy data are not available.

†When using a low occupancy factor for a room immediately adjacent to an x-ray room, care should be taken to also consider the areas farther removed from the x-ray room. These areas may have significantly higher occupancy factors than the adjacent room and may therefore be more important in shielding design despite the larger distances involved.

‡The occupancy factor for the area just outside a corridor door can often be reasonably assumed to be lower than the occupancy factor for the corridor.

amount—1000 µSv or 1 mSv (100 mrem). The main reason for this disparity lies in the fact that the occupationally exposed population is only a tiny fraction of the overall population. Therefore, the potential for detrimental radiobiologic effects in the general public as a whole as a result of the higher MPED to occupationally exposed personnel is statistically negligible. Whether the area beyond a structure is designated as controlled or uncontrolled is very significant in determining the amount of radiation shielding to be added to that structure. The following sections discuss the use of these concepts in the determination of radiation shielding requirements.

## Calculating Barrier Shielding Requirements

For each wall, door, and other barrier in an x-ray room that is to provide protection against radiation, the product of mA-minutes $\times$ U $\times$ T must be determined. The number of mA-minutes or workload is generally fixed by the overall use of the x-ray unit, whereas the use and occupancy

factors are typically different among various barriers. The protection planner also must know whether the barrier is primary or secondary and whether the area beyond the barrier is controlled or uncontrolled.

With the publication of NCRP Report No. 147,[6] entitled *Structural Shielding Design for Medical Imaging Facilities,* the objective of a shielding calculation is now described as determining the thickness of a barrier sufficient to reduce the *air kerma** in a full or partially occupied area to a value that is less than or at most equal to the ratio P/T. The quantity P refers to the permissible weekly radiation dose (note: for diagnostic x-rays, dose and dose equivalent are numerically equal) to that location and, as discussed earlier, T is the area's occupancy factor.

**Primary Barrier Calculation.** Using material from NCRP Report No. 147, the combined

---

*Recall that air kerma ($K_a$) is essentially absorbed dose in air resulting from the passage of an x-ray beam through it. Its numeric value is specified in units of gray.

mathematical and empiric relation that was briefly mentioned in the section on the ISL is introduced. For primary or direct radiation only, the relation is given by $B = P (d_p)^2/K_r UTN$, where B is by definition the broad-beam x-ray transmission factor and is in fact the ratio of $K_a$ behind a barrier of material thickness "x" to the value of $K_a$ at the same location with no intervening barrier; $d_p$ is the distance from the x-ray source to a representative location and distance behind the direct radiation barrier (e.g., one third of a meter beyond the barrier is typical); N is the expected number of patients examined in the room per week; $K_r$ is the average unshielded air kerma per patient at a reference distance of 1 m from the source; and P depends on whether the barrier is for a controlled or uncontrolled area. Once the value of B has been calculated for a particular situation, then plots of transmission factors versus attenuating material thickness supplied in Appendix B of NCRP Report No. 147 may be used to obtain the required shielding thickness for the barrier. Such a graph is shown in Figure 13-20.

The primary radiation intensity for a selected kVp at the barrier location for an x-ray suite may be determined by making air kerma measurements on the suite's x-ray unit at a reference distance (e.g., 100 cm) from the x-ray tube target with the aid of a calibrated ionization chamber. This information can then be used to determine the amount of shielding necessary to attenuate the radiation to permissible levels for that x-ray energy. The following example demonstrates determination of the primary barrier shielding requirement associated with a wall Bucky from an average-usage radiographic room.

---

Example: Let the average kVp for the x-rays striking the barrier = 100.

Let $U = \frac{1}{2}$ and $T = \frac{1}{4}$.

Let there be 100 patients per week in this x-ray room.

Let the area behind the wall be an uncontrolled area. Therefore, P = 0.02 mGy/wk.

Let the total distance from x-ray source to occupied area $d_p$ (including one third of a meter beyond the shielding barrier) be 3 m.

---

**FIGURE 13-20** Assorted plots of primary broad-beam transmission through lead.

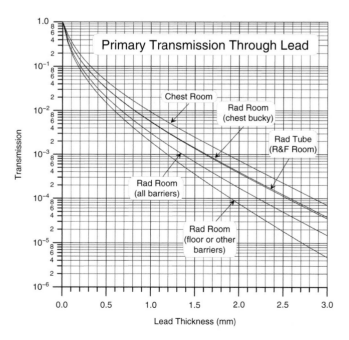

From measurements on the x-ray unit, we find that at 1 m for 100 kVp, the value of $K_r$ is 6 mGy per mA-min.

Solution: Substituting the foregoing information into the expression for the transmission factor gives:

$$B = (0.02)(3)^2/(6)(0.5)(0.25)(100)$$
$$= 0.0024$$

From the graph in Figure 13-20, using the curve for rad room chest Bucky, we obtain a shielding requirement of approximately 1.3 mm lead. Currently, in the United States shielding is specified in fractions of an inch of lead, most commonly, 1/32″ and 1/16″. If we do some metric-to-English unit conversions, we find that the standard 1/32″ is approximately 0.8 mm and the standard 1/16″ is equal to 1.58 mm. Because our calculation of shielding for our primary barrier required 1.3 mm lead, then in the United States the choice would be to conservatively install 1/16″ lead shielding for this barrier.

**Secondary Barrier Calculation.** Secondary barriers intercept both scatter and leakage radiation. No additional shielding against secondary radiation is needed for areas already protected against primary radiation. Because scatter and leakage radiation emerge in all directions, the use factor for these is always 1.

*Scatter Radiation.* The intensity and energy of the scatter radiation at the location of a barrier are generally unknown. Therefore, the following have been assumed for the determination of barrier shielding requirements:

1. The energy of the scatter radiation is equal to the primary radiation
2. The intensity of radiation scattered at 90 degrees at a distance of 1 m from its source is reduced by a factor of 1000 relative to the primary radiation for a field size of 400 cm² (approximately 20 cm × 20 cm)

The greater the x-ray field dimension at the source of the scatter radiation (usually the patient), the larger the amount of generated scatter

radiation will be. Also significant are the primary beam photon energy and the location of the x-ray beam on the patient. The ISL again plays an important role in shielding determination, but in the case of scatter radiation the distance is measured from the center of the irradiated portion of the patient, rather than from the x-ray tube target.

*Leakage Radiation.* Leakage radiation does not emerge directly from the collimator opening, but rather penetrates through the x-ray tube housing walls or through the sides of the collimator when the x-ray beam is on. Leakage radiation is therefore an additional radiation output that shielding designers must consider. Regulatory standards mandate that the maximum permissible leakage exposure rate at 1 m from the target of a diagnostic x-ray tube in all directions cannot exceed 100 mR/hour when the tube is being operated continuously at its maximal permitted kVp and mA combination.

Leakage radiation is always present when the x-ray tube is on, even if the collimator jaws are tightly closed. Because of the attenuation that occurs when leakage radiation penetrates the tube housing walls, it is essentially a monoenergetic beam; thus the concept of half-value layer (HVL) may be used at barriers to reduce leakage radiation levels to permissible values. Data tables incorporating this concept have been devised to specify the amount of shielding needed to attenuate leakage radiation sufficiently at various distances from the x-ray tube. This shielding should be compared with that necessary to attenuate scatter radiation satisfactorily. Traditionally, if both requirements do not differ substantially (i.e., are less than 3 HVLs) then the conservative decision would be to install a composite shielding that is the sum of the shielding for each radiation source. However, if the barrier shielding for the two differs substantially (i.e., more than 3 HVLs), then conservatively one can just use the larger value. The following example illustrates the method used in most existing diagnostic x-ray rooms for determining leakage radiation shielding requirements.

Example: Suppose that shielding must be added to a wall that is subject only to secondary radiation to protect a controlled area. Given the following information, find the total thickness of lead needed.

    HVL for scatter and leakage radiation
    Each = 0.2 mm lead
    Shielding requirement for scatter radiation alone for a particular barrier
    = 0.75 mm lead
    Shielding requirement for leakage radiation alone for that barrier
    = 0.3 mm lead
    Solution: The difference in barrier shielding requirements for scatter and leakage = 0.45 mm lead, which is less than 3 HVL, which = 3 × 0.2 mm lead, or 0.6 mm lead. Therefore, the conservative total shielding thickness for the barrier would be 0.75 + 0.3 = 1.05 mm lead.

## Summary for New Approaches to Shielding

At this time, the majority of installed shielding was designed according to the concepts and information in NCRP Report No. 49,[7] which was published in 1976. Despite the current trend toward decreasing the maximum dose limits and consequently making more stringent the appropriate design limits for installations, experts do not expect that retrofitting of additional shielding will be necessary in existing installations. The techniques in NCRP Report No. 49 were sufficiently conservative (in terms of overshielding) to accommodate the lower dose limits. New approaches will ensure that future installations are designed in accordance with these lower limits.

Among the new approaches to shielding design detailed in NCRP Report No. 147, a more rigorous analysis of workload incorporates the range of kVps actually used. In addition, the true role of leakage radiation in state-of-the-art equipment is now modeled explicitly, along with scatter. The traditional rule of adding an HVL if leakage and scatter barrier requirements are similar has

been abandoned in favor of exact calculations. Use factors now reflect a true percentage of the time that the beam is directed at various barriers. Some existing shielding that was generally ignored in older design calculations, such as the patient table, Bucky, and cassette holder, is included in the new designs. Finally, the suggested occupancy factors have been reevaluated to approximate more closely the percentage of the time that workers are expected to be present (see Table 13-3). In NCRP Report No. 49, a minimal occupancy factor of at least $\frac{1}{16}$ was assumed. Under the revised guidelines, occupancy factors for areas such as closets and stairways may be placed as low as $\frac{1}{40}$. Some of the changes in the revision of NCRP Report No. 49 are listed in Table 13-4.

## POSTING OF CAUTION SIGNS FOR RADIOACTIVE MATERIALS AND RADIATION AREAS

As part of a successful radiation safety program, caution signs must be posted in any room or area where "radioactive materials or radiation sources

| TABLE 13-4 | Brief Summary of National Council on Radiation Protection and Measurements Report No. 147 New Shielding Guidelines |
|---|---|
| **Item** | **New Approach** |
| Workload | More realistic use of contemporary survey data |
| Leakage and scatter | Explicit barrier calculations |
| Use factor | Adjusted for beam direction data reflecting actual usage patterns |
| Occupancy factor | Realistic assumptions of occupancy of low-occupancy areas (e.g., stairwells) |

Adapted from National Council on Radiation Protection and Measurements (NCRP): *Structural shielding design for medical imaging facilities,* Report No. 147, Bethesda, Md, 2004, NCRP.

are used or stored."[8] To ensure the safety of all persons approaching a radiation area or a container containing radioactive materials, the signs should be obvious and easy to read. The word "Caution" usually appears at the top of the sign, followed by the conventional three-blade radiation symbol and then specific words to make persons approaching the area aware of the radiation hazard present. These specific words include:

- "Radiation area"
- "High radiation area"
- "Very high radiation area"

The signs that are posted are required to have the radiation "symbol colored magenta, purple, or black on a yellow background."[8] Some examples of posting sign requirements are identified in Box 13-4.

---

**BOX 13-4 | Posting Sign Requirements**

1. A permanent sign bearing the words "Caution Radiation Area" must be conspicuously posted in any area accessible to individuals in which radiation levels could result in an individual receiving a dose equivalent in excess of 0.05 mSv in 1 hour at 30 cm from the radiation source or from any surface that the radiation penetrates.[8]
2. A permanent sign bearing the words "Caution High Radiation Area" must be conspicuously posted in any area accessible to individuals in which radiation levels could result in an individual receiving a dose equivalent in excess of 1 mSv in 1 hour at 30 cm from the radiation source or from any surface that the radiation penetrates.[8]
3. A permanent sign bearing the words "Grave Danger, Very High Radiation Area" must be conspicuously posted in any area accessible to individuals in which radiation levels could result in an individual receiving an absorbed dose in excess of 5 $Gy_t$ in 1 hour at 1 m from a radiation source or from any surface that the radiation penetrates.[8]

From *Radiation safety manual*, section 10: *Area classification and posting*, 1999, UW Environmental Health and Safety.

---

## SUMMARY

- An annual occupational effective dose of 50 mSv (5 rem) for whole-body exposure during routine operations and an annual effective dose of 1 mSv (0.1 rem) for individuals in the general population have been established.
- A cumulative effective dose (CumEfD) limits a radiation worker's whole-body lifetime effective dose to his or her age in years times 10 mSv (years × 1 rem).
- Radiation workers can receive a larger equivalent dose than the general public without altering the genetically significant dose (GSD).
- Occupational exposure must be kept as low as reasonably achievable (ALARA).
- The following methods of reducing scatter radiation also reduce the occupational hazard for the radiographer:
  - Use of beam-limitation devices, higher-kVp and lower-mA techniques, appropriate beam filtration, and adequate protective shielding.
  - Correct use of protective apparel (lead aprons, gloves, thyroid shields).
  - Reduction of repeat examinations.
- The basic principles of time, distance, and shielding can be used to minimize occupational radiation exposure.
- Pregnant radiographers can wear an additional monitoring device at waist level to ensure that the monthly equivalent dose does not exceed 0.5 mSv (0.05 rem).
- Primary and secondary protective barriers must be designed to ensure that annual effective dose limits are not exceeded.
- To protect the radiographer and the patient from leakage radiation, a lead-lined metal diagnostic-type protective tube housing must be used.
- The following practices are important in protecting the radiographer during routine fluoroscopy:
  - The radiographer, in addition to wearing appropriate protective apparel, should stand as far away from the patient as is

practical and move closer to the patient only when assistance is required.

- A spot film device protective curtain and Bucky slot shielding device must be used.
- The x-ray beam must be adequately collimated, and high-speed image receptor systems and a cumulative timing device should be used.

- The following are required to protect the radiographer during mobile radiographic examinations:
  - The radiographer must wear protective garments.
  - The radiographer should stand at least 2 m (approximately 6 feet) from the patient, x-ray tube, and useful beam.
  - The radiographer should stand at a right angle to the x-ray beam–scattering object (the patient) line.

- Limited exposure time and dose-reduction features are required to protect the radiographer during high-level-control fluoroscopy.
- Distance is the most effective means of protection from ionizing radiation.
- If the peak energy of the x-ray beam is 100 kVp, a lead apron of at least 0.25 mm lead equivalent thickness should be worn if the radiographer cannot remain behind a protective barrier. A lead apron of 0.5 or 1 mm lead equivalent thickness affords much greater protection.
  - Lead gloves, a thyroid shield, and protective glasses are sometimes required.
- Radiographers should never stand in the primary beam to hold a patient during a radiographic exposure.
- When designing diagnostic x-ray suites, equivalent dose to radiation workers, non-occupationally exposed personnel, and the general public must be taken into consideration.
  - Facilities must be equipped with radiation-absorbent barriers.
  - Occupancy factor, workload, and use factor must be considered when thickness requirements for a protective barrier

are being determined. Whether an area beyond a structure is designated as a controlled or uncontrolled area is significant in determining the amount of radiation shielding to be added to that structure.
- Caution signs must be posted in any room or area where "radioactive materials or radiation sources are used or stored."[8]

## REFERENCES

1. National Council on Radiation Protection and Measurements (NCRP): *Limitation of exposure to ionizing radiation,* Report No. 116, Bethesda, Md, 1993, NCRP.
2. Bushong SC: *Radiologic science for technologists: physics, biology and protection,* ed 10, St. Louis, 2013, Mosby.
3. Femia J: It pays off in safety to know your C-arm. *Adv Imaging Radiat Ther Prof* 20:19, 2007.
4. Marx MV: *Interventional procedures: risks to patients and personnel, in radiation risk,* Reston, Va, 1996, American College of Radiology Commission on Physics and Radiation Safety.
5. Center for Devices and Radiological Health, U.S. Food and Drug Administration: White paper: Association for Medical Imaging Management, 2011.
6. National Council on Radiation Protection and Measurements (NCRP): *Structural shielding design for medical x-ray imaging facilities,* Report No. 147, Bethesda, Md, 2004, NCRP.
7. National Council on Radiation Protection and Measurements (NCRP): *Structural shielding design and evaluation for medical use of x-rays and gamma rays with energies up to 10 meV,* Report No. 49, Washington DC, 1976, NCRP.
8. *Radiation safety manual,* section 10: *Area classification and posting,* 1999, UW Environmental Health and Safety.

## GENERAL DISCUSSION QUESTIONS

1. Why has a cumulative effective dose limit for the whole body been established for radiation workers?
2. Why can radiation workers receive a larger equivalent dose than members of the general population?

3. What can a radiographer do during a radiographic procedure to reduce scattered radiation from a patient?

4. When an additional radiation dosimeter is worn by a pregnant radiographer to monitor the equivalent dose to the embryo-fetus, where should the dosimeter be placed if a protective lead apron is worn?

5. Why is it *not* necessary to reassign a declared pregnant radiographer to a lower radiation exposure risk area?

6. Why is the control-booth barrier considered as a secondary protective barrier?

7. During a fluoroscopic procedure, when a radiographer's presence is *not* immediately required, where should this person stand until his or her services are needed?

8. How can the use of a remote control exposure device on a mobile radiographic unit reduce exposure for the radiographer?

9. Why is it best to position the image intensifier of a C-arm fluoroscope close to the patient during any x-radiation procedure?

10. How can the radiologist reduce radiation exposure for himself or herself and for assisting personnel during a high-level-control interventional procedure?

11. During a high-level-control interventional procedure, how can a record of radiation exposure be obtained?

12. When should the radiographer stand in the primary beam to restrain a patient during a radiographic exposure?

13. What factors must the shielding designer take into account to meet necessary radiation protection standards?

14. What quantity *best* describes the weekly radiation usage of a diagnostic x-ray unit?

15. What mathematical relationship plays a major role in the design of radiation safety barriers?

## REVIEW QUESTIONS

1. When performing a mobile radiographic examination, if the protection factors of distance and shielding are equal, the radiographer should stand at a _____ to the scattering object (the patient) line.
   A. 30-degree angle
   B. 45-degree angle
   C. 75-degree angle
   D. 90-degree angle

2. Diagnostic imaging personnel may receive an annual occupational effective dose of _____ for whole-body exposure during routine operations.
   A. 1 mSv
   B. 5 mSv
   C. 25 mSv
   D. 50 mSv

3. At a 90-degree angle to the primary x-ray beam, at a distance of 1 m, the scattered radiation is what fraction of the intensity of the primary beam?
   A. $\frac{1}{10}$
   B. $\frac{1}{100}$
   C. $\frac{1}{1000}$
   D. $\frac{1}{10,000}$

4. If a radiographer stands 6 m away from an x-ray tube and receives an exposure rate dose of 4.0 mGy$_a$/hr, what will the exposure rate dose be if the same radiographer moves to stand at a position located 12 m from the x-ray tube?
   A. 1 mGy$_a$/hr
   B. 2 mGy$_a$/hr
   C. 3 mGy$_a$/hr
   D. 4 mGy$_a$/hr

5. Which of the following are methods that can be used by a C-arm operator to reduce occupational exposure for himself or herself and other personnel?
   1. Collimate the x-ray beam to include only the anatomy of interest.
   2. Use the foot pedal or the hand-held exposure switch with their cables extended away from the machine as

far as possible whenever making an exposure.

3. Use magnification whenever possible to visualize body parts better.
   A. 1 and 2 only
   B. 1 and 3 only
   C. 2 and 3 only
   D. 1, 2, and 3

6. If the Bucky slot shielding device and spot film device protective curtain, or sliding panel, were *not* in the correct position during a routine fluoroscopic examination, what would the fluoroscopist do?
   A. Exceed an exposure rate dose of 1 mGy$_a$/hr at a distance of 0.6 m from the side of the x-ray table
   B. Not exceed an exposure rate dose of 1 mGy$_a$/hr at a distance of 0.6 m from the side of the x-ray table
   C. Exceed an exposure rate dose of 2.5 mGy$_a$/hr at a distance of 0.6 m from the side of the x-ray table
   D. Exceed an exposure rate dose of 5 mGy$_a$/hr at a distance of 0.6 m from the side of the x-ray table

7. Units of either mAs/wk or mA-min/wk are used to determine the _____ for a specific x-ray room.
   A. Distance factor
   B. Occupancy factor
   C. Use factor
   D. Workload

8. A Bucky slot shielding device of at least _____ must automatically cover the Bucky slot opening in the side of the x-ray table during a fluoroscopic examination when the Bucky tray is positioned at the foot end of the table.
   A. 0.25 mm aluminum equivalent
   B. 0.25 mm lead equivalent
   C. 0.5 mm aluminum equivalent
   D. 0.5 mm lead equivalent

9. For mobile radiographic units, which are not equipped with remote control exposure devices, the cord leading to the exposure switch must be long enough to permit the radiographer to stand *at least* _____ from the patient, the x-ray tube, and the useful beam to reduce occupational exposure.
   A. 1 m
   B. 2 m
   C. 3 m
   D. 5 m

10. Of the following factors, which is considered when determining thickness requirements for protective barriers?
    1. Occupancy factor (T)
    2. Workload (W)
    3. Use factor (U)
    A. 1 only
    B. 2 only
    C. 3 only
    D. 1, 2, and 3

# Radioisotopes and Radiation Protection

## OBJECTIVES

*After completing this chapter, the reader will be able to perform the following:*

- Explain what causes cancerous growths or tumors to be eliminated or controlled by irradiation.
- Describe how therapeutic isotopes may be characterized.
- Describe the process of electron capture.
- Identify the two best radiation safety practices to follow for patients having therapeutic prostate seed implants.
- Explain the process of beta decay.
- Discuss the radiation hazards that may be encountered by personnel caring for a patient who is receiving iodine-131 therapy treatment for thyroid cancer.
- Explain how radioisotopes that are used as radioactive tracers in nuclear medicine work.
- Identify the most common radioisotope used in nuclear medicine diagnostic studies.
- Identify and describe the types of radiation events that are used in positron emission tomography (PET).
- Identify the most common isotope used for PET scanning.
- Explain the benefit of the combined imaging device called a *PET/CT scanner.*

- Describe radiation safety concerns associated with the design of a PET/CT imaging suite, and explain how radiation protection has been provided.
- Discuss the reasons for concern over the use of radiation as a terrorist weapon, and identify what action most hospitals have taken for handling emergency situations involving radioactive contamination.
- Explain what a radioactive dispersal device, or "dirty bomb," is, and discuss the possible consequences of the detonation of such a device.
- Describe the procedure for external decontamination from radioactive materials.
- State the dose limit per event for individuals engaged in both nonlifesaving and lifesaving activities during a radiation emergency.
- Explain the reason why the Environmental Protection Agency (EPA) sets limits for radioactive contamination.
- Discuss the medical management of persons experiencing radiation bioeffects.
- Describe various strategies used to treat internal radiation contamination.

Copyright © 2014, Elsevier Inc.

## KEY TERMS

annihilation radiation
beta decay
computed tomography (CT)
decontamination
electron capture
Environmental Protection
  Agency (EPA)
fluorine-18 ($^{18}$F)
fluorodeoxyglucose (FDG)
Geiger-Müller (GM) detectors

half-value layer (HVL)
internal contamination
iodine-123 ($^{123}$I)
iodine-125 ($^{125}$I)
iodine-131 ($^{131}$I)
isotopes
neutrino
nuclear medicine
PET/CT scanner
positron

positron emission tomography
  (PET)
radiation emergency plans
radiation therapy
radioactive contamination
radioactive dispersal device, or
  "dirty bomb"
radioisotopes
surface contamination
technetium-99m ($^{99m}$Tc)

Atoms that have the same number of protons within the nucleus but have different numbers of neutrons are called **isotopes**. Most elements in the periodic table (see Appendix C) have associated isotopes, and quite a few of them have many. However, not all the nuclei of these isotopes represent stable configurations of protons and neutrons. Some have too many neutrons, whereas others have too many protons. Because of this, such isotopes spontaneously undergo changes or transformations to rectify the unstable arrangement. All atoms of this nature are referred to as **radioisotopes.**

This chapter provides a brief description of the use of radioisotopes in both diagnostic and therapeutic medical procedures and discusses some relevant radiation safety issues. The use of radiation as a terrorist weapon is also discussed, and the chapter includes some fundamental principles for dealing with radioactive contamination in a health care setting.

To assist the learner, both English and metric units are used in this chapter.

## MEDICAL USAGE

### Radiation Therapy

As discussed in previous chapters, well-oxygenated, rapidly dividing cells are very sensitive to damage by radiation. This causes cancerous growths or tumors to be either eliminated or at least controlled by irradiation of the area containing the growth. Radiation can be delivered internally to such regions by infusion or implantation of certain radioisotopes. These therapeutic isotopes are characterized by relatively long half-lives that are measured in terms of multiple days or multiple years and, with the exception of a few of them, by relatively high-energy radiation emissions. The radiation may be

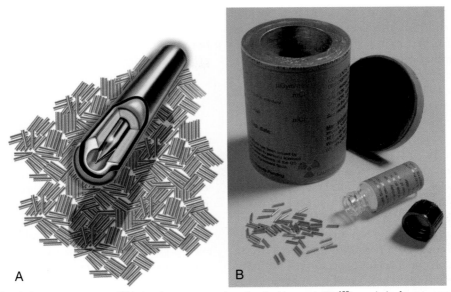

**FIGURE 14-1** **A,** Iodine-125 ($^{125}$I)-titanium–encapsulated cylindric seed. **B,** $^{125}$I seeds before encapsulation.

in the form of gamma rays* or fast electrons (beta radiation). Several of the most important therapeutic radioisotopes are briefly described here.

**Iodine-125.** Iodine-125 ($^{125}$I) is an unstable and therefore radioactive isotope of the element iodine. It has been used quite extensively since 2000 in the form of titanium-encapsulated cylindric seeds (4.5 mm long and in cross-section about the diameter of a paper clip [Fig. 14-1]) to give a tumoricidal radiation equivalent dose to cancers that are confined within the prostate gland. With the aid of computerized treatment planning and real-time ultrasound imaging, the seeds are permanently inserted into the gland in a calculated prescribed arrangement. The goal is to deliver 145 gray (Gy) to at least 90% of the prostate's volume while limiting radiation dose as much as possible to adjacent structures such as the urethra, bladder, and anterior rectal wall.

The insertion process is done in the operating room and typically takes about 2 hours. This is a same-day procedure, and the patient is usually discharged within 4 to 5 hours afterward.

$^{125}$I has 53 protons and 72 neutrons in its nucleus and has a half-life of 59.4 days. It decays by a process called **electron capture,** wherein an inner-shell electron is captured by one of the nuclear protons, followed directly by the two combining to produce a neutron. There is also the emission of characteristic energy in the form of a 27-keV x-ray generated because of the filling of the inner-electron shell vacancy by an outer low-energy electron. The nucleus now has one less proton, and thus the decay process has led to the formation of a different element called *tellurium-125* ($^{125}$Te). $^{125}$Te, which has 52 protons and 73 neutrons, is produced in an unstable excited energy state; this instability is immediately relieved as its nucleus emits energy in the form of a 35-keV gamma ray. Both the 27-keV characteristic x-rays and the 35-keV gamma rays deliver the radiation equivalent dose to the prostate gland.

Because these radiation emissions have little penetrating power, a very high percentage of the

---

*Gamma rays are high-energy photons (particles of electromagnetic radiation) that are emitted by the nucleus as a result of an unstable situation. They differ from x-ray photons, which are also particles of electromagnetic radiation, only in the method of how they are produced.

radiation energy remains concentrated in the prostate gland. All the remaining radiation is virtually absorbed by the patient, and yet some detectable radiation emerges from the patient. At a distance of 3 feet, the radiation exposure rate for virtually all prostate seed implants is less than 0.5 milliroentgens per hour (mR/hr), increasing to 15 to 20 mR/hr at the patient's lower abdominal surface.

The concepts of distance and time are the best radiation safety practices to be followed for these types of therapeutic implants. A typical safety recommendation is that patients with $^{125}$I implants should significantly limit durations of close contact (<3 feet) with small children and pregnant women for a period of 6 months (three half-lives) after the implant procedure. They may then resume completely normal behavior.

**Iodine-131.** Iodine-131 ($^{131}$I) is another unstable isotope of the element iodine, with 53 protons and 78 neutrons in its nucleus. It has a half-life of 8 days. As a consequence of its radioactive decay process (**beta decay***), it generates both electrons with an approximate mean energy of 192 keV and relatively high-energy assorted gamma rays (mean energy of 365 keV).

$^{131}$I can be joined chemically with sodium to form a radioactive compound called *sodium iodide* $^{131}$I, which can be orally administered in the form of tablets. For a patient who has thyroid cancer, it is desirable to strongly irradiate any residual thyroid tissue not removed by surgery while significantly sparing surrounding tissue and other organs. Because the thyroid gland tends to highly (but not totally) absorb any iodine in the blood, administration of $^{131}$I-labeled sodium iodide tablets is an efficient way of delivering a destructive radiation dose to a specific cancer site, in this case the remainder of the thyroid. The relatively low-energy electrons mainly cause the destruction.

Although the much more penetrating gamma rays deliver some radiation dose to more distant body sites, these rays primarily exit the body and present a radiation protection hazard to both:

- Nursing personnel
- Nuclear medicine technologists

As discussed in earlier chapters, the concepts of time, distance, and shielding should be applied. If the patient is hospitalized (usually no more than 2 days), a large, up to 1-inch-thick, rolling lead shield can be positioned between the patient and any attending personnel for protection. Such patients are also encouraged to drink lots of fluids so that as much $^{131}$I, and therefore high-energy gamma radiation, can be removed from the body by urination in as short a time as possible.

The radioiodide tablets dissolve in the bloodstream, thus permitting passage of radioactive matter through the pores of the skin. This poses yet another radiation safety hazard and a potential lengthy cleanup, or decontamination, task. Therefore, hospital rooms for $^{131}$I therapy patients are usually isolated and carefully prepared with absorbent cloths to substantially minimize radiation exposure to both personnel and visitors that results either from emitted gamma radiation from the patient or from contaminated surfaces. Only trained oncology nurses and nuclear medicine personnel should be allowed in the patient's room.

## Nuclear Medicine

**Nuclear medicine** is the branch of medicine that employs radioisotopes to study organ function in a patient, to detect the spread of cancer into bone, and to treat certain types of diseases. Diagnostic techniques in nuclear medicine typically make use of short-lived radioisotopes as radioactive tracers. These radionuclides have been attached to biologically active substances or chemicals and form radioactive compounds that diffuse predominantly into certain regions or organs where it is medically desired to scrutinize particular physiologic processes.

---

*Beta decay is the process wherein a neutron relieves an instability by a neutron transforming itself into a combination of a proton and an energetic electron (called a *beta particle*). There is also emission of another particle called a neutrino.

**Iodine-123.** One of the most common examples of this process makes use of **iodine-123** ($^{123}$I), another unstable isotope of the element iodine, which undergoes radioactive decay by the process of electron capture (described in the section on **radiation therapy**) and has an average half-life of 13.3 hours. When chemically coupled with sodium, it forms the radiotracer compound sodium iodide $^{123}$I. This compound preferentially concentrates in the thyroid gland and achieves levels of concentration that can be directly correlated with the thyroid gland's performance status. Thus measurement of radioactivity in the region of the thyroid gland, which results from the relative uptake by the thyroid of $^{123}$I-labeled sodium iodide, makes it possible to determine the thyroid's health status.

**Technetium-99m.** By far the most common radioisotope used in nuclear medicine diagnostic studies (as much as 80% of all procedures) is **technetium-99m** ($^{99m}$Tc). This isotope is produced from the radioactive decay of another unstable isotope (molybdenum-99 [$^{99}$Mo]), which relieves its instability by beta decay, during which (as discussed previously) an excess neutron transforms itself into a proton, with the emission of a fast electron from the nucleus. An additional proton within the nucleus means a change in atomic number and consequently a different element. The new element in this case is $^{99m}$Tc, with 43 protons and 56 neutrons. Because the beta decay of $^{99}$Mo produces technetium in an excited or higher-energy state than normal, it too is unstable. Most isotopes generated in this manner immediately shed their excess energy. However, some do not do so for a short period, and these relatively more enduring isotopes are given the designation *m*, which stands for *metastable* (meaning "more lasting"). $^{99m}$Tc has a half-life of 6 hours and decays primarily by emission from its nucleus of a gamma ray photon with energy of 140 keV.

$^{99m}$Tc is an extremely versatile radioisotope because it can be incorporated into a wide variety of different compounds or biologically active substances, each with a specificity for different tissues or organs of the body. For example, in combination with a tin compound, it binds to red blood cells and is useful for mapping circulatory system disorders; in combination with a sulfur compound, it is absorbed by the spleen, thus making it possible to image the structure of the spleen; in another chemical combination, it concentrates in bone and permits evaluation of potential cancer spread to bony areas; it can also be used to evaluate heart function. All these studies are possible because either a deficiency of radioisotope uptake (i.e., a cold spot in radioactivity) or an excessive uptake of radioisotope-labeled compound (i.e., hot spots of radioactivity) signals abnormal organ behavior. Because of such capabilities, nuclear medicine offers diagnostic input relating to function that goes beyond the information provided by ordinary x-ray techniques.

## Positron Emission Tomography and Computed Tomography

In Chapter 3, in which the pair production interaction is discussed, a diagnostic modality called **positron emission tomography** (PET) is also mentioned. Although this modality does not require the occurrence of pair production interactions, it does make use of the **annihilation radiation** events that are a by-product of this interaction. However, in the case of PET, the annihilation radiation is initiated by the radioactive decay of the nucleus of an unstable isotope. The instability in this case is associated with too many protons residing within the nucleus. Nuclei such as these usually spontaneously undergo a reaction in which the excess proton is transmuted into a neutron and a positively charged electron (**positron**). This conserves electric charge because the neutron has none. In order to conserve energy as well, the process includes the emission of an additional particle called the **neutrino**. A neutrino has no electric charge and almost negligible mass, but its energy of motion (kinetic energy) balances the energy of the reaction. Neutrinos almost never interact and are therefore nearly impossible to detect.

A positron, classified as antimatter, when passing close to an electron—normal matter—will interact destructively with the electron. In the process, both particles will disappear, having *annihilated* one another. Their respective masses are converted into energy that will be carried off by two photons emerging from the annihilation site in opposite directions, each with a kinetic energy of 511 keV. These energies correspond to the mass energies of the former positron and electron.

**Imaging.** If there is a volume (e.g., a human torso) in which many of these annihilation events are taking place, and if this volume is surrounded by a ring of densely packed detectors that are specifically tuned to 511-keV photon energies, then it is possible, in a manner analogous to that used in **computed tomography (CT)**, to reconstruct diagnostically useful images of the regions within the encompassed volume from which the annihilation photons are coming. This is the concept of PET scanning.

**Fluorine-18.** By far the most important isotope in PET scanning is the positron-emitter **fluorine-18** ($^{18}$F), which symbolically can be depicted as $_9$F$^{18}$. The subscript 9 is the atomic number and is equal to the number of protons within the nucleus, whereas the superscript 18 is the mass number and refers to the total number of nuclear particles. Thus nine neutrons are present in the nucleus of $^{18}$F. Nine neutrons are not enough to maintain a stable arrangement of protons and neutrons within this nucleus. More neutrons are needed, and so the unstable nucleus undergoes a change in which, as described previously, one less proton is present. This can be represented as:

$$p \rightarrow n + e^+ + v$$

where v is the symbol for a neutrino.

If the isotope as a whole is looked at, the process can be represented as:

$$_9F^{18} \rightarrow {_8}O^{18} + v + 2 \text{ annihilation energy photons}$$

where $_8$O$^{18}$ is a stable isotope of oxygen with 8 protons and 10 neutrons.

PET is an important imaging modality because it can be used to examine metabolic processes within the body. This is particularly relevant to the proliferation of cancer cells. Such cells seek to reproduce without end and in order to do so require a great deal of sugar, or glucose, to supply the energy for the unlimited growth. Therefore, if it were possible to introduce within the body a radioactive molecule that was very similar to a glucose molecule, then the presence of excessive glucose metabolism sites associated with cancer cell proliferation could be discerned by detecting areas of abnormally high radioactivity.

The great significance of $^{18}$F is that it can be attached to a glucose molecule, yielding a compound called **fluorodeoxyglucose (FDG)**. FDG is a radioactive tracer that is very similar in chemical behavior to ordinary glucose, and so it is taken up or metabolized by cancerous cells. As such it reveals the locations of these cells through its positron emission decay and subsequent generation of oppositely traveling annihilation photons. These annihilation event sites are physically localizable through the PET scanner's patient-surrounding ring of coincidence detectors.

If a PET scanner is mechanically joined in a tandem configuration (e.g., like a two-person bicycle) with a CT scanner to produce a single joint imaging device, then in essence a facility gains not only the ability to detect the presence of abnormally high regions of glucose metabolism, yielding evidence of cancer spread (metastasis) into other body areas, but also, at the same time, the means to obtain detailed information about the anatomic location and extent of these lesions or growths. Such a combined imaging device is called a **PET/CT scanner** (Fig. 14-2).

## Radiation Protection

Positron emitters result in the production of high-energy radiation. Each $^{18}$F nuclear transformation by positron decay yields two highly penetrating 511-keV photons. These cannot be shielded by an ordinary lead apron. In fact,

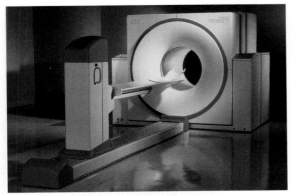

**FIGURE 14-2** Combined positron emission tomography/computed tomography (PET/CT) system.

because the thickness of lead needed to attenuate such high-energy radiation by 50% (known as the **half-value layer [HVL]**) is approximately 0.2 inch, adequate shielding at close distances would require up to an inch of lead. Therefore, the design of a PET/CT imaging suite involves significant radiation safety concerns. A discussion of the radiation safety design difficulties with respect to the PET/CT technologist for a minimal, but not zero, radiation exposure facility follows.

Unlike the usual diagnostic imaging suites in which the designer concentrates on protection from the radiation produced by an x-ray machine, the design of a PET/CT imaging suite presents unique additional radiation safety problems. In this situation, the scatter radiation generated by the CT scanner portion is the least of the designer's difficulties. Of much more importance is the high-energy annihilation photons emanating in all directions from the patient having the PET/CT scan. Furthermore, the presence of yet a third source of radiation, also of high energy, must be considered. Every patient who is to have a PET/CT scan requires what is called a "prep" time. During this time $^{18}$F, in the form of FDG with an activity usually of approximately 15 millicuries (555 megabecquerels [MBq]), is injected into the patient. The patient typically remains in the injection or prep room in a semireclining position for 45 to 60 minutes so that the FDG can be distributed throughout the body. This implies

that in order to have a smooth-flowing, coordinated patient throughput, it will be necessary that while one "hot" patient is being scanned, a second "hot" patient is reclining in a nearby room *waiting* to be scanned. Therefore, during this procedure the technologist and other personnel, as well as the general public, must be protected from at least two sources of high-energy photon radiation in addition to the scatter x-radiation from the CT scanner.

All of this makes the calculations for a practical space-limited shielding design anything but trivial. These problems are much simplified, however, when a facility can be designed from scratch instead of being retrofitted into limited existing space. Unfortunately, most often the latter is the case. Earlier it was shown that it takes a considerable amount of lead to attenuate photons with 511-keV energy. Therefore, unless other potentially mitigating factors can be applied, the amount of lead shielding needed to ensure acceptable radiation safety could become unreasonable. However, such mitigating factors do exist. They involve the concepts of weekly workload (W) and occupancy factor (T),* the decay in activity of the $^{18}$F during the prep and scan times, self-attenuation by the patient, and, significantly, the distance to each area of occupancy, also known as the *inverse square law*. Requirements for the protection of a radiographer in a new PET/CT suite are briefly considered here.

A potential workload for an average facility could be 7 PET/CT patients per daily shift, which amounts to 35 patients per week, with each patient, let us say, receiving at the start of prep time an activity of 15 mCi of $^{18}$F. The larger the weekly workload, the more shielding will be necessary in order to maintain permissible maximum equivalent dose levels to personnel and the public. $^{18}$F has a physical half-life of 110 minutes; therefore, the patient's degree of radioactivity will decrease naturally throughout the prep time, losing approximately 25% to 30% by the time

---

*Workload and occupancy factor are discussed in Chapter 13.

of scanning. This process will continue during the 45- to 50-minute scan time, with the amount of $^{18}$F decreasing through physical decay alone to approximately 50% of its initial activity at the conclusion of the scan. The patient's radioactivity is further decreased by any voiding that may take place just before the scanning procedure. The two processes taken together constitute what is known as an *effective half-life* ($T_{eff}$), which can be much less than the physical half-life of 110 minutes. Consequently, the patient's remaining radioactivity will typically be about one fourth of its initial value after the scan. This is important for radiation safety of the general public and any family members at the patient's home.

Such patients at discharge produce a measured midline surface radiation intensity of 40 to 50 mR/hr, and at a distance of 1 foot a radiation intensity of approximately 15 mR/hr. Usually, it is recommended that such patients maintain a 1-m distance from others as much as possible for the remainder of the day. After returning home, the patient is encouraged to drink plenty of fluids, so that with frequent urination and little permanent tissue retention, the patient's $T_{eff}$ will be so small that emitted radiation will be almost negligible 1 day later. After this time, the patient may resume full contact with all.

A well-designed facility should be arranged so that no areas of full occupancy are immediately adjacent to a high-energy radiation source; the prep room and scanning location of the patient are the most important of these sites from which to have distance. A secondary but less significant site is the patient's toilet, which could easily acquire some contamination.

In order to determine the equivalent dose rate (millirem [mrem]/hr or microsievert [μSv]/hr) at a particular distance from a person injected with a specific amount of $^{18}$F, the shielding planner must make use of a measured quantity called the *dose rate constant.** This value is 6.96 μSv/hr, or

*The information discussed in this paragraph is based on material presented at the 2004 American College of Medical Physics Annual Meeting in Scottsdale, Arizona, by Melissa C. Martin, MS, FACR, in a workshop entitled *PET/CT-Site Planning and Shielding Design.*

0.7 mrem/hr, at a distance of 1 m per mCi of $^{18}$F. Thus, if the patient did not self-attenuate any of the $^{18}$F radiation, then just after a 15-mCi injection the equivalent dose rate at 1 m would be approximately $0.7 \times 15 = 10.5$ mrem/hr (105 μSv/hr). At greater distances, the inverse square law can be applied to obtain a value. For example, at a distance of 4 m (approximately 13 feet), the equivalent dose rate without any shielding present diminishes to:

$$\frac{10.5}{4^2} = 0.66 \text{ mrem/hr (6.6 μSv/hr)}$$

Distance is a powerful tool of radiation protection. A well-designed facility takes good advantage of this. Returning to the injected patient, there are other facilitators of radiation protection at hand. Both the patient and nature are generators of these facilitators. It has been found that the body can absorb a substantial amount of $^{18}$F annihilation radiation.

The mean maximum equivalent dose rate at 1 m from the patient per mCi (37 MBq) injected just after the injection is not 0.7 mrem/hr (6.96 μSv/hr), as it would be for an unshielded point source of radiation; rather, it has been determined to be approximately 0.3 mrem/hr (3 μSv/hr) per mCi. At a distance of 4 m from the patient just after a 15-mCi injection, the equivalent dose rate is now given by:

$$15 \times \frac{0.3}{4^2} = 0.28 \text{ mrem/hr (2.8 μSv/hr)}$$

The contribution of nature to the radiation protection effort is that $^{18}$F has a short half-life. Therefore, the 15-mCi dose injected at 2 PM will be approximately 70% as strong at 3 PM (the approximate time that a scan will start) because of natural radioactive decay. Thus, in actuality, the equivalent dose delivered by the "hot" patient waiting during the prep time at a distance of 4 m is less than 0.28 mrem. If not this amount, then what dose equivalent would a person at this location effectively receive in 60 minutes? It must be a percentage of the whole, between 100% and

70%. Doing the mathematics of radioactive decay* yields a value of approximately 83%, or a correction factor of 0.83. Consequently, the equivalent dose at a distance of 4 m that could be received by a technologist continuously at this location (i.e., occupancy level T = 1) from a 1-hour prep patient in the absence of any added shielding is:

$$0.83 \times 0.28 \, \text{mrem} = 0.23 \, \text{mrem} \, (2.3 \, \mu\text{Sv})$$

Over the course of a week, then, with all conditions remaining the same, this person will accumulate an equivalent dose of:

$$35 \times 0.23 \, \text{mrem} = 8.1 \, \text{mrem} \, (81 \, \mu\text{Sv})$$

Over 50 weeks, this would add up to 400 mrem (4000 μSv) from prep patients alone. However, it is known that prep patients are not the only sources of high-energy radiation dose to PET/CT personnel. There is also the scan patient and, to a much lesser extent, the patient's toilet. The contributions of these sources of radiation dose also need to be factored into the facility's design and shielding plan.

Consider the scan patient in some detail. As always, it is desirable to have a good distance, if at all possible, between personnel and radiation source. That may not be possible if the facility is being fit into a preexisting area. So let it be assumed that there is a separation of only 3.3 m from the scan patient's midline to the location of the PET/CT technologist. In the absence of additional shielding, what could be the equivalent dose rate from the scan patient? The first factor to be aware of is the lesser activity in the scan patient, namely, 70% of the original 15 mCi. However, this is not the whole story. The prep patient is encouraged to void just before being scanned. What this means is that the residual $^{18}$F in the patient's body at the start of the scan is less than 70% of the original activity. If it is assumed that approximately 20% more was removed by voiding, then at the start of the scan, the activity within the patient is just 50% of the

original activity, namely, $0.5 \times 15 = 7.5$ mCi. If there were no other considerations,* then at the start of the scan the equivalent dose rate at the location of the technologist with no shielding would be:

$$\frac{7.5 \, \text{mCi} \times 0.3 \, \text{mrem/hr per mCi}}{(3.3)^2} = 0.2 \, \text{mrem/hr} \, (2 \, \mu\text{Sv/hr})$$

However, as seen previously, the radioactivity within the patient continues to decay all throughout the approximate 1 hour between voiding and his or her departure. Therefore, the equivalent dose to the technologist from the scan patient will actually be $0.83 \times 0.2$ mrem/hr, or 0.17 mrem (1.7 μSv). Over the course of a week, this amounts to $35 \times 0.17 = 6$ mrem (60 μSv). At 50 weeks, this equals 300 mrem (3 mSv). Assuming that all other sources (e.g., patient's toilet and possibly the "hot" laboratory) of radiation dose to the technologist could contribute an additional 50 mrem annually, then the unshielded technologist could receive an annual equivalent dose of 750 mrem (400 + 300 + 50) in this facility.

Shielding can be installed to decrease this amount significantly. Let us seek to reduce this value to a total of 250 mrem (2.5 mSv), or 5 mrem/wk (50 μSv/wk).

Figure 14-3 depicts a facility layout schematic that will be referred to for shielding calculations. For simplicity, these calculations will be restricted to protection of the PET/CT radiographer. In addition, the task will be further confined to reducing the contributions from the patient occupying the prep room and the patient being scanned. Beginning with the scan patient, it is required that both the viewing window and its surrounding wall be shielded so that the 300-mrem (3 mSv) annual equivalent dose contribution decreases to 100 mrem (1 mSv). As mentioned earlier, the amount of lead needed to decrease the intensity of this high-energy radiation by 50% is called its *half-value layer* (HVL). The HVL is equal to 0.2 inch of lead. One HVL

---

*Decay correction factor = 1.443 × (110/60)
$(1 - e^{-[0.693 \times 60/110]})$

*In this discussion, any shielding provided by the scanner itself is being neglected.

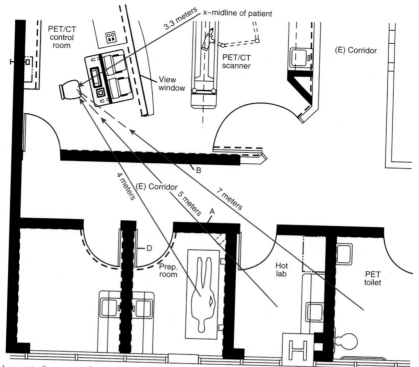

**FIGURE 14-3** Layout diagram of a positron emission tomography/computed tomography (PET/CT) imaging facility.

will bring the equivalent dose down to 150 mrem (1.5 mSv), and 2 HVLs will cut it to 75 mrem (0.75 mSv). Therefore, less than 2 HVLs would be needed. Doing the mathematics* results in:

1.56 HVLs or 1.56 × 0.2 inch of lead

$$= 0.312 \text{ inch of lead} \left( \frac{5}{16} \text{ inch} \right)$$

Thus, $\frac{5}{16}$ inch (7.9 mm) of lead must be placed in the wall surrounding the view window, and

---

*If n is the required number of HVLs, then in order to attenuate the radiation to $\frac{1}{3}$ of its value:

$$2^{-n} = \frac{1}{3}$$
$$\log 2^{-n} = \log(1/3)$$
$$-n \log 2 = \log 1 - \log 3 = -\log 3$$
$$n = \log 3 / \log 2$$
$$n = 1.56$$

the view window itself must be composed of this amount of lead acrylic to achieve the goal. This amount of lead is far more than would be required to shield the operator from the much less penetrating CT scatter radiation. Therefore, the scatter radiation does not have to be additionally accounted for. For the patient in the prep room, the goal is to interpose shielding so that the 400 mrem (4 mSv) annual equivalent dose contribution to the technologist decreases to 100 mrem (1 mSv); this decrease by a factor of 4 clearly requires 2 HVLs, or 0.4 inches (~13/32 inch or 1 cm) of lead. Examining the diagram, it is evident that this amount of shielding can be distributed between the prep room corridor wall and door (labeled A and D, respectively) and the scan suite corridor wall (labeled B). Excluding personnel other than the operator and any other circumstances, a practical solution is to place $\frac{1}{4}$ inch (6 mm) of lead in A and D and $\frac{3}{16}$ inch (~5 mm) of lead in B.

In conclusion, it is obvious that there is much to be considered when radiation shielding is designed for a PET/CT facility. Other personnel and the general public must also be protected from the high-energy radiation. Their protection involves lower permissible equivalent dose limits than for the occupationally exposed radiographer. If there is the opportunity to design the facility from scratch, then the required shielding can be greatly reduced; if not, then the calculations and the amount of needed shielding can be sizable.

## RADIATION EMERGENCIES: USE OF RADIATION AS A TERRORIST WEAPON

After the attack on the World Trade Center by hijacked airplanes on September 11, 2001, the possibility of the use of other terrorist weapons, such as radiation, became a public health concern. Today, most hospitals have **radiation emergency plans** for handling emergency situations involving **radioactive contamination**. Radiologic technologists should become aware of the radiation emergency plans that exist in the facilities in which they work. In this section, some fundamental principles of dealing with radioactive contamination in a health care environment are discussed.

## Contamination

A **radioactive dispersal device**, or "dirty bomb," is a radioactive source mixed with conventional explosives. It is intended to contaminate an area with radioactive material and thereby cause panic. The actual long-term health effects of a dirty bomb are likely to be minimal. If the radioactive material remains in a small area, few people may be affected. However, if enough explosives are used to spread the radioactive material over a broad area, then the radioactivity will be diluted and may not be much higher than background levels.

For example, it would be difficult for terrorists to accumulate as much radioactive material as existed in the Chernobyl nuclear reactor. Even if they were able to do this and were to explode the device with the same force as the explosion at Chernobyl, the actual number of radiation injuries would probably be quite small. At Chernobyl, no cases of acute radiation syndrome (ARS) were caused by exposure outside the immediate vicinity of the reactor. The only cases occurred in emergency workers, primarily firemen, who worked very near the reactor. They had little training and essentially no protective gear to prepare them for a radioactive emergency. In the United States at the present time, emergency responders are equipped to monitor and assess personnel exposure on-site in an emergency situation.

After an explosion of a dirty bomb, some individuals would be contaminated with dust and debris, some of which could contain radioactive materials. The procedure for **decontamination** is surprisingly simple. Removal of contaminated clothing and immersion in a shower comprise the best method. If a wound contains radioactive material, a simple rinse of the area is usually sufficient to allow medical personnel to provide medical attention. Most hospitals are stocked with **Geiger-Müller (GM) detectors** (described in Chapter 5), and emergency personnel are trained to provide guidance concerning contamination levels. The facility's radiation safety officer (RSO) would also be available to assess contamination levels.

It is unlikely that a dirty bomb would cause contamination with so much radioactive material that a victim could not receive medical attention. The key here is that the same personnel need not be near patients for any length of time. Most emergency room treatments do not require the staff to be near patients for as long as an hour. Even if a GM detector shows readings of two to five times natural background radiation, this means an effective dose of only 0.03 to 0.15 mSv/hr to a physician who is in direct contact with the patient. Therefore, a physician could treat this patient under these circumstances without exceeding normal dosimeter limits. In fact, normal dosimeter limits do not apply in radiation emergency situations.

The **Environmental Protection Agency (EPA)** suggests that during an emergency situation, individuals engaged in nonlifesaving activities work under a dose limit of 50 mSv per event. For individuals engaged in lifesaving activities, the dose limit rises to 250 mSv per event.[1] Because it may be difficult to monitor all workers involved in a radiation emergency, a dose rate criterion is often used. In this case, if the dose rate in the area is less than 0.1 mSv/hr, emergency personnel may enter an area to perform critical tasks. At a dose rate of 0.1 Sv/hr, emergency personnel should await specific instructions from radiation experts on how to proceed.[2]

## Cleanup of a Contaminated Urban Area

The EPA sets limits for radioactive contamination that assume that a 1-in-10,000 risk of causing a fatal cancer is unacceptable. This type of regulation requires hospitals, educational facilities, and industries to control accidental exposures so that the health of the population cannot be measurably affected. It also assumes that many other carcinogens are present and that all are regulated to a similar low level.

However, if radioactive contamination were to result from a dirty bomb, it is hoped that a more realistic evaluation of actual risk would be used. Unnecessary use of resources to clean a large inhabitable area (e.g., at the heart of a major city) to unreasonably stringent standards would be an unfortunate outcome requiring the expenditure of vast resources that could be used to benefit the public elsewhere. For example, a 1-in-10,000 probability of causing a fatal cancer corresponds approximately to a 2-mSv effective dose. Recall from Chapter 2 that the effective dose resulting from average natural background radiation is approximately 3 mSv. Therefore, cleanup of a contaminated site to levels associated with normal radiation protection

standards would require heroic measures, such as:

- Removal of topsoil
- Digging up of roadways

A practical compromise should be made to allow land use after a reasonable cleanup.

## Medical Management of Persons Experiencing Radiation Bioeffects

If **surface contamination** is suspected, personnel should wear gowns, masks, and gloves when working with the patient. The same procedures that control the spread of infection are useful to prevent the spread of radioactive contamination. The clothing of individuals who have been contaminated should be placed in plastic containers and set aside for later evaluation. Removal of surface contamination involves removal of the patient's clothing and the use of a shower to cleanse the skin.

The various stages of ARS are discussed in Chapter 8. (A complete discussion of procedures for handling acute radiation syndrome is beyond the scope of this text. The interested reader is referred to recent publications on this subject.[3,4]) In dealing with patients with ARS, some estimate of the amount of exposure they have received helps predict the clinical course of the syndrome (Table 14-1). For exposures localized to specific regions of the body, medical management involves the prevention of infection and control of pain and potential skin grafts. If beta-emitting radioactive material settles on a patient's skin, the dose is superficial, and skin grafts may be successful. Gamma-emitting materials can produce a deeper dose that could interfere with healing.

During the first 48 hours of ARS, symptoms such as nausea and vomiting occur. Medical management at this time is simply to treat the symptoms and try to prevent dehydration. The bone marrow becomes depleted (leukopenia and thrombocytopenia) after a few weeks. Bone marrow transplantation has been attempted in individuals such as severely exposed Chernobyl

| TABLE 14-1 | Dose-Effect Relation after Acute Whole-Body Radiation from Gamma Rays or X-Rays* | | |
|---|---|---|---|
| **Whole-Body (Gy$_t$)** | **Absorbed Dose Effect** | | |
| 0.05 | No symptoms | | |
| 0.15 | No symptoms, but possible chromosomal aberrations in cultured peripheral blood lymphocytes | | |
| 0.5 | No symptoms (minor decreases in white blood cell and platelet counts in a few persons) | | |
| 1 | Nausea and vomiting in approximately 10% of patients within 48 hr after exposure | | |
| 2 | Nausea and vomiting in approximately 50% of persons within 24 hr, with marked decreases in white blood cell and platelet counts | | |
| 4 | Nausea and vomiting in 90% of persons within 12 hr, and diarrhea in 10% within 8 hr; 50% mortality in the absence of treatment | | |
| 6 | 100% mortality within 30 days because of bone marrow failure in the absence of treatment | | |
| 10 | Approximate dose that is survivable with the best medical therapy available | | |
| >10-30 | Nausea and vomiting in all persons in less than 5 min; severe gastrointestinal damage; death likely in 2 to 3 wk in the absence of treatment | | |
| >30 | Cardiovascular collapse and central nervous system damage, with death in 24 to 72 hr | | |

*Data from Gusev I, Guskova AK, Mettler FA Jr, eds: *Medical management of radiation accidents,* ed 2, Boca Raton, Fla, 2001, CRC Press.

emergency workers. However, this strategy has not been successful. The current plan is to administer drugs that stimulate any remaining bone marrow.

In the event of **internal contamination,** various strategies are used, depending on the clinical and radiologic form of contamination. Some of these methods include:

- Dilution (forcing fluids)
- Blocking absorption in the gastrointestinal tract (administration of emetics, charcoal, laxatives)

If the radionuclide is iodine, administration of potassium iodide to block further uptake in the thyroid is possible if no more than a few hours have elapsed since the contamination.

The National Library of Medicine and the National Institutes of Health maintain a website that contains a wealth of information on dealing with radiation emergencies. It contains:

- Both basic and advanced methods for decontamination
- Methods to reduce exposure
- Specific medical emergency procedures for various situations

The website may be found at www.nlm.nih.gov/medlineplus/radiationemergencies.html.

## SUMMARY

- Isotopes are atoms that have the same number of protons within the nucleus but have different numbers of neutrons.
  - Some nuclei of isotopes have too many neutrons or too many protons for stability.
  - Radioactive isotopes spontaneously undergo changes or transformations to rectify their unstable arrangement.
- Rapidly dividing cells that are well oxygenated are very radiosensitive.
  - When cells are radiosensitive, cancerous growths or tumors can be either eliminated or at least controlled by irradiation of the area containing the growth.
- Therapeutic isotopes may be characterized by relatively long half-lives.
- Fast electrons are beta radiation.
- Gamma rays and x-ray photons differ only in their point of origin.
- Iodine-125 decays with a half-life of 59.4 days by a process called *electron capture.*

- The most practical radiation protection to follow for patients having therapeutic prostate seed implants is use of the concepts of distance and time.
- When iodine-131 is being administered to treat a hospitalized patient for thyroid cancer, a large, up to 1-inch-thick, rolling lead shield can be positioned between the patient and any attending personnel for protection.
- Diagnostic techniques in nuclear medicine typically make use of short-lived radioisotopes as radioactive tracers.
  - Technetium-99m is the most common radioisotope used in nuclear medicine.
- Positron emission tomography (PET) makes use of annihilation radiation events.
  - When annihilation occurs, the positron and electron interact destructively and disappear. Their respective masses convert into energy that will be carried off by two photons emerging from the annihilation site in opposite directions, each with a kinetic energy of 511 keV.
  - A neutrino is a particle that has almost negligible mass and no electric charge but carries away any excess energy from the nucleus of the atom.
  - Fluorine-18 is the most important isotope used for PET scanning.
  - PET is an important imaging modality because it can examine metabolic processes within the body.
  - Fluorodeoxyglucose (FDG) is a radioactive tracer that is taken up or metabolized by cancerous cells and that reveals their location through positron emission decay and subsequent generation of oppositely traveling annihilation photons.
  - A PET/CT scanner can detect the presence of regions of abnormally high glucose metabolism, thus providing evidence of metastasis to other body areas, and at the same time can obtain detailed information about the location and size of these lesions or growths.

- Positron emitters result in the production of high-energy radiation, and for this reason, the design of a PET/CT imaging suite involves significant radiation safety concerns.
- Most hospitals have radiation emergency plans for handling emergency situations involving radioactive contamination.
- A radioactive dispersal device, or "dirty bomb," is a radioactive source mixed with conventional explosives, the actual long-term health effects of which will most likely be minimal.
  - If radioactive material from a dirty bomb remains in a small area, only a few people may be seriously affected.
  - Conversely, if enough explosives are used to spread the radioactive material over a broad area, radioactivity will be diluted and may not be much higher than background levels.
  - If a dirty bomb were to explode with the same force as the explosion at Chernobyl, the actual number of radiation injuries could be quite small.
- The United States currently has emergency responders who are prepared and equipped to monitor and assess personnel exposure on-site in an emergency situation.
  - After an explosion of a dirty bomb, externally contaminated individuals can be decontaminated by removal of contaminated clothing and immersion in a shower.
  - Geiger-Müller (GM) detectors may be used by trained emergency personnel to monitor contamination levels.
  - During an emergency situation, individuals engaged in nonlifesaving activities are to work under a dose limit of 50 mSv per event, whereas those persons performing lifesaving activities have a dose limit of 250 mSv.
  - If surface contamination is suspected, emergency personnel should protect themselves by wearing gowns, masks, and gloves while working with the patient.

- Handling of patients with internal contamination varies depending on the clinical and radiologic form of contamination. Strategies may include dilution and blocking absorption in the gastrointestinal tract. Potassium iodide can be administered to block further uptake of radioactive iodine in the thyroid gland.

## REFERENCES

1. Mettler FA, Voelz GL: Major radiation exposure: what to expect and how to respond. *N Engl J Med* 346:1554, 2002.
2. National Council on Radiation Protection and Measurements (NCRP): *Management of terrorist events involving radioactive material,* Report No. 138, Bethesda, Md, 2001, NCRP.
3. Gusev I, et al, editors: *Medical management of radiation accidents,* ed 2, Boca Raton, Fla, 2001, CRC Press.
4. Jarrett D, editor: *Medical management of radiation casualties: handbook,* AFRRI Secial Publication 99-92, Bethesda, Md, 1999, Armed Forces Radiobiology Research Institute. (Also available at: www.afrri.usuhs.mil.)

## GENERAL DISCUSSION QUESTIONS

1. Why do isotopes that have too many neutrons or too many protons spontaneously undergo changes or transformations?
2. What causes cancerous growths or tumors to be eliminated or controlled by irradiation?
3. What difference exists between gamma rays and x-ray photons?
4. What are the best radiation safety practices to follow for patients having therapeutic prostate seed implants?
5. While caring for a hospitalized patient receiving iodine-131 therapy for cancer, what can hospital personnel do to minimize occupational exposure?
6. What radiation safety concerns are associated with the design of a PET/CT imaging suite, and how is radiation

protection provided to meet these concerns?
7. What is a radioactive dispersal device, or "dirty bomb," and what are the possible consequences if such a device is detonated?
8. If a wound contains radioactive material, what should be done to decontaminate the wound?
9. What dose level may an individual engaged in lifesaving activities during a radiation emergency receive?
10. If surface contamination is suspected, what should medical personnel wear when working with a contaminated patient?

## REVIEW QUESTIONS

1. Well-oxygenated rapidly dividing cells are:
   A. Very insensitive and are not damaged by radiation.
   B. Very sensitive to damage by radiation.
   C. Moderately sensitive to damage by radiation.
   D. Somewhat sensitive to damage by radiation.
2. Iodine-125 decays with a half-life of 59.4 days by a process called:
   A. Attenuation.
   B. Electron capture.
   C. Pair production.
   D. Photodisintegration.
3. Which of the following steps should be taken for external decontamination from radioactive materials?
   1. Removal of contaminated clothing
   2. Immersion of contaminated person in a shower
   3. Monitoring of the contaminated individual with a Geiger-Müller detector
   A. 1 and 2 only
   B. 1 and 3 only
   C. 2 and 3 only
   D. 1, 2, and 3

4. What dose level may an individual who is engaged in nonlifesaving activities during a radiation emergency safely receive?
   A. 10 mSv per event
   B. 30 mSv per event
   C. 50 mSv per event
   D. 250 mSv per event

5. The clothing of individuals that has been contaminated should be:
   A. Aired out on a clothesline to decontaminate.
   B. Burned immediately.
   C. Placed in plastic containers and set aside for later evaluation.
   D. Shaken out and put back on.

6. All of the following statements are true *except:*
   A. In dealing with patients with acute radiation syndrome (ARS), some estimate of the amount of exposure they have received helps predict the clinical course of the syndrome.
   B. If beta-emitting radioactive material settles on a patient's skin, the dose is very deep and skin grafts will not be very successful.
   C. Gamma-emitting radioactive materials may produce a deep dose that may interfere with healing.
   D. Current strategy for an ARS patient is to administer drugs that stimulate any remaining bone marrow.

7. Some of the strategies used to treat internal radiation contamination include:
   1. Dilution (forcing fluids).
   2. Blocking absorption in the gastrointestinal tract (administration of emetics, charcoal, laxatives).
   3. Administration of potassium iodide to block further uptake in the thyroid, if the radionuclide is iodine and no more than a few hours have elapsed since the contamination.
   A. 1 only
   B. 2 only
   C. 3 only
   D. 1, 2, and 3

8. A well-designed PET/CT facility should be arranged so that there are no areas of full occupancy immediately adjacent to a:
   A. High-energy radiation source.
   B. Low-energy radiation source.
   C. Patient waiting area.
   D. Public corridor.

9. Which of the following are almost impossible to detect?
   A. X-rays
   B. Gamma rays
   C. Positrons
   D. Neutrinos

10. Patients receiving iodine-125 should *significantly* limit durations of close contact (<3 feet) with small children and pregnant women for a period of:
    A. Six days after the implant procedure.
    B. Six weeks after the implant procedure.
    C. Six months after the implant procedure.
    D. Six years after the implant procedure.

# Relationships between Systems of Units

In science, as is shown throughout the text of *Radiation Protection in Medical Radiography,* various quantities are important for describing physical processes. Very familiar examples of such quantities are length, mass, force, energy, and time. If one also includes electric charge, then practically all of the fundamental constants of nature contain as part of their description combinations of these physical quantities or, more accurately, *the units associated with them.* The purpose of this appendix is to tabulate these units for the various systems that are in actual use and to show how they are related to one another.

There are three basic systems of physical units that have been in existence for a long time and that are familiar to varying degrees, depending on what part of the world one lives in and perhaps one's field of work. They are the English system, the centimeter-gram-second system (CGS system), and the MKS (SI) system. The following tables specify for each important physical quantity the corresponding associated fundamental unit in each of the three systems and the relationships among these units when possible. Boxes demonstrating calculations for conversions among units and for equivalent and effective dose are also provided.

## English System

| Quantity | Unit |
|---|---|
| Length | Foot, inch |
| Force (weight) | pound (lb) |
| Mass | slug (an object of mass 1 slug weighs 32 lb) |
| Energy | Foot-pound |
| Power | horsepower (hp) |
| Pressure | $lb/in^2$ |
| Time | second |
| Electric charge | coulomb |
| Temperature | degrees Fahrenheit (°F) |
| Absorbed dose | No specific unit |

## CGS System

| Quantity | Unit |
|---|---|
| Length | centimeter (cm) |
| Force (weight) | dyne (1 gm-cm/sec$^2$) |
| Mass | gram (g) |
| Energy | erg (1 gm-cm$^2$/sec$^2$) |
| Power | ergs per second |
| Pressure | barye (Ba) (1 Ba = 1 dyne/cm$^2$) |
| Time | second |
| Electric charge | statcoulomb or esu (esu means electrostatic unit of charge) |
| Temperature | degrees Centigrade (Celsius) (°C) |
| Absorbed dose | rad (1 rad = 100 ergs/gram) |
| Equivalent dose | rem |

## MKS (SI) System

| Quantity | Unit |
|---|---|
| Length | meter (m) |
| Force (weight) | newton (1 N = 1 kg-m/sec$^2$) |
| Mass | kilogram (kg) |
| Energy | joule (1 J = 1 kg-m$^2$/sec$^2$) |
| Power | watt (1 W = 1 joule/sec) |
| Pressure | N/m$^2$ |
| Time | second |
| Electric charge | coulomb (C) |
| Temperature | degrees Centigrade (Celsius), degrees Kelvin |
| Absorbed dose | gray (Gy) (1 Gy = 1 J/kg) |
| Equivalent dose | sievert (Sv) |

## Relationships among Units

| Quantity | Unit Conversions |
|---|---|
| Length | 1 m = 100 cm = 39.37 inches; 2.54 cm = 1 inch |
| Force (weight) | 1 N = 0.225 lb = 10$^5$ dynes |
| Mass | 1 kg = 1000 g; 1 slug = 14.6 kg |
| Energy | 1 J = 10$^7$ ergs = 0.738 ft-lb |
| Power | 1 W = 0.738 ft-lb/sec; 1 hp = 550 ft-lb/sec = 746 W = 0.746 kW |
| Pressure | 1 N/m$^2$ = 1.45(10)$^{-4}$ lb/in$^2$ =10 Ba; 1 atmosphere = 14.7 lb/in$^2$ = 1.013(10)$^5$ N/m$^2$ |
| Time | second |
| Electric charge | 1 esu = 1 statcoulomb = 3.34(10)$^{-10}$ C |
| Temperature | $T_F = \frac{9}{5} T_C + 32$ <br> $T_K = T_C + 273$ |
| Absorbed dose | 1 Gy = 100 rad, 1 cGy = 1 rad |
| Equivalent dose | 1 Sv = 100 rem |

## Conversion of Roentgens (R) to Coulombs per Kilogram (C/kg)

Example: To convert 100 R to C/kg:

1. Set up the equation: $100 R \times 2.58(10)^{-4} \frac{C/kg}{R}$

2. Cancel R: $100 \cancel{R} \times 2.58(10)^{-4} \frac{C/kg}{\cancel{R}}$

3. Obtain answer: 0.0258 C/kg
4. Write answer in standard scientific notation: 2.58(10)$^{-2}$ C/kg

## Conversion of Coulombs per Kilogram (C/kg) to Roentgens (R)

Example: To convert 100 C/kg to R:

1. Set up the equation: $100 \, C/kg \div 2.58(10)^{-4} \frac{C/kg}{R}$

   Or

   $$\frac{100 \, C/kg}{2.58(10)^{-4} \frac{C/kg}{R}}$$

2. Cancel C/kg: $100 \cancel{C/kg} \div 2.58(10)^{-4} \cancel{C/kg}/R$
3. Obtain answer: 39(10)$^4$ R or 390,000 roentgens (an enormous radiation exposure)

## Conversion of Rad to Gray (Gy)

Rule: Number of rad ÷ 100 = Number of gray
Example 1: 5000 rad = 5000 ÷ 100 rad/Gy = 50 Gy
Example 2: 5 rad = 5 ÷ 100 rad/Gy = 0.05 Gy

## Conversion of Gray (Gy) to Rad

Rule: Number of gray × 100 = Number of rad
Example 1: 15 Gy = 15 × 100 rad/Gy =1500 rad
Example 2: 50 Gy = 50 × 100 rad/Gy = 5000 rad

## Subunit Conversion of Centigray (cGy) to Rad

Rule: Number of cGy $\times$ 1 = Number of rad
Example 1: 10 cGy = 10 $\times$ 1 = 10 rad
Example 2: 75 cGy = 75 $\times$ 1 = 75 rad

## Subunit Conversions of Rad to Centigray (cGy)

Rule: Number of rad $\div$ 1 = Number of cGy
Example 1: 10 rad = 10 $\div$ 1 = 10 cGy
Example 2: 75 rad = 75 $\div$ 1 = 75 cGy

## Determining and Expressing Equivalent Dose (EqD) Using Rad and Rem

Example: An individual received the following absorbed doses: 10 rad of x-radiation, 5 rad of fast neutrons, and 20 rad of alpha particles. What is the *total* equivalent dose?

$$EqD = (D \times W_R)_1 + (D \times W_R)_2 + (D \times W_R)_3$$

(The radiation weighting factor for each radiation in question may be obtained from Table 4-2.)
   Answer:

| Radiation Type | D | X | $W_R$ | = | EqD |
|---|---|---|---|---|---|
| X-radiation | 10 rad | $\times$ | 1 | = | 10 rem |
| Fast neutrons | 5 rad | $\times$ | 20 | = | 100 rem |
| Alpha particles | 20 rad | $\times$ | 20 | = | 400 rem |
| | | | Total EqD | = | 510 rem |

## Determining and Expressing Effective Dose (EfD) in Rem

Example: The $W_R$ for x-radiation is 1 (see Table 4-2), and the $W_T$ for the gonads is 0.20 (see Table 4-3). If the gonads receive an absorbed dose (D) of 10 rad from exposure to x-radiation, what is the EfD in rem?
   Answer:

$$\begin{aligned} EfD &= D \times W_R \times W_T \\ &= 10 \times 1 \times 0.20 \\ &= 2\,rem \end{aligned}$$

## Traditional and SI Equivalents

| | |
|---|---|
| 1 roentgen (R) equals | 1. $2.58 \times 10^{-4}$ C/kg of air |
| 1 milliroentgen (mR) equals | 1. $\frac{1}{1000}$ R or $10^{-3}$ R |
| 1 rad equals | 1. 100 erg/g |
| | 2. $\frac{1}{100}$ J/kg |
| | 3. $\frac{1}{100}$ Gy |
| | 4. 1 cGy |
| 1 millirad equals | 1. $\frac{1}{1000}$ rad |
| 1 rem equals | 1. $\frac{1}{100}$ J/kg (for x-radiation, Q = 1) |
| | 2. $\frac{1}{100}$ Sv |
| | 3. 1 cSv |
| | 4. 10 mSv |
| 1 millirem equals | 1. $\frac{1}{1000}$ rem |

# Standard Designations for Metric System Lengths, Electron Volt Energy Levels, and Frequency Spectrum Ranges

**Metric System Equivalents for Length**

| Length | Symbol | Power of 10 Fractional Form | Power of 10 Decimal Form | Scientific Notation |
|--------|--------|----------------------------|--------------------------|---------------------|
| Yottameter | Ym | 1,000,000,000,000,000,000,000,000 | 1,000,000,000,000,000,000,000,000 | $10^{24}$ (m) |
| Zettameter | Zm | 1,000,000,000,000,000,000,000 | 1,000,000,000,000,000,000,000 | $10^{21}$ (m) |
| Exameter | Em | 1,000,000,000,000,000,000 | 1,000,000,000,000,000,000 | $10^{18}$ (m) |
| Petameter | Pm | 1,000,000,000,000,000 | 1,000,000,000,000,000 | $10^{15}$ (m) |
| Terameter | Tm | 1,000,000,000,000 | 1,000,000,000,000 | $10^{12}$ (m) |
| Gigameter | Gm | 1,000,000,000 | 1,000,000,000 | $10^{9}$ (m) |
| Megameter | Mm | 1,000,000 | 1,000,000 | $10^{6}$ (m) |
| Kilometer | km | 1000 | 1000 | $10^{3}$ (m) |
| Hectometer | hm | 100 | 100 | $10^{2}$ (m) |
| Dekameter | dam | 10 | 10 | $10^{1}$ (m) |
| Meter | m | 1 | 1 | $10^{0}$ (m) |
| Decimeter | dm | 1/10 | 0.1 | $10^{-1}$ (m) |
| Centimeter | cm | 1/100 | 0.01 | $10^{-2}$ (m) |
| Millimeter | mm | 1/1000 | 0.001 | $10^{-3}$ (m) |
| Micrometer | μm | 1/1,000,000 | 0.00001 | $10^{-6}$ (m) |
| Nanometer | nm | 1/1,000,000,000 | 0.000000001 | $10^{-9}$ (m) |
| Picometer | pm | 1/1,000,000,000,000 | 0.000000000001 | $10^{-12}$ (m) |
| Femtometer | fm | 1/1,000,000,000,000,000 | 0.000000000000001 | $10^{-15}$ (m) |
| Attometer | am | 1/1,000,000,000,000,000,000 | 0.000000000000000001 | $10^{-18}$ (m) |
| Zeptometer | zm | 1/1,000,000,000,000,000,000,000 | 0.000000000000000000001 | $10^{-21}$ (m) |
| Yoctometer | ym | 1/1,000,000,000,000,000,000,000,000 | 0.000000000000000000000001 | $10^{-24}$ (m) |

**Electron Volt Common Energy Designations.** The abbreviation *eV* stands for *electron volt*; 1 eV is defined as the energy acquired by an electron when it is moved through a 1-V potential difference by a battery or some other mechanism.

The following terms designate various powers of 10 multiples of 1 eV:

$$1 \text{ KeV} = 1000 \text{ eV} = 10^3 \text{ eV}$$
$$1 \text{ MeV} = 1{,}000{,}000 \text{ eV} = 10^6 \text{ eV}$$
$$1 \text{ GeV} = 1{,}000{,}000{,}000 \text{ eV} = 10^9 \text{ eV}$$

The following terms designate various powers of 10 fractions of 1 eV:

$$1 \text{ meV} = 0.001 \text{ eV} = 10^{-3} \text{ eV}$$
$$1 \text{ } \mu\text{eV} = 0.000001 \text{ eV} = 10^{-6} \text{ eV}$$
$$1 \text{ neV} = 0.000000001 \text{ eV} = 10^{-9} \text{ eV}$$

**Common Frequency Spectrum Designations.** The abbreviation *Hz* stands for *hertz*, which is the standard unit for frequency; 1 Hz is by definition equal to one repeatable cycle of a phenomenon or event (e.g., a water wave rising from flat to crest, descending to trough, and returning to flat) occurring in 1 second. Ten hertz corresponds to 10 such cycles occurring every second, whereas 0.1 Hz corresponds to only $\frac{1}{10}$ of a cycle occurring each second.

The following terms designate frequency ranges that constitute various powers of 10 multiples of 1 Hz:

$$1 \text{ KHz} = 10^3 \text{ Hz}$$
$$1 \text{ MHz} = 10^6 \text{ Hz}$$
$$1 \text{ GHz} = 10^9 \text{ Hz}$$
$$1 \text{ THz} = 10^{12} \text{ Hz}$$
$$1 \text{ PHz} = 10^{15} \text{ Hz}$$
$$1 \text{ EHz} = 10^{18} \text{ Hz}$$

# Periodic Table of Elements

# Periodic Table of the Elements

**Legend (example):**

- 11 — Atomic number
- Na — Element symbol
- Sodium — Element name
- 22.990 — Atomic weight

**Categories:**
- Alkali metals
- Alkaline earth metals
- Lanthanides
- Actinides
- Transition metals
- Unknown properties
- Post-transition metals
- Metalloids
- Other nonmetals
- Halogens
- Noble gases

| Period | 1 / 1A | 2 / 2A | 3 / 3B | 4 / 4B | 5 / 5B | 6 / 6B | 7 / 7B | 8 / 8B | 9 / 8B | 10 | 11 / 1B | 12 / 2B | 13 / 3A | 14 / 4A | 15 / 5A | 16 / 6A | 17 / 7A | 18 / 8A |
|---|---|---|---|---|---|---|---|---|---|---|---|---|---|---|---|---|---|---|
| 1 | 1 H Hydrogen 1.0078 | | | | | | | | | | | | | | | | | 2 He Helium 4.0026 |
| 2 | 3 Li Lithium 6.938 | 4 Be Beryllium 9.0122 | | | | | | | | | | | 5 B Boron 10.806 | 6 C Carbon 12.009 | 7 N Nitrogen 14.006 | 8 O Oxygen 15.999 | 9 F Fluorine 18.998 | 10 Ne Neon 20.180 |
| 3 | 11 Na Sodium 22.990 | 12 Mg Magnesium 24.305 | | | | | | | | | | | 13 Al Aluminum 26.982 | 14 Si Silicon 28.084 | 15 P Phosphorus 30.974 | 16 S Sulfur 32.059 | 17 Cl Chlorine 35.446 | 18 Ar Argon 39.948 |
| 4 | 19 K Potassium 39.098 | 20 Ca Calcium 40.078 | 21 Sc Scandium 44.956 | 22 Ti Titanium 47.867 | 23 V Vanadium 50.942 | 24 Cr Chromium 51.996 | 25 Mn Manganese 54.938 | 26 Fe Iron 55.845 | 27 Co Cobalt 58.933 | 28 Ni Nickel 58.693 | 29 Cu Copper 63.546 | 30 Zn Zinc 65.38 | 31 Ga Gallium 69.723 | 32 Ge Germanium 72.63 | 33 As Arsenic 74.922 | 34 Se Selenium 78.96 | 35 Br Bromine 79.904 | 36 Kr Krypton 83.798 |
| 5 | 37 Rb Rubidium 85.468 | 38 Sr Strontium 87.62 | 39 Y Yttrium 88.906 | 40 Zr Zirconium 91.224 | 41 Nb Niobium 92.906 | 42 Mo Molybdenum 95.96 | 43 Tc Technetium 98.9062 | 44 Ru Ruthenium 101.07 | 45 Rh Rhodium 102.91 | 46 Pd Palladium 106.42 | 47 Ag Silver 107.87 | 48 Cd Cadmium 112.41 | 49 In Indium 114.82 | 50 Sn Tin 118.71 | 51 Sb Antimony 121.76 | 52 Te Tellurium 127.60 | 53 I Iodine 126.90 | 54 Xe Xenon 131.29 |
| 6 | 55 Cs Cesium 132.91 | 56 Ba Barium 137.33 | 57–71 Lanthanides | 72 Hf Hafnium 178.49 | 73 Ta Tantalum 180.95 | 74 W Tungsten 183.84 | 75 Re Rhenium 186.21 | 76 Os Osmium 190.23 | 77 Ir Iridium 192.22 | 78 Pt Platinum 195.08 | 79 Au Gold 196.97 | 80 Hg Mercury 200.59 | 81 Tl Thallium 204.38 | 82 Pb Lead 207.2 | 83 Bi Bismuth 208.98 | 84 Po Polonium (209) | 85 At Astatine (210) | 86 Rn Radon (222) |
| 7 | 87 Fr Francium (223) | 88 Ra Radium (226) | 89–103 Actinides | 104 Rf Rutherfordium (261) | 105 Db Dubnium (262) | 106 Sg Seaborgium (266) | 107 Bh Bohrium (264) | 108 Hs Hassium (269) | 109 Mt Meitnerium (268) | 110 Ds Darmstadtium (268) | 111 Rg Roentgenium (268) | 112 Cn Copernicium (268) | 113 Uut Ununtrium (268) | 114 Fl Flerovium (268) | 115 Uup Ununpentium (268) | 116 Lv Livermorium (268) | 117 Uus Ununseptium (268) | 118 Uuo Ununoctium (268) |

**Lanthanides**

| 57 La Lanthanum 138.91 | 58 Ce Cerium 140.12 | 59 Pr Praseodymium 140.91 | 60 Nd Neodymium 144.24 | 61 Pm Promethium (145) | 62 Sm Samarium 150.36 | 63 Eu Europium 151.96 | 64 Gd Gadolinium 157.25 | 65 Tb Terbium 158.93 | 66 Dy Dysprosium 162.50 | 67 Ho Holmium 164.93 | 68 Er Erbium 167.26 | 69 Tm Thulium 168.93 | 70 Yb Ytterbium 173.04 | 71 Lu Lutetium 174.97 |
|---|---|---|---|---|---|---|---|---|---|---|---|---|---|---|

**Actinides**

| 89 Ac Actinium (227) | 90 Th Thorium 232.04 | 91 Pa Protactinium 231.04 | 92 U Uranium 238.03 | 93 Np Neptunium (237) | 94 Pu Plutonium (244) | 95 Am Americium (243) | 96 Cm Curium (247) | 97 Bk Berkelium (247) | 98 Cf Californium (251) | 99 Es Einsteinium (252) | 100 Fm Fermium (257) | 101 Md Mendelevium (258) | 102 No Nobelium (259) | 103 Lr Lawrencium (262) |
|---|---|---|---|---|---|---|---|---|---|---|---|---|---|---|

*Source: Tate K: Periodic table of the elements. www.LiveScience.com.*

# Chance of a 50-KeV Photon interacting with Atoms of Tissue as it travels through 5 cm of Soft Tissue

Let $N_0$ be the number of x-ray photons incident on a uniform slab of tissue of thickness "y." The probability that there will be an interaction of any sort between a photon and an atom within the slab is, in the simplest case, proportional to the slab thickness and the number of incident photons and the mean target size presented by a slab atom to an x-ray photon.

**Mathematically, One May Proceed as Follows:**

1. Let dN be the change in the number of photons in the x-ray beam after the beam has passed through an infinitesimal distance dy. Because the number of photons decreases with every interaction, dN is a negative quantity.
2. At any depth within the phantom, the number of interactions that will occur in the next incremental thickness dy is proportional to the remaining number of photons N at that depth and the distance of penetration dy. In mathematical terms:

$$dN = -\mu N dy$$

where the symbol $\mu$ is the constant of proportionality and is known as the *linear attenuation coefficient*. It is defined by the previous equation and has the following unit: 1/cm.

3. Rearranging the previous equation, one performs the following integration:

$$\int_{N_0}^{N} dN/N = -\mu \int_0^y dy$$

which leads to the following relation:

$$\ln(N/N_0) = -\mu y$$

4. If one uses the properties of logarithms and raises both sides of the last equation to the power e, the x-ray attenuation equation is as follows:

$$N = N_0 e^{-\mu y}$$

5. For 50-KeV photons passing through 5 cm of soft tissue:

$$\mu_{\text{soft tissue}} = 0.214 \text{ and } y = 5$$

Substituting these values into the last equation and rearranging the equation a bit, the following is obtained:

$$N/N_0 = e^{-(0.214 \times 5)} = 0.34$$

which shows that only 0.34, or 34%, of the initial number of photons in the 50-KeV beam remain (i.e., have not undergone an interaction) after traversing a 5-cm slab of tissue. In other words, 66% of the incident x-ray beam has interacted with a tissue atom.

# Relationship among Photons, Electromagnetic Waves, Wavelength, and Energy

Before 1900, all attempts to use current theories and concepts in physics to explain the measured energy distribution of radiation from a heated body failed grievously. In that year, a German physicist, Max Planck, introduced the concept of a "quantum," or discrete unit of energy, to resolve these discrepancies. According to Planck's theory, whenever radiation is emitted or absorbed by a hot object, the energy of that radiation is not emitted or absorbed continuously but rather in discrete amounts, which he called *quanta*.

Mathematically, a single such amount or energy quantum is given by the following equation:

$$E = hf$$

where f is the frequency of the radiation and h is a proportionality constant called, appropriately, *Planck's constant*. This quantum of energy has since received the name *photon*. Thus the energy of a photon varies directly as the frequency of the associated radiation. Because the frequency f and the wavelength w of any type of radiation are related by the simple expression

$$c = fw$$

where c is the speed of light (300,000,000 m/sec in a vacuum), then

$$E = hf = hc/w$$

This result shows that the energy of a photon decreases as the wavelength of the radiation increases (e.g., photons of infrared light are less energetic than those of ultraviolet light because infrared wavelengths are longer than ultraviolet wavelengths). Einstein used these ideas to explain the emission of electrons from a metallic surface when visible light radiation was directed at it. This is called the *photoelectric effect*. The light-produced electrons, or photoelectrons, were found to have *energies that depended on the wavelength of the focused light* but were completely independent of the intensity or brightness of that light. This phenomenon could not be explained by traditional physics. However, it was fully explicable in terms of the new concept of radiation energy (quanta or photons) and the energy relation given in the last equation. That relation contains no reference to the brightness of the light. For his work in this area, Einstein received the Nobel Prize in Physics in 1921.

To summarize, photons are the particles associated with the electromagnetic (EM) radiation spectrum (within which visible light and x-rays are included). When energy is transferred from an EM wave through interaction with matter, the energy is transferred by photons in discrete, or integral, amounts. Each such discrete amount is directly proportional to the frequency of the EM radiation.

# Electron Shell Structure of the Atom

Other than the hydrogen atom, all atoms contain more than one electron. The purpose of this appendix is to describe, without delving too extensively into the details of modern physics, specifically quantum mechanics, how electrons are arranged—that is, ordered—in multielectron atoms. To do so we must introduce two discovered principles that serve as the foundations for our discussion. These are, simply, that electrons in undisturbed or stable atoms are always distributed in the lowest overall energy configuration or energy states and that no two electrons can ever occupy the exact same energy level (in more precise terminology, no two electrons in an atom can exist in the exact same quantum state). The latter restriction was postulated from careful analysis of observed atomic spectral lines by the German physicist Wolfgang Pauli in 1925 and has since been known as the Pauli Exclusion Principle.

Early in the twentieth century it was discovered that the distribution of electrons within an atom relative to the nucleus is not continuous or equally spaced but rather is specifically "discrete." This means that atomic electrons do not locate in a uniform way about the nucleus as marbles in a bowl or stack up one right after the other according to distance from the nucleus. Rather it was determined that their "most probable" allowable locations are in certain concentric "shells" of limited capacity that radially fan out from the nucleus. The existence of these electron shells was first determined experimentally from x-ray absorption studies—that is, missing spectral lines (absent wavelengths or frequencies) that are observed as black segments in an atom's energy spectrum after a beam of x-rays is passed through samples of various elements. These missing wavelengths ($\lambda$) or frequencies ($\nu$) are directly related to the energies of x-ray photons ($E = h\nu = hc/\lambda$) that have been absorbed by the atoms within the target samples. Through examination of such spectra in detail, it became possible to map out the actual pattern of electron energy levels within various atoms. This led to a direct correlation between the Bohr solar system model of the atom, in which groups of electrons were believed to orbit the nucleus at certain distances, and the concept of electron shells that were formed by these orbiting electron groups. Each electron shell was associated with a particular orbital radius at which some electrons were most likely to be found. The smaller the radius, the more tightly were these electrons held in their orbits about the nucleus, or in terms of energy the greater was their binding energy and consequently the effort needed to free them from the attraction of the nucleus. For electron groups or electron shells farther away from the nucleus, the binding energies progressively decreased with distance until one reached the outermost shell, in which electrons needed only a few electron volts of additional energy to escape the atom. These electrons are therefore the predominant category of atomic electrons removed by ionizing radiation and also, quite importantly, the electrons most often involved in chemical reactions. For this reason they are given the name "valence" electrons.

The electron shells were labeled in order of increasing distance from the nucleus with capital letters beginning with the letter $K$, designating the innermost electron shell, and progressing through *L, M, N, O, P,* and *Q.* Again from spectral analysis, it was found that each electron shell except for the K shell was composed of multiple subshells labeled with lowercase letters *s, p, d, f, g, h,* and *i,* and these subshells were limited in

the maximum number of electrons they could contain (s, 2; p, 6; d, 10; f, 14; g, 18; h, 22; i, 26). The theoretical rules that govern this are beyond the scope of this appendix. The following table demonstrates the electron shell occupancies for a number of atoms.

| Atom | Atomic Number | Electron Shells | Electron Subshells and Electron Occupancy | |
|---|---|---|---|---|
| Hydrogen | 1 | K | s | 1 |
| Helium | 2 | K | s | 2 |
| Lithium | 3 | K | s | 2 |
| | | L | s | 1 |
| Carbon | 6 | K | s | 2 |
| | | L | s | 2 |
| | | | p | 2 |
| Oxygen | 8 | K | s | 2 |
| | | L | s | 2 |
| | | | p | 4 |
| Sodium | 11 | K | s | 2 |
| | | L | s | 2 |
| | | | p | 6 |
| | | M | s | 1 |
| Argon | 18 | K | s | 2 |
| | | L | s | 2 |
| | | | p | 6 |
| | | M | s | 2 |
| | | | p | 6 |
| Calcium* | 20 | K | s | 2 |
| | | L | s | 2 |
| | | | p | 6 |
| | | M | s | 2 |
| | | | p | 6 |
| | | N | s | 2 |
| Krypton | 36 | K | s | 2 |
| | | L | s | 2 |
| | | | p | 6 |
| | | M | s | 2 |
| | | | p | 6 |
| | | | d | 10 |
| | | N | s | 2 |
| | | | p | 6 |

*Because the electrons in an unexcited atom will always be arranged in the lowest overall energy configuration, there will be situations in which small subshells of higher shells will begin filling up before large subshells of lower shells are completely filled.

# Compton Interaction

The principle of conservation of mass-energy is that for an isolated system (i.e., a system on which no external energy source or energy drain is active), the total mass plus energy of all the particles comprising the system remains constant. This restraint, however, does not prevent mass-energy transfers between individual particles.

The *linear momentum* of a particle is defined as the product of its mass and its velocity. A photon, which is the particle associated with electromagnetic radiation, moves at the speed of light; consequently, according to Einstein's theory of relativity, a photon must be a massless entity. Because of the equivalence between mass m and energy E given by the famous relation

$$E = mc^2$$

where c is the speed of light in a vacuum, one can associate a mass equivalent with the photon given by

$$E/c^2$$

Then the photon can be considered to have a linear momentum given by the product of the "mass equivalent" and the velocity of the

*Linear momentum = mass times velocity

Photon mass equivalent = $E/c^2$
Magnitude of photon velocity = speed of light c
Photon linear momentum p therefore is given by:
$$p = (E/c^2)c$$
$$= E/c$$

From Appendix E we have that: E = hc/w where w is the wavelength of the photon.
Therefore:

$$P = \frac{(hc/w)}{c} = h/w$$

photon.* The principle of conservation of linear momentum states that, for an isolated system, the sum of the linear momenta of all its particles is constant. Exchanges of linear momentum between particles within the system can, of course, occur.

The Compton interaction is, most simply, a collision between an incident x-ray photon and the weakly bound outer electron of a target atom. Application of the principles of the conservation of mass-energy and the conservation of linear momentum to the x-ray photon and outer electron system leads to equations that can be used to predict the energies and angles of scattering of both particles after their collision. If the energy of the incident photon is E, the following energy balance relation can be written:

$$E = E' + K$$

where E' is the photon's energy after the collision and K is the recoil energy of the "struck" electron.

Several important types of Compton interactions will now be described. These effects depend on the size of E and the angle at which the photon interacts with the electron.

**Case 1:** The photon makes a head-on collision with the electron.
   *Result:* The electron travels or scatters directly forward, and the photon travels or scatters backward (180-degree scatter angle).
   *Energy Situations:*
   a. E ≪ 511 keV (low energy range):
      E' is approximately equal to E
      K is almost zero

b.  E = 511 keV:
   E′ = E/3
   K = (2/3) E
c.  E ≫ 511 keV (high energy range):
   E′ is approximately zero
   K = E to good approximation

**Case 2:** The photon grazes the electron.

*Result:* The photon emerges from the collision nearly undeflected from its initial direction, and the electron scatters at right angles.

*Energy Situation:*
   E′ is approximately equal to E
   K is approximately zero

Collisions of this nature, in which the incident photon loses little or no energy, are especially important in the planning of radiation shielding for therapeutic x-ray suites.

# APPENDIX H

# Revision of 10 CFR Part 35*

**§ 35.50 Training for Radiation Safety Officer.** Except as provided in § 35.57, the licensee shall require an individual fulfilling the responsibilities of the Radiation Safety Officer (RSO) as provided in § 35.24 to be an individual who:

(a) Is certified by a specialty board whose certification process includes all of the requirements in paragraph (b) of this section and whose certification has been approved by the Commission or;

(b) (1) Has completed a structured educational program consisting of both:

(i) 200 hours of didactic training in the following areas:

(A) Radiation physics and instrumentation;

(B) Radiation protection;

(C) Mathematics pertaining to the use and measurement of radioactivity;

(D) Radiation biology; and

(E) Radiation dosimetry; and

(ii) One year of full-time radiation safety experience under the supervision of the individual identified as the RSO on a Commission or Agreement State license that authorized similar types(s) of use(s) of byproduct material involving the following:

(A) Shipping, receiving, and performing related radiation surveys;

(B) Using and performing checks for proper operation of dose calibrators, survey meters, and instruments used to measure radionuclides;

(C) Securing and controlling byproduct material;

(D) Using administrative controls to avoid mistakes in the administration of byproduct material;

(E) Using procedures to prevent or minimize radioactive contamination and using proper decontamination procedures; and

(F) Disposing of byproduct material; and

(2) Has obtained written certification, signed by a preceptor RSO, that the requirements in paragraph (b) (1) of this section have been satisfactorily completed and that the individual has achieved a level of competency sufficient to independently function as an RSO for medical uses of byproduct material; and

(3) Following completion of the requirements in paragraph (b) of this section, has demonstrated sufficient knowledge in radiation safety commensurate with

*Training is the same as described in current 10 CFR Part 35.

the use requested by passing an examination given by an organization or entity approved by the Commission in accordance with Appendix A of this part; or

(c) Is an authorized user, authorized medical physicist, or authorized nuclear pharmacist

identified on the licensee's license and has experience with the radiation safety aspects of similar types of use of byproduct material for which the individual has RSO responsibilities.

# Consumer-Patient Radiation Health and Safety Act of 1981*

## SUBTITLE I—CONSUMER-PATIENT RADIATION HEALTH AND SAFETY ACT OF 1981

### Short Title

[42 USC 10001.] note
**SEC. 975.** This subtitle may be cited as the "consumer-patient radiation health and safety act of 1981."

### Statement of Findings

[42 USC 10001.]
**SEC. 976.** The congress finds that ...
(1) it is in the interest of public health and safety to minimize unnecessary exposure to potentially hazardous radiation due to medical and dental radiologic procedures;
(2) it is in the interest of public health and safety to have a continuing supply of adequately educated persons and appropriate accreditation and certification programs administered by state governments;

(3) the protection of the public health and safety from unnecessary exposure to potentially hazardous radiation due to medical and dental radiologic procedures and the assurance of efficacious procedures are the responsibility of state and federal governments;
(4) persons who administer radiologic procedures, including procedures at federal facilities, should be required to demonstrate competence by reason of education, training, and experience; and
(5) the administration of radiologic procedures and the effect on individuals of such procedures have a substantial and direct effect upon United States interstate commerce.

### Statement of Purpose

[42 USC 10002.]
**SEC. 977.** It is the purpose of this subtitle to—
(1) provide for the establishment of minimum standards by the federal government for the accreditation of education programs for persons who administer radiologic procedures and for the certification of such persons; and
(2) ensure that medical and dental radiologic procedures are consistent with rigorous safety precautions and standards.

---

*Modified from Consumer-Patient Radiation Health and Safety Act of 1981, Chapter 107, Secs. 10001-8 (Aug. 13, 1981).

# Definitions

[42 USC 10003.]

**SEC. 978.** Unless otherwise expressly provided, for purposes of this subtitle, the term—

(1) "radiation" means ionizing and nonionizing radiation in amounts beyond normal background levels from sources such as medical and dental radiologic procedures;

(2) "radiologic procedure" means any procedure or article intended for use in—

    (A) the diagnosis of disease or other medical or dental conditions in humans (including diagnostic x-rays or nuclear medicine procedures); or

    (B) the cure, mitigation, treatment, or prevention of disease in humans that achieves its intended purpose through the emission of radiation;

(3) "radiologic equipment" means any radiation electronic product that emits or detects radiation and is used or intended for use to—

    (A) diagnose disease or other medical or dental conditions (including diagnostic x-ray equipment); or

    (B) cure, mitigate, treat, or prevent disease in humans that achieves its intended purpose through the emission or detection of radiation;

(4) "practitioner" means any licensed doctor of medicine, osteopathy, dentistry, podiatry, or chiropractic who prescribes radiologic procedures for other persons;

(5) "persons who administer radiologic procedures" means any person, other than a practitioner, who intentionally administers radiation to other persons for medical purposes and includes medical radiologic technologists (including dental hygienists and assistants), radiation therapy technologists, and nuclear medicine technologists;

(6) "Secretary" means the Secretary of Health and Human Services; and

(7) "State" means the several states, the District of Columbia, the Commonwealth of Puerto Rico, the Commonwealth of the Northern Mariana Islands, the Virgin Islands, Guam, American Samoa, and the Trust Territory of the Pacific Islands.

# Promulgation of Standards

[Regulation. 42 USC 10004.]

**SEC. 979.**

(a) Within 12 months after the date of enactment of this act, the Secretary, in consultation with the Radiation Policy Council, the Administrator of Veterans' Affairs, the Administrator of the Environmental Protection Agency, appropriate agencies of the States, and appropriate professional organizations, shall by regulation promulgate minimum standards for the accreditation of educational programs to train individuals to perform radiologic procedures. Such standards shall distinguish between programs for the education of (1) medical radiologic technologists (including radiographers), (2) dental auxiliaries (including dental hygienists and assistants), (3) radiation therapy technologists, (4) nuclear medicine technologists, and (5) such other kinds of health auxiliaries who administer radiologic procedures as the Secretary determines appropriate. Such standards shall not be applicable to educational programs for practitioners.

[Regulation.]

(b) Within 12 months after the date of enactment of this act, the Secretary, in consultation with the Radiation Policy Council, the Administrator of Veterans' Affairs, the Administrator of the Environmental Protection Agency, interested agencies of the States, and appropriate professional organizations, shall by regulation promulgate minimum standards for the certification of persons who administer radiologic procedures. Such standards shall distinguish between certification of (1) medical radiologic technologists (including radiographers), (2) dental auxiliaries (including dental hygienists and assistants), (3) radiation therapy technologists, (4) nuclear medicine technologists, and (5) such other kinds of health auxiliaries who administer radiologic procedures as the Secretary determines appropriate. Such standards shall include minimum certification criteria for individuals with regard to accredited education, practical experience, successful passage of required examinations, and such other criteria as the Secretary shall deem necessary for the adequate qualification of individuals to administer radiologic procedures. Such standards shall not apply to practitioners.

## Model Statute

[42 USC 10005.]
**SEC. 980.** In order to encourage the administration of accreditation and certification programs by the states, the Secretary shall prepare and transmit to the states a model statute for radiologic procedure safety. Such model statute shall provide that—
(1) it shall be unlawful in a state for individuals to perform radiologic procedures unless such individuals are certified by the state to perform such procedures; and
(2) any educational requirements for certification of individuals to perform radiologic procedures shall be limited to educational programs accredited by the state.

## Compliance

[42 USC 10006.]
**SEC. 981.**
(a) The Secretary shall take all actions consistent with law to effectuate the purposes of this subtitle.
(b) A state may utilize an accreditation or certification program administered by a private entity if—
(1) such state delegates the administration of the state accreditation or certification program to such private entity;
(2) such program is approved by the state; and
(3) such program is consistent with the minimum federal standards promulgated under this subtitle for such program.

(c) Absent compliance by the states with the provisions of this subtitle within 3 years after the date of enactment of this act, the Secretary shall report to the Congress recommendations for legislative changes considered necessary to ensure the states' compliance with this subtitle.
[Report to Congress.]
(d) The Secretary shall be responsible for continued monitoring of compliance by the states with the applicable provisions of this subtitle and shall report to the Senate and the House of Representatives by January 1, 1982, and January 1 of each succeeding year the status of the states' compliance with the purposes of this subtitle.
(e) Notwithstanding any other provision of this section, in the case of a state that has, prior to the effective date of standards and guidelines promulgated pursuant to this subtitle, established standards for the accreditation of educational programs and certification of radiologic technologists, such state shall be deemed to be in compliance with the conditions of this section unless the Secretary determines, after notice and hearing, that such state standards do not meet the minimum standards prescribed by the Secretary or are inconsistent with the purposes of this subtitle.

## Federal Radiation Guidelines

[42 USC 10007.]
**SEC. 982.** The Secretary shall, in conjunction with the Radiation Policy Council, the Administrator of Veterans' Affairs, the Administrator of the Environmental Protection Agency, appropriate agencies of the states, and appropriate professional organizations, promulgate Federal radiation guidelines with respect to radiologic procedures. Such guidelines shall—
(1) determine the level of radiation exposure due to radiologic procedures that is unnecessary and specify the techniques, procedures, and methods to minimize such unnecessary exposure;

(2) provide for the elimination of the need for retakes of diagnostic radiologic procedures;

(3) provide for the elimination of unproductive screening programs;

(4) provide for the optimum diagnostic information with minimum radiologic exposure; and

(5) include the therapeutic application of radiation to individuals in the treatment of disease, including nuclear medicine applications.

## Applicability to Federal Agencies

[42 USC 10008.]

**SEC. 983.**

(a) Except as provided in subsection (b), each department, agency, and instrumentality of the executive branch of the federal government shall comply with standards promulgated pursuant to this subtitle.

[Regulations.]

[38 USC 101 *et seq.* ]

(b) (1) The Administrator of Veterans' Affairs, through the Chief Medical Director of the Veterans' Administration, shall, to the maximum extent feasible consistent with the responsibilities of such Administrator and Chief Medical Director under subtitle 38, United States Code, prescribe regulations making the standards promulgated pursuant to this subtitle applicable to the provision of radiologic procedures in facilities over which the Administrator has jurisdiction. In prescribing and implementing regulations pursuant to this subsection, the Administrator shall consult with the Secretary in order to achieve the maximum possible coordination of the regulations, standards, and guidelines, and the implementation thereof, which the Secretary and the Administrator prescribe under this subtitle.

[Report to congressional committees.]

(2) Not later than 180 days after standards are promulgated by the Secretary pursuant to this subtitle, the Administrator of Veterans' Affairs shall submit to the appropriate committees of Congress a full report with respect to the regulations (including guidelines, policies, and procedures thereunder) prescribed pursuant to paragraph (1) of this subsection. Such report shall include—

(A) an explanation of any inconsistency between standards made applicable by such regulations and the standards promulgated by the Secretary pursuant to this subtitle;

(B) an account of the extent, substance, and results of consultations with the Secretary respecting the prescription and implementation of regulations by the Administrator; and

(C) such recommendations for legislation and administrative action as the Administrator determines are necessary and desirable.

[Publication in Federal Register.]

(3) The Administrator of Veterans' Affairs shall publish the report required by paragraph (2) in the Federal Register.

# IMAGE CREDITS AND COURTESIES

Abelin T, Egger M, Ruchti C: *Fallout from Chernobyl. Belarus increase was probably caused by Chernobyl*, BMJ 12:1298, 1994
Figure 9-11

Allen CW: *Radiotherapy and phototherapy including radium and high frequency currents*, New York, 1904, Lea Brothers
Figure 9-8

Ballinger PW, Frank ED: *Merrill's Atlas of Radiographic Positions and Radiologic Procedures*, ed 9, St Louis, 1999, Mosby
Figure 11-12

Ballinger PW, Frank ED: *Merrill's Atlas of Radiographic Positions and Radiologic Procedures*, ed 10, St Louis, 2003, Mosby
Figures 3-10A, 11-7

Betsy Shields, Presbyterian Hospital, Charlotte, North Carolina, in Bushong SC: *Radiologic science for technologists: physics, biology and protection*, ed 10, St Louis, 2013, Elsevier/Mosby
Figure 11-18

Brown P: *American martyrs to science through the roentgen rays*, Springfield, Ill, 1936, Charles C Thomas
Figures 4-4A and 4-5

Burndy Collection at the Huntington Library, San Marino, California
Figure 4-1

Bushong SC: *Radiologic science for technologists: Physics, biology and protection*, ed 10, St Louis, 2013, Elsevier/Mosby
Figures 6-13, 11-21, 11-22, 11-23

Carestream Health, Inc.
Figure 4-2

Carolyn Caskey Goodner, Identigene, Inc.
Figure 8-11

Fluke Biomedical
Figures 12-7, 12-8, 12-10, 13-8

Frank ED, Long BW, Smith BS: *Merrill's Atlas of Radiographic Positioning & Procedures*, ED 12, St. Louis, 2012, Mosby
Figures 1-2, 1-5A, 3-4D, 3-10B, 11-8, 11-19, 12-5, 12-15A, 14-2

Glasser O: *William Conrad Roentgen and the early history of the roentgen rays*, London, 1933, John Bale, Sons, and Danielsson, Ltd.
Figure 4-3

Greenpeace/Clive Shirley
Figure 2-8

Hendee WR, Ritenour ER: *Medical imaging physics*, ed 4, Chicago, 2002, John Wiley & Sons
Figures 4-8, 7-1, 11-17

Implant Sciences Corporation
Figure 14-1

Ken Bontrager
Figure 4-5

Ken Graham Photography
Figures 2-7A, 8-2, 9-12

Landauer, Inc, Glenwood, Ill.
Figures 5-2, 5-3, 5-4, 5-7

Magnum Photos
Figure 9-9

Mark Rzeszotarski
Figure 11-25, 11-26, 13-16

National Council on Radiation Protection and Measurements [NCRP]: *Structural shielding design for medical x-ray imaging facilities,* Report No. 147, Bethesda, 2004
Figure 13-20

National Council on Radiation Protection and Measurements [NCRP]: *Ionizing radiation exposure of the population of the United States,* Report No. 160, Bethesda, 2009
Figure 2-2

Oak Ridge Associated Universities
Figure 2-4

Pennsylvania State University Engineering Library
Figure 2-6A

PhotoAssist, Inc.
Figure 8-3

*Radiobiology and Radiation Protection: Mosby's Radiographic Instructional Series,* St. Louis, 1999, Mosby
Figures 1-5B, 1-6, 3-11, 6-1, 6-8, 6-9, 6-11, 7-3, 7-15 8-4, 8-5, 8-6, 9-5, 9-6, 11-15, 11-24, 12-12

Riegh R: *Am J Roentgenol* 89:182, 1963
Figure 9-14

Sinclair WK: *Radiation protection recommendations on dose limits: the role of the NCRP and the ICRP and future developments,* J Radiat Oncol Biol Phys 131:387, 1995
Figure 9-10

Thibodeau A: *Anatomy and physiology,* ed 5, St Louis, 2003, Mosby
Figure 6-10

Thibodeau GA, Patton KT: Anatomy and physiology, ed 6, St Louis, 2007, Mosby
Figure 8-8

*U.S. Department of Energy,* Nevada Operations Office, Las Vegas, Nev
Figures 2-5, 2-6B, and 2-7B and C

*U.S. Environmental Protection Agency,* Washington, DC
Figure 2-3

Victoreen, Inc, Cleveland
Figure 5-11

# INDEX

Page numbers followed by "f" indicate figures, "t" indicate tables, and "b" indicate boxes.